GRAHAM'S
Principles and Applications of
RADIOLOGICAL PHYSICS

SEVENTH EDITION

GRAHAM'S

Principles and Applications of
RADIOLOGICAL PHYSICS

MARTIN VOSPER, BSc (Hons), PgDip, MSc, HDCR
Senior Lecturer, Division of Radiography, University of Hertfordshire, Hatfield, UK and
Lecturer, Division of Midwifery and Radiography, City University, London

ANDREW ENGLAND, BSc (Hons), PgCert, MSc, PhD, FHEA
Senior Lecturer in Radiography, School of Allied Health Professions, Keele University, Staffordshire, UK

VICTORIA MAJOR, MSc, PgCert, DCR(R), DRI, FHEA
Paul Strickland Scanner Centre, Mount Vernon Cancer Centre, Northwood, UK

ELSEVIER

ELSEVIER

Notice

Practitioners and researchers must always rely on their own experience and knowledge in evaluating and using any information, methods, compounds or experiments described herein. Because of rapid advances in the medical sciences, in particular, independent verification of diagnoses and drug dosages should be made. To the fullest extent of the law, no responsibility is assumed by Elsevier, authors, editors or contributors for any injury and/or damage to persons or property as a matter of products liability, negligence or otherwise, or from any use or operation of any methods, products, instructions, or ideas contained in the material herein.

ISBN: 978-0-7020-6816-4

Printed in Poland

Content Strategist: Trinity Hutton
Senior Content Development Specialist: Helen Leng
Senior Project Manager: Manchu Mohan
Design: Margaret Reid
Illustrations: Narayanan Ramakrishnan
Marketing Manager: Ed Major

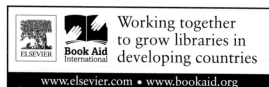

Last digit is the print number: 9 8 7 6 5 4 3 2 1

CONTENTS

PREFACE

Back in 1981, at a time when magnetic resonance imaging and even computed tomography were quite recent innovations, Robin Wilks authored the first edition of *Principles of Radiological Physics*. We remember that this textbook became a welcome addition to the market for anyone working in medical imaging who wanted a book that was neither too basic nor too complex. It became a valuable resource for us and many of our colleagues during training. We agree with Robin Wilks's belief that there really is a point to physics in medical imaging practice because it underpins technology, dosimetry, technique choice and image appearances. In 2011, steered by Donald Graham and Paul Cloke, the sixth edition was renamed *Principles and Applications of Radiological Physics*, to reflect the fact that physics is not merely theoretical but is the carriage on which all clinical medical imaging rides. This conviction is carried forwards into the present edition.

As of 2020, we find that advanced techniques in medical imaging have further expanded and developed to an extent which would have amazed Wilhelm Roentgen; hence the later chapters of the book have been developed to reflect these advances. Conventional or 'plain' X-ray imaging is still essential but is now based entirely on digital methods, with film being of historical interest only. The authors have retained several chapters concerned with key physics principles but have relegated topics that are now less applicable to modern practice. As before, there is use of insight boxes and diagrams, rather than too much complex mathematics. This seventh edition focuses on medical imaging rather than on radiotherapy, simply because there are specialist textbooks on radiotherapy physics available. However medical imaging is of great importance in radiotherapy for localisation, planning and treatment monitoring. We trust that this book will continue to be of interest to anyone training in medical imaging, whether they are radiographers, technologists, radiologists, physicists or radiotherapists.

Martin Vosper
Andrew England
Victoria Major

ACKNOWLEDGEMENTS

The authors would like to acknowledge the contributions of Robin Wilks, Donald Graham and Paul Cloke, who developed the previous editions of this textbook. Much of their material remains fundamental to radiological physics. We would also like to recognise the students and colleagues, too many to name, who provided feedback and suggestions. Thanks are due to Warrington & Halton Hospitals NHS Foundation Trust for providing some of the clinical images.

To our loved ones—to Julie who finds joy in each new day's discoveries,
also to Anna, Alicia, Evie and Neil

GRAHAM'S
Principles and Applications of
RADIOLOGICAL PHYSICS

Fundamentals

Principles of medical imaging

CHAPTER CONTENTS

1.1   AIM

This chapter considers the principles of medical imaging, with some reference to radiotherapy and radiation protection. The chapter also considers the historical development of the imaging methods which are in use today, as well as their capabilities. The physics of medical imaging, although often regarded as a 'dry' and academic topic, underpins much of what we do in radiology and radiography. Without a knowledge of physics, it would be hard to understand the choice of imaging methods for different diseases, the workings of imaging equipment, the selection of suitable radiation exposure factors or the concept of radiation doses.

1.2   MEDICAL IMAGING AND RADIOTHERAPY

Modern medical imaging involves the use of a wide range of energetic emissions from specialist scanners – such as X-rays, gamma rays, radio waves, magnetism and sound. This book will not consider the use of medical photography or thermography (heat imaging), which could also be regarded as forms of medical imaging in the broadest use of the term. Medical imaging is chiefly involved in diagnosis, the investigation of the person's illness or physical state through the production of images. However, it can also be used to guide medical 'interventions', which are mainly forms of treatment.

Radiotherapy involves the use of large quantities of ionising radiations, such as X-rays, gamma rays, electrons and protons, to kill cancerous tissues while sparing surrounding normal tissues as much as possible. Radiotherapy will not be considered in any detail within this book because there are other more specialist texts available.

Table 1.1 provides an overview of some key dates in the development of medical imaging and radiotherapy.

1.2.1   Medical imaging

The introduction of medical X-ray imaging in the late 19th century, together with later developments (see Table 1.1), was revolutionary because it enabled us to explore the inner structures and workings of the living human body in a noninvasive way. Before this, diagnosis of disease was mainly possible only via clinical examination, surgery or at postmortem. Medical imaging may be referred to both as radiography, which is the process of taking radiographs, and radiology, which is the medical practice of using radiographic images for the diagnosis of disease. However, there is some overlap between the roles of radiographer and radiologist in many countries. The overall quality of a medical imaging service can be judged in several ways. It is possible to obtain physical measurements of the quality of the images themselves, using concepts such as resolution (the size of the smallest objects that can be visualised), contrast (signal differences between structures) and noise (random variations in signal). However, clinicians are often more interested in measures of diagnostic accuracy,

TABLE 1.1   Some key dates in the development of medical imaging and radiotherapy

Date	Event
1839	Daguerre used silver compounds to produce permanent photographic images. This technology would later develop into film that could be used for X-ray imaging
1878	Crookes, using an evacuated glass tube containing an anode and cathode, showed the existence of cathode rays (a stream of electrons) between the two electrodes when a voltage was applied
1895	Roentgen discovered X-rays while experimenting with a variant of the Crookes tube
1896	Becquerel discovered radioactivity while working with some uranium salts and photographic film
1896	First clinical use of X-ray images, by Hall-Edwards
1897	First use of X-rays to treat skin cancers
1897	Edison developed luminescent intensifying screens to amplify X-ray images—this evolved into both static and moving (fluoroscopic) imaging
1898	The Curies developed theories of radioactivity and discovered new radioactive elements such as radium
1901	Pierre Curie suggested that a radioactive source could be placed inside a tumour to treat it—a technique termed brachytherapy
1912	Marie Curie founded the Radium Institute in Paris, which pioneered the use of radioactive sources for cancer treatments
1913	Coolidge created an improved vacuum tube which was the forerunner of all later X-ray tube designs
1913	Following the deaths of some early radiologists, the Roentgen Society published guidelines on safety for medical radiation workers
1920s	Use of orthovoltage X-ray tubes at voltages of 200–500 kilovolt (kV) to treat deep tumours with external beam radiotherapy
1928	The International Commission on Radiological Protection (ICRP) was created to address safety concerns in medical imaging and radiotherapy
1942	Dussik undertook the first human ultrasound procedure
1956	Use of the linear accelerator (LINAC) to produce X-rays of megaelectron volt (MeV) energies for external beam radiotherapy
1957	Anger created the gamma camera, which is widely used in radionuclide imaging
1973	Hounsfield developed the first clinical computed tomography (CT) scanner
1973	The first clinical positron emission tomography (PET) scanner
1977	The first human magnetic resonance imaging (MRI) scan, by Damadian
1987	Fuji introduced a digital plate technology for X-ray imaging, designed to replace film and termed computed radiography (CR)
2000	Townsend and Nutt developed a combined PET-CT scanner
2007	Kodak developed digital direct radiography (DR) for X-ray imaging

such as sensitivity, which is the percentage probability of detecting disease when it is present, and specificity, which is the percentage probability of excluding disease when it is absent. More generally, a healthcare provider would want to know the effectiveness of an imaging service. For example, is it cost effective, is it safe, is it timely, does it influence treatment, does it improve health outcomes for patients?

Modern medical imaging provides a wide range of techniques, which are often termed 'modalities', for imaging human anatomy and pathology, such as conventional (or 'plain') X-ray, computed tomography (CT), magnetic resonance imaging (MRI), ultrasound and radionuclide imaging. Medical imaging may be used to screen for the presence of disease, classify disease, determine the extent of disease, test for response to treatment or check for disease recurrence. A general principle of medical imaging is that no procedure should be undertaken unless the likely benefit to the patient exceeds the likely risk. In the case of ionising radiations, this principle is incorporated in legal regulations, which include the tenet that all radiation exposures should be as low as reasonably achievable (the ALARA principle). In the case of diagnostic X-ray exposures, the possible radiation effects, such as cancer, are almost entirely stochastic (governed by chance), meaning that harm is not inevitable and is unlikely at low exposure levels. The so-called non-ionising radiation procedures, such as ultrasound and MRI, are not thought to present cancer risks, although MRI can present severe safety hazards in some circumstances.

Fig. 1.1 shows a radiographer preparing the equipment for a common diagnostic X-ray examination.

Light is a form of electromagnetic radiation (see Chapter 9) and it seems logical to suggest that if we can obtain photons of electromagnetic radiation, which have higher energies than light photons, these may have sufficient energy to penetrate body tissues and allow us to visualise internal organs. X-rays are in this part of the electromagnetic spectrum and so will penetrate body tissues and allow us to image internal organs. Unfortunately, the retina of the eye cannot detect X-rays and so we cannot see an image of a structure just by directing an X-ray beam on it. This means that the X-rays, which have passed through the body, must be made to strike an image receptor that will produce a visible image, for example, an imaging plate.

The principal interactions involved in the basic requirements for the formation of a radiographic image are shown in Fig. 1.2.

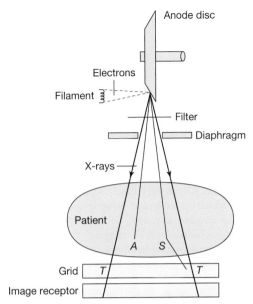

Fig. 1.2 The principal interactions involved in the production of a radiographic image. *A* represents absorbed photons, *S* represents scattered photons and *T* represents transmitted photons.

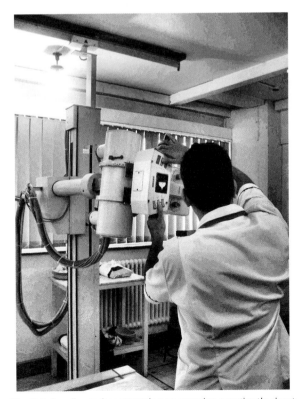

Fig. 1.1 A radiographer preparing to examine a patient's chest.

Conventional X-ray radiography and CT are examples of 'transmission' imaging techniques, whereby rays pass through a patient's body and are collected by detectors on the opposite side. Images are created by the fact that rays are differentially absorbed in the patient, being removed from the beam when passing through denser body structures. This creates image contrast, which is a difference in signal intensities.

Radionuclide imaging (RNI) is a form of 'emission' imaging, which studies the uptake of gamma-ray emitting radioactive atoms in the human body. The intention is that these gamma rays should pass through the body tissues and into detectors, without much absorption in the body. Note that this is a completely different aim from that of transmission imaging techniques such as CT. As a result RNI does not provide detailed anatomical depiction of body structures and this is assisted by the relatively high energy of the gamma rays.

Ultrasound is an example of 'reflection' imaging, employing reflections of high frequency sound waves at tissue boundaries to return signals, which are termed 'echoes'. Unlike X-rays and gamma rays, which travel at the speed of light (300,000 kilometres per second!) and are relatively little impeded by the human body, sound waves travel at much slower speeds (300–3000 metres per second) in body tissue and require a 'medium' containing molecules to be transmitted. Sound waves are very heavily impeded by dense body structures such as bone.

MRI also returns signal 'echoes' but is not a reflection-imaging technique. Although the physics of MRI signal production is complex, involving interactions between magnetic and electromagnetic fields as well as altered nuclear spin states, it could for our purpose here be simply termed an 'absorption and reemission' technique. This simply refers to a process by which radiofrequency energy is received by hydrogen nuclei in body tissues, exchanged and reemitted as a radiofrequency signal.

Conventional X-ray radiography and CT are primarily anatomical imaging methods, being very good at depicting body structures but relatively poor at displaying physiology and function. RNI is very much a physiological imaging method, which is excellent at showing function but weak at displaying detailed anatomy. CT and RNI may be combined in so-called 'hybrid imaging' techniques, which provide an 'anatometabolic' capability when their images are fused together. Examples of this are positron emission tomography (PET)-CT and single-photon emission (SPECT)-CT scanners, as well as PET-MRI. This type of imaging is especially useful in showing the metabolic activity and location of cancers. Ultrasound and MRI in isolation as 'stand-alone' methods have anatomical as well as physiological imaging capabilities, with MRI providing the widest range of subtechniques of any imaging modality.

Imaging methods may be reported to be 'gold standards' for the diagnosis of stated diseases, meaning that they provide the highest possible levels of sensitivity and specificity. For example, CT would be regarded as a gold standard method for lung disease. Often however, the choice of imaging modality might be affected by local availability, expertise, preference, cost and patient safety. A claustrophobic person would be unlikely to tolerate an MRI scan, whereas a pregnant woman would not be referred for abdominal or pelvic CT except in an emergency situation. Imaging methods may also be termed 'complementary', which means they are capable of providing additional information when working together to provide a complete diagnosis.

In all of these situations, the suitability of each imaging method is determined by physics principles, for it is the physics of imaging which gives each approach the ability (or not) to depict body tissues and diseases.

1.2.2 Radiotherapy

Radiotherapy will now be mentioned briefly, although it is not covered in detail within this textbook. In radiotherapy, we are not trying to produce images but are using the biological effects of radiation to kill tumour cells. At the same time, we try to cause as little damage as possible to the healthy cells in the body. Radiotherapy irradiates tissues with such large doses of ionising radiation that cell death, because of breakage of both strands of DNA in cell nuclei, results. Radiotherapy makes use of X-rays in the megaelectron volt (MeV) energy range, which have the effect of giving enhanced radiation doses to deep tissues and sparing superficial tissues such as the skin. These X-rays are produced by linear accelerators (LINACs), which employ advanced physics to accelerate electrons to speeds close to that of light, thereby producing high energy X-rays when these electrons strike a tungsten target. External beam radiotherapy may also use lower energy X-rays in the kiloelectron volt (keV) range, as well as gamma rays. Medical imaging is also a key part of radiotherapy processes. Imaging is used to identify, localise and stage cancers, as well as in treatment verification, simulation and planning. So it can be seen that imaging and radiotherapy work together closely within cancer treatment. CT scanners in particular are often found within radiotherapy departments.

There are four main methods of cancer treatment: surgery, chemotherapy, alteration of the hormone balance and radiotherapy. They may be used in isolation or together to give the optimum treatment regime for a given cancer in a given patient. The treatment may be radical or palliative. The former is an all-out effort to achieve a cure and the latter is used to relieve pain and other distressing symptoms when no cure for the disease is possible. This is normally in the terminal stages of the disease.

The relative success of radiotherapy in the management of cancer lies in the fact that malignant cells are more sensitive to radiation than healthy cells in the same organ. This is because cells are sensitive to radiation damage during cell division and cancer cells are usually more rapidly dividing. In addition, DNA repair mechanisms may be impaired in cancer cells. Although targeting of radiotherapy beams has improved, a number of healthy cells are affected by radiation and so must be given time to recover. Thus the radiation dose is delivered as a number of treatments rather than as a single dose. This technique is known as *fractionation* and may mean that a patient has 15 to 30 treatments over a period of 3 to 6 weeks.

1.3 METHODS OF RADIATION TREATMENT

A detailed description of the different methods of radiation treatment is beyond the scope of this introductory chapter and the reader is directed to some of the more specialised texts on the subject. In considering the overview of radiation treatment methods, we can, however, identify some distinct types, which we will discuss further. These are:

- teletherapy
- brachytherapy
- nuclear medicine.

1.3.1 Teletherapy

Here an external source of radiation (normally X-rays or gamma rays) is directed at the tumour. The technique is also termed external beam therapy. The aim is to give the maximum dose to the tumour and the minimum dose to the healthy tissue. This is often achieved by treating the tumour with a number of fields (see Fig. 1.3). The areas in the patient that receive doses of equal value are joined by lines called 'isodose lines'. The shape and the position of these lines may be altered by the use of absorbing wedges and compensators and also by altering the energy and shape of the treatment beam. Once the treatment plan has been produced, the positions of the treatment fields on the patient are checked in a simulator where the treatment angles can be set up and the fields marked. In areas of the patient around the head and the neck, accurate positioning and immobilisation are achieved by placing this part in a specially prepared clear plastic shell.

1.3.2 Brachytherapy

When we use external radiation beams, the radiation must travel through healthy tissue to reach the tumour. There are

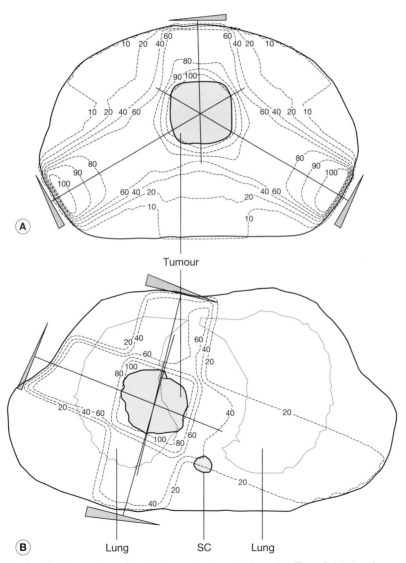

Fig. 1.3 Grossly simplified examples of radiotherapy treatment plans. (A) Three-field plan for a pelvic tumour. (B) Three-field plan for a mediastinal tumour (note how the fields minimise dose to the spinal cord (SC) on the plan).

some situations where tumours are relatively accessible from the body surface or are in body cavities where sealed radioactive sources may be inserted. This technique is known as *brachytherapy*. The technique can often mean that a large dose can be delivered to the tumour while a much smaller dose strikes the surrounding tissues because of the effects of the inverse square law (see Section 14.8). If the sources were implanted directly by the oncologist or radiotherapist, the dose to the hands of the operator could be quite large. This is overcome by inserting a number of guides into the correct position and mechanically inserting the sources over the guides for the required treatment. This technique is called 'afterloading' and is often used in the treatment of pelvic cancers.

1.3.3 Nuclear medicine

A third possibility is that the radiation can be delivered to the tissue by allowing the tissue to absorb a certain radionuclide. This is probably best illustrated by considering the treatment of an overactive thyroid gland. The activity of the gland can be reduced by surgical removal of part of the gland, or some of its tissue may be destroyed using radiation. To allow the thyroid to produce the required hormones, it must absorb iodine. The patient may be given sodium iodide (where the iodine is in the form of ^{131}I) as a capsule or in an oral solution. Some of this isotope (see Section 2.3) is taken up by the gland and the rest is secreted in the urine. ^{131}I is a beta particle emitter (see Section 10.5) and this results in a radiation dose to the thyroid tissue, which reduces its metabolic rate to normal. Because of the limited range of the beta particles produced, there is less radiation dose to structures around the thyroid than there would be if we used an external radiation beam. ^{131}I also has a relatively short half-life of 8 days and so the radiation hazard posed by the patient to others can be minimised. Note that the term 'nuclear medicine' strictly refers to the use of radioactive isotopes to treat disease, although diagnostic radionuclide imaging departments are sometimes incorrectly termed 'nuclear medicine departments'.

1.4 RADIATION PROTECTION

All ionising radiation of the cells which make up our bodies carries a risk of damage to those cells. It is also true that some tissues are more sensitive to radiation than others. The use of ionising radiation in medicine is of great value to humans, but it is the largest single factor which contributes to the artificial radiation dose received by humans. The contribution of the various radiation sources is shown in Fig. 1.4. It should be noted that for most people, natural background radiation provides a much greater annual dose than artificial radiation.

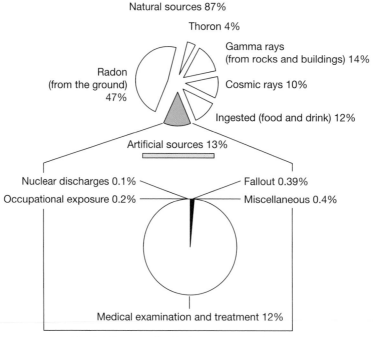

Fig. 1.4 Sources of radiation exposure to humans.

Nevertheless, because all doses of radiation, no matter how small, can be potentially harmful, we have a duty to minimise the dose to our patients and colleagues and so minimise the risk of radiation damage. The radiation dose is composed of primary radiation (the beam itself) and secondary radiation (scattered rays), and so we will need to look at the ways in which these are produced and absorbed. Because of the known hazards of radiation, there are certain statutory requirements for radiation protection and monitoring in diagnostic and therapy departments. In terms of assessing the risk, it is important to know the dose received by both patients and radiation workers and this is assessed by radiation dosimetry. There are annual dose limits for staff, but not for patients. This is because patients must continue to receive radiation procedures so long as these are 'justified', which means that benefit exceeds risk. However patient doses are monitored and must be minimised, to be as low as reasonably achievable while achieving an adequate diagnosis or treatment.

SUMMARY

This brief overview should enable the reader to understand certain physical principles which underpin medical imaging and radiotherapy.

FURTHER READING

Joiner, M., & van der Kogel, A. 2018. *Basic Clinical Radiobiology.* 5th edn. CRC Press.

Klein, A., Vinson, E., Brant, W., & Helms, C. 2018. *Brant and Helms' Fundamentals of Diagnostic Radiology.* 5th edn. Lippincott Williams & Wilkins.

Symonds, P., Deehan, C., Meredith, C., & Mills, J. 2012. *Walter's and Miller's Textbook of Radiotherapy: Radiation Physics, Therapy and Oncology.* 7th edn. Edinburgh: Churchill Livingstone.

Atoms and matter

CHAPTER CONTENTS

2.1   AIM

The aim of this chapter is to introduce the reader to the key components of an atom and to the structure of matter. Atoms are the smallest chemical components of matter and consist of positively charged atomic nuclei surrounded by shells of negatively charged electrons. Instabilities of atomic nuclei result in the phenomenon of radioactivity (see Chapter 10), which is employed in radionuclide imaging. Disturbances in the electron shells of atoms occur during X-ray production (see Chapter 11) and X-ray attenuation (see Chapter 13).

2.2   INTRODUCTION

Any attempt to understand the universe around us must start with the fundamental question: what is matter made of? The atom as the fundamental building block of matter has been the subject of a great deal of both theoretical debate and experimental study by physicists. Many of the modern theories concerning atomic and subatomic structures are extremely complex and are the subject of a number of textbooks in their own right. Most of the phenomena which we encounter in medical imaging can be explained using a relatively simple planetary model of the atom. In this model, there are particle-like electrons orbiting a particle-like nucleus—some phenomena can also be explained using the quantum physics model, and where this is appropriate this model will be referred to in Insights.

The planetary model of the atom was first described by Rutherford in 1911. It describes an atom consisting of a small, positively charged central nucleus (containing protons and neutrons) around which negatively charged electrons move in defined shells. This model can be used to illustrate the carbon atom, as shown in Fig. 2.1.

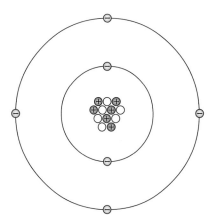

Fig. 2.1 The basic structure of a carbon atom. At the centre of the atom is a nucleus which contains 6 protons (positively charged) and 6 neutrons (zero charge); that is, the nucleus contains 12 nucleons. Six electrons (negatively charged) orbit the nucleus in defined orbitals. As the atom contains equal numbers of positive and negative charges, the whole atom is electrically neutral.

As we can see from the diagram, the nucleus of this atom consists of 12 particles—6 protons and 6 neutrons. These particles are bound together in a small volume of extremely high density – about three billion, a million times greater than the density of water. The protons in the nucleus carry a positive charge and the electrons in the atomic shells carry an equal negative charge, so this atom is electrically neutral; the neutrons carry no charge. The electrons are arranged in shells called K, L, M ... starting from the orbital closest to the nucleus. The K-shell can contain only two electrons, and, in the case of the carbon atom, the L-shell contains the remaining four. Different atoms contain different numbers of protons and neutrons in the nucleus and different numbers of electron configurations; this will be discussed later in this chapter. The particles which make up the atom are very tiny, and the atom consists largely of empty space. For example, if an atom were to be enlarged until it was the size of a house, the size of the nucleus would be about the size of a pin head, although it contains 99.95% of the total mass of the atom.

The masses and charges of the subatomic particles which will be considered in this and later chapters are summarised in Table 2.1.

TABLE 2.1   Masses and charges of the main subatomic particles

Particle	Symbol	Rest mass		Rest energy	Charge[b]	Comments
		kg	**AMU[a]**	**MeV**		
Proton	p	1.672×10^{-27}	1.007	938	+1	Nucleon, i.e., present in the atomic nucleus
Neutron	n	1.675×10^{-27}	1.009	939	0	Nucleon, i.e., present in the atomic nucleus
Alpha-particle	α	6.645×10^{-27}	4.003	3718	+2	Two protons and two neutrons Ejected in α decay
Electron	e^- or β^-	9.109×10^{-31}	0.00055 or 1/1820	0.511	−1	Form stable discrete orbits around nuclei Ejected from nucleus in β decay
Positron	e^+ or β^+	9.109×10^{-31}	0.00055 or 1/1820	0.511	+1	Antiparticle of the electron—produces annihilation radiation when both meet
Pi-meson	π^+	2.480×10^{-28}	0.150	139	+1	Binds the nucleus together (π^0 and π^- also exist)
Neutrino	ν	0	0	0	0	Emitted during β decay and electron capture Very weak attenuation by matter
Photon or quantum	h_ν	–	–	–	0	Travels at 3×10^8 m.s^{-1} Forms part of the electromagnetic spectrum

[a]1 amu is 1 atomic mass unit which is 1/12 of the mass of a neutral $^{12}_{6}$C atom.
[b]A charge of +1 is $+1.602 \times 10^{-19}$ coulomb.

2.3 THE ATOMIC NUCLEUS

The numbers of protons and neutrons in the atomic nucleus determine both the mass and the charge of the nucleus and the configuration of the electron shells of the atom. There are several important terms, which we will use in this and following chapters of this text, that require definition at this stage. These terms, which will help us to understand atomic structure, are defined in Table 2.2.

We can now consider the use of some of the terms in the tables. The most common naturally occurring stable isotope of carbon has six protons and six neutrons, as shown previously in Fig. 2.1. The atomic number (Z) of this isotope is 6 and the atomic mass number is 12. The whole atom can be written as $^{12}_{6}C$. Thus $^{12}_{6}C$ is an example of a nuclide—one which contains six protons and six neutrons. In general, an element E is written as $^{A}_{Z}E$. An isotope of carbon, which is also naturally occurring but less abundant, has seven neutrons in its nucleus and may be written as $^{13}_{6}C$. An isotope of a chemical element has a constant number of protons in the atomic nucleus (because this defines the element) but a different number of neutrons in the nucleus and thus a different atomic mass.

Note that it is not necessarily the case that isotopes of an element are radioactive, as shown by this example; $^{12}_{6}C$ and $^{13}_{6}C$ are both isotopes of carbon but neither is radioactive.

An isotope of carbon which is radioactive is $^{14}_{6}C$ —the well-known carbon-14, which is used in archaeology to date ancient organic materials. This again contains the six protons which identify it as a carbon nucleus, but this time it contains eight neutrons. $^{14}_{6}C$ is an example of a radionuclide or a radioactive isotope. It decays, as we shall see in Chapter 10, by beta decay to form $^{14}_{7}N$ (nitrogen) as the daughter product.

TABLE 2.2	Terms used to describe a nucleus	
Term	**Symbol**	**Definition**
Nucleon		A proton or neutron within a nucleus
Atomic number	Z	The number of protons in the nucleus
Atomic mass number	A	The total number of nucleons in the nucleus
Neutron number	N	The number of neutrons within the nucleus
Nuclide		A nucleus with a specific value of Z and A
Element	E	A nucleus with a given value of Z
Isotope (of an element)		Any nucleus which contains the same number of protons as the given element but has a different mass number
Isobar		Any nucleus which has the same atomic mass number as another nucleus (i.e., has the same value of A)
Radionuclide or radioisotope		Any nuclide or isotope which is radioactive

2.3.1 The stability of the nucleus

At first sight the atomic nucleus would appear to be inherently unstable because the neutrons are uncharged and the protons have a positive charge and so would electrostatically repel each other. This would suggest that the nucleus should fly apart because of the electrostatic forces between the protons.

In practice, some nuclei are so stable as to possess no measurable radioactivity ($^{12}_{6}C$ is an example; see Section 10.11) whereas others decay with a half-life (see Chapter 10) which may vary from less than a second to many years. The nucleus must be considered as a dynamic rather than a static structure where there are opposing forces acting—forces which tend to hold the nucleus together and forces which tend to disrupt the nucleus. A stable nucleus is one where the disruptive forces never win, and an unstable nucleus is one where they do succeed. The unstable nucleus is said to undergo radioactive decay. It is not possible to predict the exact moment when any particular nucleus will decay, as it is a matter of probability rather than certainty. However, if there are a large number of unstable nuclei in a sample, the law of radioactive decay is obeyed.

The forces which hold the nucleus together are quite unlike the other forces (such as gravity) with which we are familiar. They are known as *short-range nuclear forces* and act over distances of about 10^{-15} metres, over which range they are much more powerful than the electrostatic forces between the protons. These forces are shown diagrammatically in Fig. 2.2. A strong force of attraction is evident below 10^{-15} m, and this changes to a force of repulsion at about 10^{-16} m. The energy expended in keeping the nucleus together is known as the *nuclear binding energy* (NBE). If the NBE is divided by the number of nucleons within the nucleus, then a figure of about 8.4 MeV is obtained for most nuclei. This is known as the *binding energy per nucleon*. The binding energy between the nucleons is provided by the transformation of some of the nuclear mass into energy, as given by Einstein's equation $E = mc^2$. Each nucleon has a mass of approximately 931 MeV per atomic mass unit (amu), of which about 8.4 MeV is used for its NBE to nearby nucleons. Because of this, the mass of the nucleus is always less than the sum of the masses of the nucleons.

Considering the graph in Chapter 10 (Fig. 10.2), it can be seen that, for low atomic number elements, the presence of roughly equal numbers of protons and neutrons in the nucleus produces high stability. As nuclei become larger, with a greater excess of neutrons over protons, the force that holds the nucleus together is less effective, and so high atomic number elements such as uranium and radon tend to have unstable nuclei which decay by the emission of alpha-particles and other radiations.

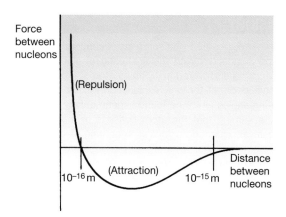

Fig. 2.2 If the separation of the nucleons is between 10^{-15} and 10^{-16} metres, then a force of attraction exists between the nucleons which helps to hold the nucleus together. If the separation is greater or less than this distance, then the force is a repulsive force.

INSIGHT

The pi (π)-meson is a type of boson, a particle with a mass between that of an electron and a nucleon and is thought to be responsible for the forces holding the nucleus together. The short-range forces are known as *exchange forces* and result in (for example) an adjacent proton and a neutron changing continually into a neutron and a proton and back again. This interchange may be written as:

$$p_1 + n_1 \rightarrow n_2 + \pi^+ + n_1 \rightarrow n_2 + p_2$$

The π^+-meson has left the original proton p_1, leaving it as a neutron n_2, and then forms a proton p_2 by combining with the original neutron n_1. The proton and the neutron are continuously exchanging their positions. Negative and neutral π-mesons also exist and are exchanged between nucleons.

2.4   ELECTRON SHELLS

Consider an atom of hydrogen, as shown in Fig. 2.3. It is assumed in the planetary model of the atom that the solitary electron is on a circular path (path 1) around the nucleus. It may be shown that a body moving in a circle of radius r at a velocity V has an acceleration of V^2/r towards the centre of the circle. According to classical physics, such acceleration would result in the emission of electromagnetic radiation from the electron so that the electron is continuously losing energy and would eventually collide with the nucleus (see path 2). Electrons do not behave in

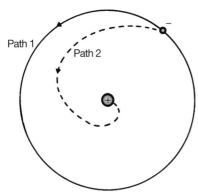

Fig. 2.3 A stable, discrete electron orbital (path 1) compared with a 'decaying electron' (path 2), as predicted by the laws of classical physics.

Principal quantum number or shell number (n)	Shell letter	Maximum number of electrons	$2n^2$
1	K	2	2
2	L	8	8
3	M	18	18
4	N	32	32

TABLE 2.3   **Numbers of electrons in atomic shells**

this manner, or atoms as we know them would not exist. The electrons orbit in stable paths (path 1)—discrete electron orbitals. Further, these orbitals are grouped in 'shells' where there is a particular number of electrons of approximately the same energy in each shell. The electrons fill up the inner shells first because the energies of the inner shells are less than the outer shells.

At this point it would be useful to consider the differences between electron shells and orbitals. 'Shells', such as *K*, *L*, *M* and so on, in increasing distance from the nucleus, are the major structure into which atomic electrons are organised. There are usually large energy differences between electron shells. 'Orbitals' are a form of subdivision of electrons within each shell, with smaller energy differences between them. An orbital describes the three-dimensional volume within which an electron can be found. There are spherical orbitals, termed 's orbitals', and dumbbell-shaped orbitals, termed 'p orbitals', as well as more complex d and f orbitals. The *K*-shell consists of a single s orbital, with two contained electrons, whereas the *L*-shell is occupied by a single s orbital and three p orbitals, containing eight electrons in total.

Table 2.3 shows the maximum number of electrons in each shell from the inner *K*-shell to the *N*-shell. The shell number, *n*, starts from $n = 1$ for the *K*-shell and is known as the *principal quantum number*. The chemical properties of an element are controlled by the electron configuration of its atoms. Atoms with filled outer electron shells are chemically inert—neon ($Z = 10$) has full *K*- and *L*-shells, as illustrated in Fig. 2.4, and so is a chemically inert gas. Fluorine ($Z = 9$), where the *K*-shell contains two electrons and the *L*-shell contains seven, is a chemically active electron acceptor (the electron fills the vacancy in the *L*-shell). Sodium ($Z = 11$), where the *K*-shell contains

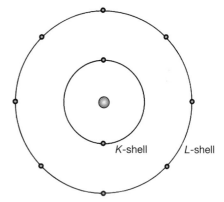

Fig. 2.4 An atom of neon, showing both *K*- and *L*-shells containing their maximum number of permitted electrons. This means that the neon atom is chemically inert.

two electrons, the *L*-shell contains eight electrons and the *M*-shell contains one, is a chemically active electron donor (the electron in the *M*-shell is donated, resulting in a filled *L*-shell).

The outer electron shells may contain subshells within them. Argon ($Z = 18$) has two electrons in its *K*-shell, eight electrons in its *L*-shell and eight electrons in the *M*-shell. The *M*-shell has a maximum complement of electrons of 18 and yet argon is chemically inert. An outer subshell of eight electrons is particularly chemically stable, a fact which is confirmed by the next inert gas, krypton, which has an electron configuration of 2, 8, 18, 8.

2.5   THE PERIODIC TABLE OF ELEMENTS

If the elements are arranged in order of increasing atomic number, it may be shown that their chemical properties, such as valency, and their physical properties, such as specific heat, tend to occur in a periodic manner. Arranging

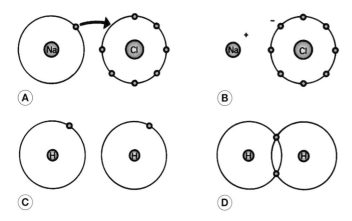

Fig. 2.5 An ionic valency bond (or electron valency) is caused by the transfer of an electron from one atom to another—Na to Cl in (A) and (B). A covalent bond (covalency) is formed when two atoms share electrons in the same orbital, as shown between two hydrogen atoms in (C) and (D).

these elements in these similar groups produces a periodic table as shown in Table E. Chemical similarities of the elements in each group may be explained by reference to their electron structure as shown in Table F, the electron configuration of the elements. It has already been noted that the number of electrons increases with atomic number and that each electron takes an orbital of the lowest possible energy. This means that the inner shells are filled before the outer shells accommodate electrons. There are two rules which determine the way in which the electron shells are gradually built up as the atomic number increases:

1. An electron shell, n, cannot contain more than $2n^2$ electrons, where n is the shell number.
2. The outer shell cannot contain more than eight electrons.

These rules are known as the *Bury–Bohr rules* after their codiscoverers and ensure that the orbitals of minimum energy are filled first.

One additional constraint is required in order that electrons may fill orbitals in the correct manner. This is known as the *Pauli exclusion principle* and states that 'no two electrons may have precisely the same orbital'. The two K-shell electrons of an atom, for example, are not at precisely the same energy level because they orbit the atom in opposing directions. These two electrons complete the K-shell so that the electrons must start to fill up the L-shell (see lithium in Table F) at a greater distance from the nucleus and so at a higher energy. These L-shell electrons all have slightly different energies from each other, and the shell is complete when it has eight electrons—neon satisfies these conditions where $n = 2$ and so $2n^2 = 8$.

The K- and L-shells are thus completed in sequence but the M-shell (which from the $2n^2$ formula can contain up to 18 electrons), when it reaches nine electrons (argon), then obeys the rule that the outer shell cannot contain more than eight electrons and the ninth electron is placed in the N-shell (see potassium in Table F). This process is repeated each time there are eight electrons in the outer orbital (see rubidium, caesium, francium, etc.).

As mentioned earlier in Section 2.4, the number of electrons in the outer orbital determines the chemical activity of the element. The ability of one atom to join another is called *valency* and the electron linkage between the atoms is called the *valency bond*. There are two types of valency bond:

1. Ionic bonds (see Fig. 2.5A and B): this type of bond is created when one or more electrons are transferred from one atom to another, forming charged atoms (or ions) which are attracted toward each other by electrostatic attraction forming the bond. After the electron exchange, the shells of each ion appear to be closed.
2. Covalent bonds (see Fig. 2.5C and D): formed by the apparent sharing of electrons such that each atom appears to increase its number of electrons forming an apparently closed shell.

2.6   ELECTRON ORBITAL CHANGES

The previous sections of this chapter have shown that electrons may only take up fixed or discrete orbitals around an atomic nucleus. We have also discussed the fact that the inner orbitals are filled before the outer orbitals, because this constitutes the lowest energy state of the whole atom. An atom in this state is said to be in its ground state because it cannot have an electron configuration which will produce a lower energy. However this is not to say that any particular atom at a given moment of time will be at its ground state, because interatomic collisions or interactions with electromagnetic radiations may have raised the energy of one of its electrons so that it is able to take up an orbital of higher

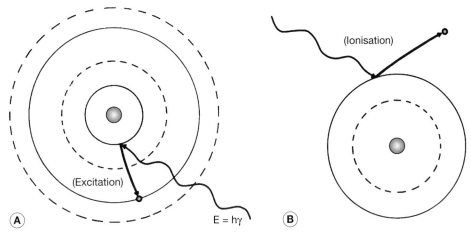

Fig. 2.6 An incoming photon interacts with an orbiting electron of an atom. In (A) this photon has sufficient energy to cause excitation and in (B) the photon causes ionisation.

energy—the electron will move further away from the nucleus. This process is called *excitation* of the atom. The excited electron is able to return to its original orbital and releases a quantum of electromagnetic radiation in the process. The energy of this quantum is equal to the energy difference between the excited state and the ground state. Alternatively, an orbiting electron may receive sufficient energy to be able to escape from the atom completely—this might happen as a result of the interaction of a photon with the electron. This process is called *ionisation* because the remaining atom will now form a positive ion. Both processes are shown diagrammatically in Fig. 2.6.

2.7 BINDING ENERGY OF THE ELECTRON SHELLS

Because the various electron shells are positioned at different distances from the atomic nucleus, they experience different forces of attraction from the nucleus. The K-shell is closest to the nucleus and so experiences the greatest force of attraction from the nucleus. It is therefore most difficult to remove an electron from the K-shell—the K-shell has the highest electron binding energy. The electron binding energy of a shell is the amount of work which must be done to remove an electron from that shell (it is normally stated in KeV or eV). The L-shell is further away from the nucleus and so experiences less force of attraction. It also experiences some repulsion from the electrons in the K-shell. For this reason, the binding energy of the electrons in the L-shell is less than the binding energy of the K-shell for a particular atom. Thus we can say that there

is a reduction in the binding energy as we move from the K-shell to the L-shell to the M-shell, and so on, within a particular atom.

The reason for the existence of the binding energy is the electrostatic attraction between the nucleus and the electrons in the shells. Thus we would expect to find an increase in the K-shell binding energy with an increase in the atomic number of the element. This is found to be the case in practice.

A knowledge of the binding energy of the various electron shells in different elements is important in radiation physics for the following reasons:
- A knowledge of the binding energies of the different shells allows us to predict the energies of the characteristic radiations which the atom might produce (see Chapter 11 for further details).
- A knowledge of the binding energies of different electron shells within an atom of an element will allow us to determine the likely position of absorption edges during photoelectric absorption (see Chapter 13 for further details).
- If we know the energy of the characteristic radiation from an element and we know the position of absorption edges when radiation is attenuated by this material, then this allows us to explain why elements are relatively transparent to their own characteristic radiation (see Section 18.4 for further details).

Although the binding energy of an electron orbital increases as we move closer to the nucleus, its potential energy reduces. Thus if an electron moves from the L-shell to the K-shell, it must lose energy (normally in the form of a photon of characteristic radiation).

2.8   THE STRUCTURE OF MATTER

So far in this chapter the discussion has focused on the properties of atoms. However, atoms are typically combined within molecules, which consist of two or more atoms, chemically bound together. Compounds consist of atoms from more than one element, present in fixed ratios. Compounds may consist of discrete molecules, as in the case of water, H_2O, or extended arrays of atoms, as in the case of crystalline structures such as common salt, NaCl. Some molecules, such as hydrogen, H_2 and oxygen, O_2, are not termed compounds, because they are composed of atoms of one element only.

2.8.1   Molecular compounds

Molecular compounds consist of discrete molecules, containing atoms that are covalently bound, sharing electrons in the bonds between atoms because the electron affinities (the tendency to hold on to electrons) of those atoms are similar. These compounds include organic (i.e., carbon-based) molecules in our body tissues, such as proteins, fats and carbohydrates. Other molecular compounds include water, which comprises about 50% to 70% of our human body weight, oil, which is used to cool X-ray tubes, and also contrast agents, used to enhance body tissues in computed tomography (CT) and magnetic resonance imaging (MRI).

2.8.2   Crystalline compounds

Crystalline compounds consist of atoms that are have ionic bonds, transferring electrons from one atom to another because the electron affinities of those atoms are very different. Thus the atoms are held together by the electrostatic attraction that exists between ions of positive and negative charge. These compounds tend to exist as extended arrays or 'lattices' of atoms. A good example for medical imaging is caesium iodide, CsI, which consists of Cs^+ and I^- ions. Iodine, being highly 'electronegative', attracts an electron away from a neighbouring caesium atom. Caesium iodide is known as a '*phosphor*' material because it emits light when struck by electromagnetic radiations such as X-rays. This is the result of temporary excitation of electrons in atomic shells. Many other inorganic phosphorescent materials, often containing rare earth elements, are employed in computed radiography (CR) and digital radiography (DR). The inorganic crystals found in bone, such as hydroxyapatite $Ca_5(PO_4)_3OH$, contain calcium and phosphorus and give bone its relatively high average atomic number relative to soft tissue.

2.8.3   Single element materials

Carbon, silicon and germanium can form extensive covalently bound structures consisting of just a single element. Carbon can exist as diamond and as graphite, the latter being used as a heat-radiating material in some X-ray tube rotating anode discs. Carbon fibre, used in X-ray couches, consists of carbon atom tubules, similar in chemical composition to graphite but much stronger. Silicon and germanium, often with added impurity atoms, are very important in X-ray circuits (see Chapter 7) because they act as semiconductors, being able to conduct electricity in response to an applied stimulus such as a voltage. This 'on-off' capability makes them very useful for tasks such as switching.

2.8.4   Inert gases

Inert or 'noble' gases are unusual because they consist of atoms that are chemically unreactive, owing to a filled outer electron shell. Thus they are 'monoatomic' in nature, consisting of lone unbound atoms. Examples are helium, used in liquid form in MRI scanners at about −269° C to maintain superconductivity; krypton and xenon, which may be used in radionuclide imaging for lung imaging; and radon, which seeps out of rocks and contributes greatly to our natural background radiation dose.

2.8.5   Metals

Metals have the properties of being lustrous, malleable and electrically conductive. They may be used as alloys (containing more than one element) or in a pure single element state. The structures are held together by metallic bonds, attributed to electrostatic attractions between positively charged metal ions and electrons which are able to move freely about and are 'shared' between the ions. The metal ions are arranged in lattice structures, similar to those found in crystalline materials. These ions are immersed in a 'sea' of electrons, which can flow in response to an applied electrical potential difference, resulting in electrical current. Copper is widely used as an electrical conductor in imaging equipment. Tungsten, because of its high atomic number and melting point, is employed in X-ray production. Aluminium is a widely used X-ray filtration material, whereas lead is able to absorb X-rays well and is a good radiation protection barrier. Titanium, resulting from its nonmagnetic properties, is employed for orthopaedic body implants, because it permits people to have MRI scans.

2.8.6   States of matter

The three common states of matter are gases, liquids and solids. Matter may typically transform in state according to temperature. In gases, the molecules are essentially isolated from each other and there are no bonds between them. Air, because of its low density, absorbs X-rays to a negligible extent and thus provides good image 'contrast' when adjacent to soft tissue in medical imaging. This can be useful for showing the lungs. Gases can also be used to depict the bowel and soft tissue infections. Ionisation of air molecules is employed in X-radiation dosimetry. Gas-filled X-ray or gamma-ray detectors have also been used historically in some scanners.

In liquids such as water, the molecules are mobile but weakly bound, especially by 'hydrogen bonds'. These are weak electrostatic attractions that occur between polar molecules. For example, in water, the oxygen atom is slightly negatively charged, and the hydrogen atoms are slightly positively charged. In MRI, the relative mobility of water in different body tissues affects the amount of signal that can be obtained from the water molecules' hydrogen atoms. Highly 'bound' water returns little signal whereas 'free' water returns a strong signal (see Chapter 25). Also the diffusion speed of water molecules is important in diffusion weighted MRI. The X-ray absorption properties of water and soft tissue are surprisingly similar, because their densities and average atomic numbers are comparable. In ultrasound, the speed of sound in water is greater than that in solids, giving acoustic impedance differences which provide signal at tissue boundaries (see Chapter 24).

Solids contain atoms or molecules that are strongly bound together, by ionic, covalent or metallic bonds. Dense solids such as bone and most metals (except aluminium) are strong absorbers of X-rays. This provides improved image contrast when viewing bone–soft tissue boundaries and also permits metals to be used as X-ray filters. Also most modern X-ray and gamma-ray detectors used in medical imaging are 'solid state'. In MRI, crystalline solids tend to return little or no signal, because any water molecules within them are rigidly bound. In ultrasound, dense solids provide barriers to the transmission of sound waves.

SUMMARY

In this chapter, you should have learnt the following:
- The main subatomic particles found within atoms.
- A planetary model of the atom which consists of a nucleus containing protons and neutrons and has electrons in specific orbitals around this nucleus.
- The structure of the atomic nucleus and the reasons for its stability or otherwise.
- The configuration of electron shells for differing atoms and the factors which determine the maximum number of electrons in a shell.
- The structure of the periodic table of elements and the electron configuration of elements.
- The meaning of the term *ground state* when applied to an atom and the consequences of raising the energy of the electrons above the ground state.
- An explanation of the term *binding energy* and a brief outline of areas where a knowledge of the binding energy of electron shells is of importance in radiation physics.
- The structure of matter and its relevance to medical imaging.

FURTHER READING

Ball, J.L., Moore, A.D., & Turner, S. 2008. *Ball and Moore's Essential Physics for Radiographers.* 4th edn. London: Blackwell Scientific. (Chapter 4.)

Bushong, S. 2016. *Radiologic Science for Technologists: Physics, Biology, and Protection.* 11th edn. Mosby. (Chapter 2.)

3

Classical physics principles—energy, force, matter and heat

CHAPTER CONTENTS

3.1   AIM

This chapter introduces the reader to some of the laws of 'classical physics'. An understanding of these laws will aid in understanding some of the later chapters of the book. Concepts such as energy, force, matter and heat are key to X-ray production in the X-ray tube, for example. Classical physics is based on principles such as mechanics and was capable of explaining most phenomena up until the late 19th century. However, observations such as the dual nature of electromagnetic radiations, which could be considered both as particles and as waves, brought about the advent of 'modern' physics after 1900. Modern physics principles are covered in Chapter 8 and provide an explanation of phenomena such as the photoelectric effect (the emission of 'free' electrons when electromagnetic radiation is absorbed) and Compton scatter. The discovery of X-rays and radioactivity at the end of the 19th century contributed to the need for more 'modern' physics explanations.

3.2   LAW OF CONSERVATION OF MATTER (MASS)

3.2.1   Statement of the law

Matter is neither created nor destroyed, but it may change its chemical form as the result of a chemical reaction.

This law tells us that the total mass of the ingredients after a chemical reaction is equal to their mass before the reaction.

INSIGHT

Consider the reaction: $H_2O \rightarrow OH^- + H^+$.

Here a molecule of water has been ionised by radiation. Matter has neither been created nor destroyed by the reaction.

3.3   LAW OF CONSERVATION OF ENERGY

3.3.1   Statement of the law

Energy can neither be created nor destroyed but can be changed from one form to another. The amount of energy in a system is constant.

This law tells us that energy is never used up but changes from one form to another.

INSIGHT

When an electron is released from the filament of an X-ray tube, it has potential energy. As it is accelerated across the tube, this potential energy is converted to kinetic energy. When it makes contact with the target of the tube, this kinetic energy is converted to heat and X-ray energy. At any time, the sum of all the energies remains constant.

Some of the common forms of energy are
- chemical
- potential
- electrical
- kinetic
- heat
- radiation.

These two laws of conservation of mass and energy are combined into one law by modern physics (see Chapter 8).

3.4   LAW OF CONSERVATION OF MOMENTUM

3.4.1   Statement of the law

The total linear or rotational momentum in a given system is constant.

This law is important when we consider collisions between two bodies.

INSIGHT

There are two types of collision that occur: elastic and inelastic. An elastic collision is one where all kinetic energy is conserved, as in the case of a 'perfect' billiard ball colliding with a similar but stationary billiard ball; the moving ball stops, while the ball which was previously stationary moves with the same velocity as the first ball had before collision. In an inelastic collision, the total kinetic energy is not conserved, as in the case of two billiard balls colliding with a glancing blow, so that both continue to move after the collision. In both cases, the momentum is conserved, although the velocities of the bodies in each case will be different.

In radiographic science, conservation of momentum is mainly concerned with the interactions of X-rays with matter; these will be dealt with in Chapter 13.

3.5   NEWTON'S LAWS OF MOTION

Newton's laws of motion can be derived from the above laws, but they are so important that they merit a separate section. They are defined as follows:

3.5.1   Law 1

A body will remain at rest or will travel with a constant velocity unless acted upon by a net external force.

3.5.2   Law 2

The rate of change of momentum of a body is proportional to the applied force.

3.5.3   Law 3

The action of one body on a second body is always accompanied by an equal and opposite action of the second body on the first.

The terms *velocity* and *momentum* in the first two laws imply direction, as both are vector quantities (see Chapter 4).

A body of mass m and velocity u has a force F applied to it. After a time t, its velocity has changed to v. Then the second law of motion can be stated as:

$$\frac{(mv - mu)}{t} \propto F$$
$$\frac{m(v - u)}{t} \propto F$$

Now $(v - u)/t$ is the rate of change of velocity or the acceleration, a, of the body (see Chapter 4). So, we can say that:

$$ma \propto F \text{ or } F = kma$$

where k is the constant of proportionality (see Appendix A).

If we choose suitable units, it can be arranged that k is equal to 1 and we finally have:

$$F = m \times a \qquad \textbf{Equation 3.1}$$

In the International System of Units ([SI]; see Chapter 4), F is measured in newtons, m is measured in kilograms and a is measured in m.s^{-2}. This makes Equation 3.1 the familiar mathematical statement of Newton's second law and can also be used as the basis for the definition of the newton ($1\ N = 1\ kg \times 1\ m.s^{-2}$).

INSIGHT

As an illustration of the use of this law, we are now in a position to calculate the kinetic energy of a body of mass, m, travelling with a velocity, v. If we apply a steady force, F, in the opposite direction to that of v, the body will slow down and eventually come to rest. The work done in bringing the body to rest must be equal to its kinetic energy. We can state this mathematically as:

$$E = -F \times s \qquad \textbf{Equation 3.2}$$

where s is the distance taken for the body to come to rest. (The force, F, and its associated acceleration, a, are regarded as negative as they are applied in the opposite direction to v.)

From Equation 3.1 we can now change Equation 3.2 as follows:

$$E = -m \times a \times s \qquad \textbf{Equation 3.3}$$

The acceleration, a, is the change in velocity per unit time. Stated mathematically, this is:

$$-a = \frac{(v - 0)}{t}$$

$$a = \frac{-v}{t}$$

Because the action of the force is consistent throughout the deceleration, the time taken for the body to stop can be calculated by dividing the distance travelled by the average velocity ($v/2$). So:

$$t = \frac{s}{\frac{1}{2}v} = \frac{2s}{v}$$

Thus we get:

$$a = \frac{-v}{t}$$

$$= \frac{-v}{(2s / v)}$$

$$= \frac{-v^2}{2s}$$

If we now consider Equation 3.3, this can be rewritten:

$$E = \frac{-m(as)}{\frac{1}{2}}$$

$$= -m\left(-\tfrac{1}{2}v^2\right) \qquad \textbf{Equation 3.4}$$

$$E = -\tfrac{1}{2}mv^2$$

Newton's third law is usually paraphrased as 'To every action there is an equal and opposite reaction'. There are many examples of this in everyday life, such as a hammer hitting a nail, but it is important to realise that there need not necessarily be physical contact between the two bodies for one to act on the other. If we take two charged bodies and bring these close together (but not actually touching), the forces between the two bodies will be equal and opposite. The significance of this in the design of the cathode of the X-ray tube will be considered in Chapter 12.

3.6 AVOGADRO'S HYPOTHESIS, THE MOLE AND AVOGADRO'S NUMBER

As we saw in Chapter 2, all substances consist of atoms or molecules. These may react chemically with the atoms or molecules of other substances. These reactions occur with fixed proportions to produce a given chemical compound, and it is possible to predict the number of molecules of the compound from knowledge of the number of molecules of the original elements or compounds, for example:

$$2H_2 + O_2 = 2H_2O$$

In the case of gases, Avogadro's hypothesis postulated that equal volumes of gases at the same temperature and pressure contain equal numbers of molecules. This hypothesis was first postulated in the early nineteenth century and has been verified by a number of experiments since then.

This is taken one stage further within the SI system in the more general statement that the number of molecules per mole is the same for any substance. The mole is the SI unit of the amount of substance and is defined as:

DEFINITION

The mole is the amount of substance which contains as many elementary particles as there are atoms in 0.012 kg of carbon-12.

Carbon-12 is used as the standard for technical experimental reasons. From this, we can predict the number of atoms or molecules in a substance by knowing its atomic mass number and comparing this with carbon-12. For example, if we consider cobalt-60, then there will be the same number of atoms in 0.06 kg of cobalt-60 as there will be in 0.012 kg of carbon-12 because each constitutes one mole of substance. The number of molecules in a mole is given by Avogadro's number (or constant) and is 6×10^{23} molecules.

3.7   HEAT

We are familiar with the feelings of hot and cold; indeed, we are crucially dependent on our body temperature staying within a very limited range to survive. Compared with the vast ranges of temperature which exist across the universe, our experience of hot and cold is very limited indeed.

To investigate heat further, we must use objective measures of heat and cold, as described in the following sections.

3.8   HEAT ENERGY AND TEMPERATURE

When heat is given to a body, its atoms or molecules are given increased kinetic energy in the form of increased lattice vibration (this is the reason why substances expand when heated). A body whose atoms have a higher kinetic energy than those of another body is said to be hotter or at a higher temperature. If two bodies are placed in contact, then heat will be transferred from the hotter body to the cooler body by collisions between the molecules at the point of contact. The molecules of the cooler body receive a net increase in kinetic energy and so its temperature rises. The molecules of the hotter body have lost kinetic energy and so its temperature falls. This process continues until the two bodies are at the same temperature when no further exchange of energy takes place. The bodies are now in a state of thermal equilibrium. Notice that the thermal energy is always transferred from the body at the higher temperature to the body at the lower temperature, irrespective of the size of the bodies. Also note that the temperature existing at thermal equilibrium will always lie somewhere between the initial temperatures of the two bodies.

3.8.1   Temperature scales

There are two temperature scales used in modern physics: Celsius (also called centigrade) and kelvin. The Celsius scale is defined as 0° C at the temperature of melting ice, and 100° C at the temperature of boiling water at an atmospheric pressure of 1.01×10^5 newtons per square metre (76 mm of mercury). On this scale, the temperature of absolute zero (see previous Insight) is approximately −273.15° C. This temperature is zero on the kelvin scale (0 K) whereas the temperature of melting ice is 273.15 K. From this, we can see that the units of temperature are the same on both scales but the scales have different starting points, that is, one unit on the Celsius scale is equivalent to one unit on the kelvin scale. Note that temperature on the kelvin scale does not have the degree symbol in front of the K. It is a convenient approximation to assume that 0° C = 273 K, so that the simple conversion formula may be used:

$$T°C = (T + 273)K \qquad \textbf{Equation 3.5}$$

where T is temperature.

3.8.2 Units of heat energy, specific heat capacity and thermal capacity

If heat is given to a body, then its molecules will have a higher kinetic energy and its temperature will rise. Hence, it is convenient to express a quantity of heat in terms of the temperature change it produces in a given body. Consider the situation where we wish to apply an amount of energy, Q, which will raise the temperature of a body by 1 kelvin unit (for simplicity, assume that this does not change the state of the body, i.e., it does not change from a solid to a liquid). This will be affected by the mass and the type of material of the body. It also seems logical to assume that we would need twice the amount of heat to raise the temperature of the body by 2 kelvin units. If we take all these factors together, we can write the equation:

$$Q = mc(T_2 - T_1) \qquad \textbf{Equation 3.6}$$

where Q is the heat energy required to raise the temperature of a body of mass m from T_1 to a temperature T_2. The factor c is approximately constant for a particular material and is known as the *specific heat capacity* of the material. We can rearrange Equation 3.6 to get:

$$c = \frac{Q}{m(T_2 - T_1)} \qquad \textbf{Equation 3.7}$$

so that c, the specific heat capacity, is in units of c joules per kilogram per kelvin ($J.kg^{-1}.K^{-1}$). Specific heat capacity can be defined thus:

> **DEFINITION**
>
> The specific heat capacity of a body is the energy in joules required to raise the temperature of 1 kilogram of the body by 1 kelvin unit.

The specific heat capacity of a substance is thus unique to that substance and it allows us to predict the behavior of different masses of the same substance.

> **EXAMPLE**
>
> The specific heat capacity of water is about 4.2 ($J.kg^{-1}.K^{-1}$). How much heat energy is required to raise a mass of 10 g of water from 280 K to 285 K? (Remember that the unit of energy is the joule and the unit of mass is the kilogram.)
>
> Using Equation 3.6, we have:
>
> $$Q = mc(T_2 - T_1)$$
> $$= 10^{-2} \times 42 \times 10^3 \times (285 - 280)$$
> $$= 210\,J$$

In the situations considered so far, we have considered the amount of heat required to raise the temperature of 1 kg of the material. Another unit of heat energy, which is useful in practice, is the thermal capacity.

> **DEFINITION**
>
> The thermal capacity of a body is the heat energy in joules which is required to raise the temperature of the body by 1 kelvin unit.

Note that this definition differs from the previous one for specific heat capacity in that no mention is made of unit mass. Thus the thermal capacity refers to the whole of the body and not just 1 kg of it. It should also be noted that the thermal capacity of a body is the specific heat capacity of the body multiplied by the mass of the body. The units of thermal capacity are joules per kelvin.

> **EXAMPLE**
>
> The anode discs of two X-ray tubes are made of the same material but one has twice the mass of the other. If the same amount of heat is applied to each anode, which will have the higher temperature rise at the end of the exposure?
>
> The thermal capacity is the product of the mass and the specific heat. Thus, the larger anode will have twice the thermal capacity of the smaller one. If the same amount of heat is applied to each, the smaller one will experience twice the temperature rise of the larger one. The importance of this will be considered when we consider the rating of the X-ray tube (see Chapter 12).

3.9 TRANSFER OF HEAT

As mentioned at the beginning of this chapter, heat can be given to a body from some other structure with greater thermal energy than the body. Similarly, if a body can be isolated from its environment or is in a state of thermal equilibrium with its surroundings, there is no net gain or loss of heat from the body.

The mechanisms of heat transfer form an important part of the study of radiography because of the large amounts of heat energy produced at the target of the X-ray tube. The mechanical and thermal stresses associated with this make it possible to damage the X-ray tube unless adequate precautions are taken. The anodes of all X-ray tubes must therefore be designed to transfer heat away from the focal spot area as quickly as possible to minimise the temperature rise in this

TABLE 3.1   Thermal conductivity of materials

Material	Thermal conductivity (W.m^{-1}.K^{-1})	Comments
Copper	386	Excellent conductor—used as the anode material in the stationary anode tube
Tungsten	202	Fairly good conductor—used as the target material in stationary X-ray tubes
Molybdenum	147	Relatively poor conductor—used as the anode stem in the rotating anode tube, to encourage heat loss from the anode by heat radiation
Glass	1.0	Poor conductor—involved in the transfer of heat to the oil in the tube housing
Rubber	0.05	Very poor conductor
Air	0.02	Very poor conductor—removes heat from the housing of the X-ray tube by convection

region. The practical application of this knowledge to the design of X-ray tubes will be considered in Chapter 12. However, we must first understand the different mechanisms of heat transfer: these are conduction, convection and radiation.

3.9.1 Conduction

Conduction is the transfer of heat between bodies by physical contact of those bodies and results in a transfer of kinetic energy by interatomic collision, thus forming the main process by which heat is transferred through a solid. If heat is applied to one end of a metal bar, the atoms at this end of the bar receive copious supplies of kinetic energy. These atoms, because of their increased vibrational energy, collide with neighbouring atoms and so kinetic energy is gradually transferred along the bar. This method of heat flow along the bar is known as *conduction of heat*.

We can find by experiment that the rate of flow of heat, q (joules per second), by conduction is controlled by a number of things:

- $Q \propto A$ (the cross-sectional area of the rod)
- $q \propto (T_1 - T_2)$ (the temperature difference between the ends of the rod; this is known as the *temperature gradient*)
- $q \propto (1/l)$ (where l is the length of the rod)
- q depends on the material of the rod.

Combining all these factors, we have:

$$q \propto \frac{A(T_1 - T_2)}{l}$$

$$q = \frac{kA(T_1 - T_2)}{l}$$

Equation 3.8

Here k is the constant of proportionality and this is a constant for any given material. It is known as the *thermal conductivity* of the material. Materials are classed as 'good'

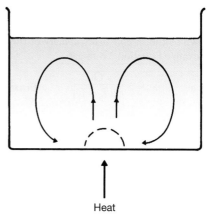

Fig. 3.1 Principles of convection. Applied heat causes the broken-line region of fluid to expand, become less dense and rise, being replaced by cooler parts of the fluid. This sets up convection currents.

or 'bad' conductors depending on the value of k. Typical values of k are shown in Table 3.1.

Note that the rate of flow of heat along a bar can be changed by altering the length, the cross-sectional area and the temperature gradient, as well as by altering the material.

3.9.2 Convection

Convection is the main process by which heat is transferred in fluids (i.e., liquids and gases). Consider heat being applied to a liquid in a beaker (Fig. 3.1). The liquid near the source of heat has thermal energy transferred to it by conduction. This increase in thermal energy causes the liquid to expand and become less dense than the surrounding liquid. The heated liquid rises (because of hydrostatic pressure) and, as it rises, it transfers heat to the surrounding molecules by conduction. The temperature of the small section of heated liquid returns to the same temperature as the surrounding liquid and so sinks back into the beaker, to be heated a second time. Thus, convection currents are established, as shown in Fig. 3.1. The overall effect is that the whole volume of fluid is heated and not just the region where the heat is applied.

Some interesting points emerge from this:

- Convection can occur only where the molecules are free to move through the medium, that is, in liquids and gases.
- It is not possible to have convection currents without some conduction.
- It is necessary to have a gravitational field for the convection currents to be initiated because the warm fluid moves in the opposite direction to the gravitational force, by hydrostatic pressure.

3.9.3   Radiation

In this process, heat is lost from a body with high thermal energy in the form of electromagnetic radiations. Radiation is the only heat transfer process that will take place through a vacuum. The most obvious and striking example is the heat we can feel from our sun where the radiation must pass through a near-perfect vacuum for 93 million miles (approximately 150 million km) to reach us. Light and heat also reach us from other stars but we are only able to discern the light, as we are not sufficiently sensitive to small amounts of heat (although the latter can be detected with infrared sensors).

We are able to feel heat by radiation because it imparts kinetic energy to molecules of our tissues, which we discern as an increase in temperature. Heat radiations occur in a band of energies just beyond the red part of the visible spectrum (see Chapter 9 for further detail of the electromagnetic spectrum). This band of energies is known as *infrared radiations*. All bodies radiate electromagnetic energies if their temperature is above absolute zero. This does not necessarily mean that we can discern the radiations, as we perceive only a narrow band of energies extending from violet light to infrared. Bodies of different colours and different surface compositions radiate somewhat differently and so it is conventional to consider black-body radiation. This we will do next.

3.9.3.1   Black-body radiation

A body looks black because very little of the light incident upon it is reflected or transmitted. A black body is defined as one that will absorb 100% of all radiations at all frequencies incident upon it. If such a black body is in a state of thermal equilibrium with its surroundings, equal amounts of radiation must be absorbed and emitted per second.

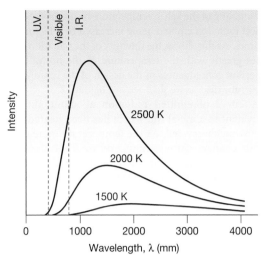

Fig. 3.2 The spectrum of electromagnetic radiation emitted by a black body at different temperatures. The total intensity (I) is a function of the kelvin temperature ($I \propto T^4$). *IR*, Infrared *UV*, ultraviolet.

From this it can be deduced that the black body must radiate more energy than any other type of body because no other body absorbs 100% of the energy incident upon it. The foregoing statements can be summarised thus:

- All bodies are capable of emitting radiation.
- A black body absorbs 100% of all radiations incident upon it.
- A black body is the most efficient emitter of radiation of any body.

We now need to know in more detail the spectrum of radiations emitted by a black body. Fig. 3.2 shows such a spectrum for a black body at different temperatures. The following should be noted from the graph:

- The wavelength corresponding to the peak radiation progressively decreases as the temperature of the body increases.
- The height of the graph (intensity of radiation) is very sensitive to changes in temperature.
- The spectrum of the radiation is a smooth curve, of which we perceive only a small part (violet to infrared).
- The total intensity of the radiation emitted by a body at a given temperature is the sum of the intensities at each wavelength. This is related to the area under the curve in each case. *Stefan's law* states that the total intensity of the emitted radiation is proportional to the fourth power of the kelvin temperature. Thus:

$$I \propto T^4$$
$$\text{or} \quad I = \sigma T^4 \qquad \textbf{Equation 3.9}$$

where σ is Stefan's constant.

Doubling of the kelvin temperature results in the amount of heat radiation emitted being increased by a factor of $2^4 = 16$ times. As this shows, the intensity of the radiation emitted varies greatly with the temperature of the body. This has important consequences in the design of the rotating anode X-ray tube disc, as we shall see in Chapter 12.

A curve of emitted radiation at about 1000 K is equivalent to a metal rod which has been heated until it is glowing cherry-red. As the temperature increases, the colour changes through light red to white because an increasing amount of the violet end of the spectrum is emitted along with the red (see 2000 K and 2500 K lines in Fig. 3.2). At higher temperatures, objects emit white light. This is true of the filament of an electric light bulb or the anode disc of the rotating anode tube after a large exposure.

INSIGHT

The mechanism that causes the emission of radiation is the acceleration and deceleration of the charged particles, which make up the atoms or molecules of the body involved. An example particularly relevant to radiography is the sudden deceleration of electrons when they strike the anode of the X-ray tube—the Bremsstrahlung or braking radiation. Here, some (or all) of the kinetic energy of the electron is transformed into an X-ray photon (see Chapter 11). Another example is the production of radio waves, where electrons are forced to oscillate at high frequencies in a radio-transmitting aerial.

The interactions of energetic atoms produce a broad band of emitted quanta wavelengths because of the range of interactions that are possible. All of these radiations form part of the electromagnetic spectrum. A narrow range of frequencies (in the infrared part) is capable of being absorbed by the whole atom (as opposed to the electron shells or the nucleus) and so these atoms gain kinetic energy. This increase in the kinetic energy of the atoms is in the form of heat. Higher frequencies of radiation interact with the electrons in the orbitals and even higher frequencies will interact with the atomic nuclei.

3.10   THERMAL EXPANSION

Most substances expand when heated, owing to the increased kinetic energy of the atoms. The linear expansivity is a measure of this thermal expansion, defined as the fractional change in unit length per unit change in kelvin temperature. The thermal expansion of different parts of

the X-ray tube is an important design consideration as the tube is subject to large temperature variations during its working life. If materials of very different thermal expansivity are used, this can cause mechanical stress that could result in fracture of one of the components. A particularly weak point in this respect is the seal between the glass and the copper anode in a stationary anode tube. A special type of glass with a thermal expansivity very similar to copper is chosen. This reduces the mechanical stress and thus the chances of fracture of the glass envelope and loss of vacuum in the tube.

3.11   EVAPORATION AND VAPORISATION

We are all familiar with the evaporation of liquids that occurs when heat is applied to them (e.g., boiling kettles). Evaporation is caused by the loss of whole atoms from the surface of the liquid. Some of the atoms are given sufficient kinetic energy to escape from the forces of attraction of their neighbours near the surface of the liquid and produce a vapour in the free space above this surface.

Whole atoms may also be liberated from the surfaces of solid materials under the action of heat. There is a stronger force of attraction between the atoms in a solid compared with a liquid and so liberation of the atoms is more difficult to accomplish. This means that in a solid the atoms require higher kinetic energy for liberation, that is, solids need to be subjected to a higher temperature. The tungsten at the target and in the filament of the X-ray tube is subjected to such high temperatures that a certain amount of vaporisation takes place. The tungsten vapour can condense to form a thin layer of tungsten on the inside of the glass of the envelope. A major effect of this is to reduce the electrical insulation provided by the glass, as tungsten is a reasonable conductor of electricity. This can produce an effect called a 'gassy tube', which renders the X-ray tube inoperable. Fortunately, this does not occur readily as tungsten has a low vapour pressure and so does not readily vaporise at its normal working temperatures.

SUMMARY

In this chapter you should have learnt:
- The laws of conservation of matter, energy and momentum
- Newton's laws of motion
- Avogadro's hypothesis, the mole and Avogadro's number
- Principles of heat, which are relevant to the operation of X-ray tubes.

FURTHER READING

Further reading on the laws of classical physics can be found in most textbooks which are used in schools for study of AS level or A2 level physics. In addition, the following may prove useful:

Ball, J.L., Moore, A.D., & Turner, S. 2008. *Ball and Moore's Essential Physics for Radiographers.* 4th edn. London: Blackwell Scientific. (Chapters 1 and 2.)

Bushong, S.C. 2016. *Radiological Science for Technologists: Physics, Biology and Protection.* 11th edn. New York: Mosby. (Chapter 1.)

Units of measurement

CHAPTER CONTENTS

4.1   AIM

This chapter introduces the reader to the main units that are used in measurement in medical imaging science. Medical imaging involves numerical values that range from the very small (such as the sizes of atoms, measured in thousand millionths of a metre) to the very large (such as the frequencies of radio waves used in magnetic resonance imaging (MRI), measured in millions of cycles per second).

4.2   UNITS OF MEASUREMENT

Science makes use of observations and measurements to record numerical values, test hypotheses and develop theories. This is the basis of experimentation. In clinical imaging we might not regard every examination as an experiment, but we do gather a large amount of observational data in many forms, such as signal intensity, signal frequency and electrical current. Also true experimentation is undertaken when measuring equipment performance, for example, using phantoms and test objects. In many imaging situations we assume that there are direct or even linear relationships between factors, such as between X-radiation exposure and signal intensity. Such situations require the recording of numerical values.

Problems arise when making experimental measurements as to what quantities to measure and how to measure them. In particular, the units in which these quantities are expressed must be defined so that when two people take the same measurement they get the same results. Also, there are obvious advantages if one set of units is universally adopted as the basis for all measurements.

Each of the base units discussed in the next section relies on the appropriate standard to which each measurement is compared. Thus there are units of standard length, standard mass, standard time interval and so on. Without such standards, no accurate measurements could be made, and it would be difficult to develop adequate theories, or models, of the physical world.

4.3   THE INTERNATIONAL SYSTEM OF UNITS BASE UNITS

There is a wide range of units of measurement used throughout the world. The International System of Units, or Système Internationale (SI) attempts to replace this with seven standard units. These standards are termed *SI units* (see Table 4.1) and represent the fundamental measurements that we might wish to make of a body:

- What is its size? (unit of *length – metre*)
- How massive is it? (unit of *mass – kilogram*)
- How bright is it? (unit of *luminous intensity – candela*)
- How much electrical current flows through it? (unit of *electrical current – ampere*)

- How many elementary particles does it contain? (unit of *amount of substance – mole*)
- How hot is it? (unit of *temperature – Kelvin*)
- How do all the quantities vary with time? (unit of *time – second*)

The very precise definitions of the units are not required for the rest of this text, but if you wish to see them, they are given in Appendix D.

The base units of mass, length and time are termed *fundamental* or *base units* because one or more of them is always involved in the measurement of any other quantity.

These seven SI base units may be combined to give derived units, as described in the next section.

4.3.1   Derived SI units

A number of derived SI units can be formed by the combination of the seven base units. Some of these are sufficiently important to be given their own names and they are listed in Table 4.2 and discussed in the rest of this chapter.

Further derived units are of a more specialised nature (e.g., absorbed radiation dose) and will be discussed in the specific chapters which require such measurement.

INSIGHT

For some quantities, we can consider a body moving between two points. For certain measurements, it is important to know how far the body has travelled between the two points, in other words, the magnitude of travel. In other cases, we wish to know not only how far it has travelled but also the direction it has travelled. Measurements where the direction is important are termed *vector quantities*, whereas those where only the magnitude and not the direction are recorded are known as *scalar quantities*.

TABLE 4.1	The International System of Units base units	
Quantity	**Unit of measurement**	**Symbol**
Length	Metre	m
Mass	Kilogram	kg
Luminous intensity	Candela	cd
Electric current	Ampere	A
Amount of a substance	Mole	mol
Temperature	Kelvin	K
Time	Second	s

TABLE 4.2	Derived International System of Units and their definitions		
Quantity	**Definition**	**SI unit**	**Scalar/vector**
Speed	Distance travelled in unit time	Metre per second ($m.s^{-1}$)	Scalar
Velocity	Distance travelled in unit time in a given direction	Metre per second ($m.s^{-1}$)	Vector
Acceleration	Change of velocity in unit time	Metre per second ($m.s^{-2}$)	Vector
Force	The application of unit force to unit mass produces unit acceleration	Newton (N) ($kg.m.s^{-2}$)	Vector
Pressure	Force applied per unit area	Pascal (Pa) ($N.m^{-2}$)	Vector
Weight	Force acting on a body because of gravity	Newton (N) ($kg.m.s^{-2}$)	Scalar
Work	Product of the force acting on a body times the distance the body moves	Joule (J) (N.m)	Scalar
Energy	Kinetic energy: work which can be done by a system because of its velocity	Joule (J)	Scalar
Potential energy	Work which can be performed because of the position or state of a system	Joule (J)	Scalar
Power	Rate of doing work	Watt (W) ($J.s^{-1}$)	Scalar
Momentum	Product of mass and the velocity of the body	($kg.m.s^{-1}$)	Vector

SI, International System of Units.

4.3.2   Speed and velocity

The speedometer in a car may be calibrated in terms of kilometres per hour (kph). This records the *speed*, which means distance travelled in unit time.

In SI units, speed (*S*), distance (*d*) and time (*t*) are related by the equation:

$$S = \frac{d}{t} \qquad \textbf{Equation 4.1}$$

where *d* is in metres, *t* is in seconds and *S*, therefore, is in metres per second (m.s^{-1}). The speedometer in a car gives no indication of the direction in which the car is moving so we can see that speed is a scalar quantity. Velocity is measured in the same units as speed (m.s^{-1}) but this time the direction of movement is also measured. Thus, a car travelling at a constant speed around a roundabout is continuously changing its velocity.

4.3.3   Acceleration

Acceleration implies a change in velocity and is defined as the change in velocity per unit time (a vector quantity).

For example, the acceleration attributed to gravity is approximately 9.8 metres per second per second (9.8 m.s^{-2}). This means that for a free-falling body, the velocity increases by 9.8 m.s^{-1} after each second. Thus if a body is dropped, its downward velocity is 9.8 m.s^{-1} after the first second, 19.6 m.s^{-1} after the next second and so on.

The acceleration attributed to gravity causes a free-falling body to increase its velocity, but if the accelerating force is in the opposite direction to the direction of movement of the body, then it will cause it to lose velocity. This force causes a negative acceleration or a deceleration.

Also, notice that acceleration is a vector quantity as the acceleration has direction (a vector measurement).

4.3.4   Force

Newton's second law of motion (see Chapter 3) shows that the net force acting on a body is proportional to the mass of the body multiplied by the acceleration produced on the body. The unit of force is therefore kg.m.s^{-2} in SI units. However, this quantity is sufficiently important to be given its own special name and is known as the *newton*. This can be defined as follows:

DEFINITION

A net force of 1 newton acting on a body of mass 1 kg causes it to have an acceleration of 1 m.s^{-2}.

Force is a vector quantity as it has direction. The acceleration produced by the action of the force (also a vector quantity) is in the same direction as the force.

4.3.5   Pressure

Pressure is defined as the force exerted per unit area. The units of pressure would therefore be N.m^{-2}. Again, it is sufficiently important to merit its own unit, known as the *pascal*, and is defined as follows:

DEFINITION

The pressure acting on a body is 1 pascal if 1 newton of force is applied per square metre of body surface.

INSIGHT

The difference between force and pressure can be readily appreciated if one considers crossing some snow wearing either shoes or skis. In both cases, the force is the same, but this force is applied to a smaller area in the case of shoes (the pressure on the snow is greater) so they tend to sink into the snow.

4.3.6   Weight and mass

As we have already seen, mass is a base SI unit, is defined as the amount of matter in a body and is defined against the standard kilogram. This is sometimes confused with the mole (the amount of substance in a body) and so it is possibly easier to understand the concept of mass if we consider it in terms of inertia. We know that a force acting on a body will produce an acceleration and that the force, the mass and the acceleration are linked by the equation $F = m \times a$ (see Equation 3.1) so that inertia can be defined as the body's resistance to acceleration. From the equation, it can be seen that as the mass of the body increases, so the force required to produce a given acceleration also increases, that is, the inertia of the body increases with mass.

The weight of a body is the downward force on the body attributed to the gravitational attraction of Earth. Hence the weight of a body is expressed in newtons, not in kilograms. An equation similar to Equation 3.1 links weight (*w*), mass (*m*) and gravity (*g*):

$$w = m \times g \qquad \textbf{Equation 4.2}$$

From this discussion and equation, we can see that a body always has mass but it only has weight in the presence of a gravitational field. Hence, a body in deep space has no weight (because of the zero gravitational field) but it has mass as it still requires a force to cause it to change its velocity (i.e., it has inertia).

4.3.7   Work and energy

Both *work* and *energy* are measured using the same units. A force is said to do work if it moves its point of application in the same direction as the applied force. This can be expressed as:

$$W = F \times d \qquad \textbf{Equation 4.3}$$

where W is work, F is force and d is distance.

Thus the units of work are newtons and metres (N.m). Again, the concept of work is sufficiently important to merit its own unit, which is the joule.

DEFINITION

1 joule of work is performed when a force of 1 newton moves its point of application through a distance of 1 metre.

Energy can be considered as the capacity of a body to do work. There are two types of energy that we need to consider separately:

1. Kinetic energy.
2. Potential energy.

4.3.7.1   Kinetic energy

Kinetic energy is energy that a body possesses by virtue of its motion. This motion may be translational (movement along a path) or rotational, or a combination of both types. The kinetic energy is simply the work that must be done in the process of bringing the body to rest. We have already looked at this when we considered Newton's laws of motion and established an equation (Equation 3.4) for the kinetic energy of a body of mass m having a velocity of v.

$$E = \frac{1}{2}mv^2 \qquad \textbf{Equation 4.4}$$

INSIGHT

Consider an electron, which has been accelerated across the X-ray tube and is travelling with a velocity v at the point when it starts to collide with the atoms of the target.

It has a kinetic energy $(= \frac{1}{2}mv^2)$ and then starts to liberate some of that energy in the form of X-ray photons. The energy of X-ray photons is measured in electron volts (eV).

4.3.7.2   Potential energy

Potential energy (PE) is energy possessed by a body (or a system) by virtue of its condition or state. Thus, a stationary body has PE if it is in a condition that allows it to release its stored energy. The PE of the system can be thought of as the work that the system will perform in bringing its PE to zero. If we consider a body of mass m,

which is at a height h above the ground, then we can apply Equation 4.3 to this situation.

$$W = F \times d$$

The force at work here is the weight of the body (mg) and the distance it can move its height above the ground (h), so we now have the equation for the PE:

$$PE = mg \times h \qquad \textbf{Equation 4.5}$$

INSIGHT

Consider the case of a hospital lift sitting at the ground floor. Attached to this lift, over a pulley system, is a counterweight. This counterweight has PE because of its position. If the brakes on the lift are released, it will assist in moving the lift up to the top floor (i.e., the counterweight performs work).

Work and energy are both scalar quantities because they do not have direction.

4.3.8   Power

A particular car may reach a speed of 60 mph in 6 s while another car of the same mass does the same speed in 20 s. The first car is said to be more powerful than the second. Assuming that the cars are travelling in the same direction, then their velocity is the same and so their kinetic energy $(= \frac{1}{2}mv^2)$ is the same, but the first car reached that energy more quickly. Hence, power can be expressed as the rate at which energy is expended and, because energy and work are basically the same thing, we can say that:

DEFINITION

Power is the rate at which work is done.

Thus power is measured in joules per second (J.s^{-1}) but is again an important enough concept to merit its own unit, the watt. Thus:

$$\text{watts} = \frac{\text{joules}}{\text{seconds}}$$

or 1 watt is 1 joule of work per second.

4.3.9   Momentum

In everyday speech, momentum expresses the ability of a moving body to 'keep going'. This depends on the mass of the body and its velocity, and so momentum is defined:

The momentum of a body is the product of its mass and its velocity.

We have already, briefly, come across the concept of momentum in the law of conservation of momentum (Chapter 3).

Consider the situation where a projectile (e.g., a bullet) strikes a barrier. The depth to which it penetrates the barrier is dependent on the mass of the projectile and its velocity at the point of impact. This fits in with our concept of momentum as the ability of a body to keep going.

4.4 UNITS USED IN MEDICAL IMAGING

Many derived SI units (such as the joule, coulomb, etc.) are used in imaging science. However, other units that do not strictly adhere to the SI system are especially useful to medical imaging and are unlikely to be discontinued, because of their practical convenience. These are shown and defined in Table 4.3.

4.4.1 mA and mAs

X-rays are produced in an X-ray tube when electrons from the cathode, with high kinetic energy, strike the anode. If we assume that each electron has a chance of producing X-rays, then the intensity of X-ray production is proportional to the number of electrons striking the anode per second. The number of electrons flowing per second is related to the current flowing through the tube. The SI unit of current is the ampere (A), as we saw earlier in this chapter, and it is equivalent to a current of 6×10^{18} electrons per second. This unit of current is too large a unit for radiography so current is measured in milliamperes (1 mA $= 10^{-3}$ A).

We wish the tube to produce X-rays only in sufficient quantity to produce the image on the recording medium (e.g., a digital plate) and so an exposure time is selected by the operator. It can be seen that, all other factors remaining constant, the amount of signal received by the plate will be

Unit	Definition
	TABLE 4.3 Units used in medical imaging
mA	The average electrical current passing through an X-ray tube during an exposure (measured in milliamperes).
mAs	The average electrical current passing through the tube during an exposure multiplied by the exposure time in seconds (1 mAs = 1 millicoulomb).
keV	The energy imparted to an electron when accelerated through a potential difference of 1 kV in a vacuum.
kVp	The peak (maximum) kilovoltage across an X-ray tube during an exposure.
EI	The 'exposure index'. A dimensionless scale of relative X-ray exposure received by an image. Different manufacturers have adopted different terms and scales for the EI.
Gy	The Gray. A derived SI unit of absorbed radiation dose. 1 Gy = 1 joule of energy absorbed per kilogram of tissue.
Sv	The Sievert. A derived SI unit of radiation dose equivalence. 1 Sv = the dose in Gy multiplied by the radiation weighting factor (the ionising ability of a type of radiation), which is 1 for X-rays and gamma rays. The Sv is also used to express the 'effective dose' which takes account of the tissue weighting factor (the radiation sensitivity of body tissues).
R	The rad. An older unit of absorbed radiation dose. 1 Gy = 100 rad.
C/kg	A derived SI unit of radiation exposure in air. 1 coulomb of charge per kilogram of air.
Bq	The becquerel. 1 radioactive disintegration per second. The SI-derived unit of radioactivity.
Ci	The curie. An older unit of radioactivity. 1 Ci = 3.7×10^{10} disintegrations per second.
T	The tesla. A derived SI unit of magnetic field strength, used in MRI.
G	The gauss. An older unit of magnetic field strength. 1 tesla = 10,000 gauss.
Hz	The hertz. A derived SI unit of wave frequency. 1 Hz = 1 cycle per second. Used a lot in ultrasound and MRI.

MRI, Magnetic resonance imaging; *SI*, International System of Units.

determined by the number of X-rays leaving the tube. From these arguments, this is determined by the total number of electrons striking the anode of the tube. The total number of electrons striking the target (and hence the X-ray output) is determined by the number of electrons flowing in unit time (related to the mA) and the length of time for which the current flows (the exposure time in seconds, s). The X-ray output from a tube (if all other factors remain unaltered) is determined by the mAs.

Any combination of mA and time which produces a given mAs will result in the same quantity of X-rays being emitted by the tube. If 60 mAs was required to produce an acceptable image, this could be delivered in the ways listed in Table 4.4.

The mAs is equivalent to the millicoulomb (10^{-3} C), which is the unit of electrical charge. The mAs is, however, used in preference to the millicoulomb as it makes it more obvious that this can be altered by altering the tube current (mA) or the exposure time (s).

4.4.2 keV

As we have already seen in this chapter, energy is measured in joules. When we come to consider the energies involved in the atom or the energies of the photons of the X-ray beam, the coulomb is an extremely large unit. The electron volt (eV) and the kiloelectron volt (keV = 10^3 eV) are much more convenient units of measurement for such energies.

DEFINITION

If an electron is accelerated from rest across a potential difference of 1 volt in a vacuum, it gains a kinetic energy of 1 electron volt.

TABLE 4.4 Different combinations of mA and time to produce a given mAs

Current (mA)	Exposure time (s)	mAs
20	0.5	10
50	0.2	10
100	0.1	10
200	0.05	10
500	0.02	10

Note how a larger mA permits a shorter exposure time. This is useful for 'freezing' patient movement but puts more heat stress on the target of an X-ray tube.

Similarly, an electron accelerated from rest across a potential difference of 1 kilovolt in a vacuum gains a kinetic energy of 1 kiloelectron volt. The energy (E) in joules can be calculated from the equation:

$$E = e \times V \qquad \textbf{Equation 4.6}$$

In this equation, e is the charge on the electron (1.6×10^{-19} C) and V is the potential difference measured in volts. Thus:

$$1 \text{ eV} = 1.6 \times 10^{-19} \text{ J}$$
$$1 \text{ keV} = 1.6 \times 10^{-16} \text{ J}$$

INSIGHT

If 75 kVp is selected by an operator for a specific exposure, then some of the electrons travelling across the X-ray tube will have a kinetic energy of 75 keV when they strike the anode. If we assume that some of these electrons give up all their energy as a single X-ray photon, then the energy of this photon will be 75 keV and it will represent the maximum photon energy in this beam. Thus by altering the kVp, the operator can alter the maximum photon energy of the beam.

4.5 PREFIXES AND POWERS

A prefix is a term placed before a unit to express the numerical quantity of that unit in a way which is universally understood. For example, kilo is a prefix which means 'a thousand', whereas milli is a prefix which means 'a thousandth'. Commonly used prefixes are presented in Table 4.5.

A power, or exponent, is a mathematical way to express a numerical value and is usually based on the figure 10 (on a 'base' of 10). It then represents the number of times which 10 is multiplied by itself. For example, 10 to the power 2 is 'ten squared' (i.e., 10 multiplied by 10, or 100) and is expressed as 10^2. Or 10 to the power 3 is 'ten cubed' (i.e., 10 multiplied by 10 multiplied by 10, or 1000) and is expressed as 10^3. Powers are a convenient way of expressing large or small numbers without needing to write a lot of noughts. Commonly used powers are presented in Table 4.5.

TABLE 4.5   Prefixes and powers

Prefix and symbol	Power	Example
exa E	10^{18}	Diagnostic X-ray frequencies up to 30 exahertz.
peta P	10^{15}	Visible light frequency: 0.3 to 0.8 petahertz.
tera T	10^{12}	Terabyte: computer hard drive.
giga G	10^{9}	Gigahertz: computer processor speeds.
mega M	10^{6}	42 megahertz precessional frequency for hydrogen nuclei at 1 tesla field strength in MRI.
kilo k	10^{3}	30 to 150 kiloelectron volt X-ray energies.
hecto h	10^{2}	Rarely used. A hectare is a square with sides of 100-metre length.
deci d	10^{-1} (i.e., 0.1)	A decilitre is 100 millilitres.
centi c	10^{-2}	Centigray: absorbed radiation doses.
milli m	10^{-3}	Millisievert: effective radiation doses.
micro μ	10^{-6}	Best X-ray image resolution about 50 micrometres.
nano n	10^{-9}	Atomic size: 0.1 to 0.3 nanometres. X-ray wavelengths: 0.1 nanometres.
pico p	10^{-12}	Atomic size: 100 to 300 picometres.
femto f	10^{-15}	Atomic nucleus size: 1 to 15 femtometres.

MRI, Magnetic resonance imaging.

SUMMARY

In this chapter, we considered the following factors related to units of measurement:
- The SI base units for length, mass, luminous intensity, electric current, amount of substance, temperature and time.
- The SI derived units for speed, velocity, acceleration, force, pressure, weight, work, energy, power and momentum.
- Units of measurement used in radiography.

FURTHER READING

Ball, J.L., Moore, A.D., & Turner, S. 2008. *Ball and Moore's Essential Physics for Radiographers*, 4th edn. London: Blackwell Scientific. (Chapter 1.)

Bushong, S. 2016. *Radiologic Science for Technologists: Physics, Biology, and Protection* 11th edn. St. Louis: Mosby. (Chapter 1.)

5

Electricity

CHAPTER CONTENTS

5.1   AIM

This chapter is concerned with the science of static electrical charges (electrostatics) and flowing electrical charges (electricity). The application of these concepts to medical imaging will be discussed. The accumulation of electrical charge can be found in many instances within the science of medical imaging, for example, in ionisation chambers, X-ray detectors and capacitors. Flowing electricity powers X-ray circuits and other imaging equipment. Electrostatics and electricity are based on the negative charges possessed by electrons, which may flow through conductive circuits and also accumulate in some circumstances, providing a 'charge buildup'. Although we may consider the idea of 'positive charges', this is a rather abstract concept because positive charge is caused by the absence of electrons. So a positive charge is like an 'electron hole', which may nevertheless flow through a material, as it does in semiconductors. Before electrons were discovered, the flow of electrical current was regarded as a flow of positive charge, although it was later realised that it is the flow of electrons in the opposite direction which constitutes electrical current. Note that although protons in the atomic nucleus are positively charged, they do not flow within an electrical circuit. However, positively charged ions (atoms or molecules which have lost electrons) may flow in liquids or gases.

5.2   ELECTROSTATICS

Electrostatics, as the name implies, is the study of static electrical charges. We are familiar with many examples of electrostatics from our ordinary lives, from sparks which may occur from our clothes when undressing, to the large discharges of electricity which occur during lightning strikes. Much of the early experimentation with electricity involved electrostatics. It was discovered at an early stage that there were two types of electrical charge, one called negative and the other positive. Although it is mathematically convenient to regard charge in this way, it does not explain what electrical charge actually is and how it behaves.

5.3   PROPERTIES OF ELECTRICAL CHARGES

The general properties of electrical charges are as follows:
- Charges can be considered as being of two types: positive and negative. But it is flow of negative charge which is the basis of electricity.
- The smallest unit of negative charge which can exist in isolation is that possessed by an electron.

- Electrical charges exert forces on each other even when they are separated by a vacuum. The forces are mutual, equal and opposite, as expected by Newton's third law (see Section 3.5).
- Like charges (for example, two negative charges) repel each other whereas unlike charges (for example, a positive and a negative charge) attract each other.
- The magnitude of the mutual forces between the charges is influenced by:
  - the magnitude of the individual charges
  - the medium in which they are embedded, being greatest when the medium is a vacuum
  - the inverse square of the distance between the charged bodies—this is another application of the inverse square law (see Section 14.8).
- Electrical charges may be induced in a material by the proximity of a charge, leading to a force of attraction between the two.
- Electrical charges may flow easily in some materials (called *electrical conductors*) and not in other materials (called *electrical insulators*). Both types of material are capable of having charges induced in them.
- When electrical charges move, they produce a magnetic field.

5.4   FORCE BETWEEN TWO ELECTRICAL CHARGES IN A VACUUM

Consider two charges, q_1 and q_2, separated by a distance, d, in a vacuum, as shown in Fig. 5.1.

If we assume that both charges are of the same sign, then q_1 will exert a force of repulsion (F) on q_2 and q_2 will exert the same force of repulsion on q_1. As we have already stated, it can be shown that:

$$1.\ F \propto q_1$$
$$2.\ F \propto q_2$$
$$3.\ F \propto \frac{1}{d_2}$$

Thus F is proportional to the magnitude of each charge and to the inverse square of the distance separating them.

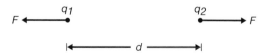

Fig. 5.1 The forces (F) between two electrical charges, q_1 and q_2, separated by a distance (d) are equal and opposite.

If we combine the factors in (1), (2) and (3), we can produce the equation:

$$F \propto \frac{q_1 q_2}{d^2} \qquad \textbf{Equation 5.1}$$

If q_1 and q_2 both have the same sign, then F will be positive and will represent a force of repulsion. If the charges have opposite signs, then F will be negative and will represent a force of attraction.

If we wish to replace the proportionality sign in Eq. 5.1 by an equals sign, then we need to introduce a constant of proportionality (see Appendix A). This equation now reads:

$$F = \frac{q_1 q_2}{4 \pi \varepsilon_0 d^2} \qquad \textbf{Equation 5.2}$$

This equation is often referred to as *Coulomb's law of force* between two charges and has a constant of proportionality, $\frac{1}{4}\pi\varepsilon_0$, where ε_0 is the permittivity of a vacuum and has a value of 6.85×10^{-12} Fm^{-1}. The charges q_1 and q_2 are expressed in coulombs, the separation d is in meters and the force F is in newtons.

The coulomb corresponds to the charge carried by 6×10^{18} electrons or protons. An alternative (and more practical) definition of the coulomb is:

DEFINITION

A charge of 1 coulomb is possessed by a point if an equal charge placed 1 metre away from it in a vacuum experiences a force of repulsion of $\frac{1}{4}\pi\varepsilon_0$ newton.

INSIGHT

The influence of the inverse square law on the force between charged bodies may be understood if we assume that charged bodies produce lines of force in all directions, similar to the light emission from a point source of light obeying the inverse square law. The number of such lines is proportional to the magnitude of the charge (analogous to the brightness of the light source). This is shown diagrammatically in Fig. 5.2, where the arrows point in the direction of force experienced by a positive charge if placed at that point. There will be further discussion of lines of force in the section of this chapter dealing with electrical field strength (see Section 5.6).

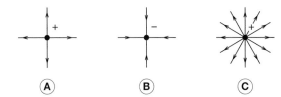

Fig. 5.2 Electric 'lines of force' associated with (A) a weak positive charge, (B) a weak negative charge and (C) a strong positive charge.

5.5 PERMITTIVITY AND RELATIVE PERMITTIVITY (DIELECTRIC CONSTANT)

Equation 5.2 holds true only when the charges are in a vacuum, as ε_0 is the permittivity of a vacuum. In any other medium, the equation requires to be modified to:

$$F = \frac{q_1 q_2}{4 \pi \varepsilon d^2} \qquad \textbf{Equation 5.3}$$

where ε is the permittivity of the medium.

It is, however, often convenient to compare the permittivity of the medium relative to that of a vacuum, that is, if the permittivity of the medium is twice that of a vacuum, then the relative permittivity (K) is 2. This can be obtained from the simple formula:

$$K = \frac{\varepsilon}{\varepsilon_0}$$

or by cross-multiplying:

$$\varepsilon = \varepsilon_0 K \qquad \textbf{Equation 5.4}$$

so Equation 5.3 may be rewritten as:

$$F = \frac{q_1 q_2}{4 \pi \varepsilon_0 K d^2} \qquad \textbf{Equation 5.5}$$

K is known as the *dielectric constant* of the medium and so we can see that the relative permittivity and the dielectric constant are the same. Note that as the dielectric constant is a comparative number, it does not have any units. The dielectric constant is further discussed in Section 5.11 later where we consider its importance in capacitors.

5.6 ELECTRICAL FIELD STRENGTH

We have already seen that an electrical charge is capable of influencing other charges placed at a distance from it. This influence on other charges at a distance is known as a *field* and, for the purpose of comparing electrical charges, E is measured in units of newton/coulomb. Consider the electrical field around a point charge. If we wish to know the field strength at a point, we simply place a unit of positive charge at that point and measure the magnitude and direction of the force exerted upon it. If we consider Eq. 5.5 and have $q_2 = 1$ (unit charge), then we can say:

$$E = \frac{q_1 \times 1}{4\pi\varepsilon_0 K d^2}$$

$$E = \frac{q_1}{4\pi\varepsilon_0 K d^2}$$

Equation 5.6

We have already considered a diagrammatic representation of a field around a point charge (Fig. 5.2). The arrows represent the direction of the force acting on a unit positive charge (if placed at that point) and the line density represents the intensity of the electrical field.

5.7 ELECTROSTATIC INDUCTION OF CHARGE

As mentioned earlier (Section 5.3), a charge may be induced on an electrical conductor or on an insulator. Each will now be considered.

5.7.1 Induction of a conductor

The situation that exists if an electrically charged body (B) is placed close to a conductor (A) is shown in Fig. 5.3. A conductor is a body which will allow a flow of electrons. The positive charge on B attracts electrons to it and leaves equal numbers of positive charges on the opposite surface of A. Notice that the opposite charge is induced on the surface of the conductor closest to the inducing charge and that equal numbers of positive and negative charges are induced. Eventually a state of equilibrium is reached where the electrons on the surface of A experience an equal force of attraction from the two sets of positive charge. When this happens, no further electron flow takes place.

The charge distribution results in a net force of attraction as the unlike charges are closer to the charged body than the like charges.

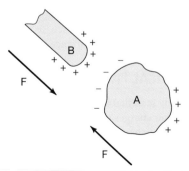

Fig. 5.3 Induction of a charge on a conducting body, A, results in a force of attraction, F, with the inducing body, B.

Withdrawal of the charged body results in uniform distribution of the charges in A.

5.7.2 Induction of an insulator (dielectric)

If we bring a charged body close to an insulator, a similar force of attraction occurs—this can be demonstrated by running a comb through your hair and then holding it close to a small piece of paper, which will be attracted to it. This result is somewhat surprising, as electrons cannot move as freely through an insulator as a conductor. Some insulators are more efficient at producing induced charges than others and it is found that this varies with the dielectric constant (see Section 5.5) of the material.

5.8 ELECTRICAL POTENTIAL

There are a number of similarities between electrical potential and potential energy. In the case of potential energy, this represents the work done raising a body to a height from a zero level. Similar concepts will now be discussed for electrical potential.

5.8.1 Zero electrical potential

There is zero electrical potential at a point at which the force exerted by the charged body on unit charge would be zero. It is often stated that 'the Earth is at zero potential'. The Earth is assumed to be electrically neutral in that it contains equal numbers of positive and negative charges. Thus there is no force on an electron within the neutral Earth. Hence no work is done and the electrical potential of Earth or any other neutral body is zero.

5.8.2 Absolute potential and potential difference

From the discussion so far, we may define the absolute electrical potential at a point as follows:

> **DEFINITION**
>
> The absolute electrical potential at a point is the work done moving a unit positive charge from infinity to that point.
>
> In practice, it is more convenient to compare the potential at one point relative with another than to know its absolute potential. If the potential at point A is V_A and the potential at point B is V_B, then the potential difference (PD) between A and B is $V_A - V_B$ and represents the difference in the work done moving unit positive charge from infinity to point A and from infinity to point B. It can be seen that this is the same as the work which would be required to move a unit positive charge to point B. This leads to the definition of PD.

The PD between two points is the work done on a unit positive charge in moving it from one point to the other.

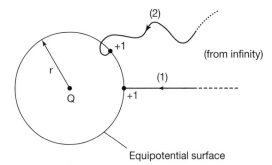

Fig. 5.4 The electrical potential energy of a point charge, Q.

Note that traditional definitions of electrical potential and PD are based on the concept of positive charge. This is because these definitions predate the discovery of the negatively charged electrons which are in fact responsible for charge accumulation and electrical current flow.

5.8.3   The volt

The volt is the International System of Units (SI) unit of potential and is defined as:

1 volt of potential exists at a point if 1 joule of work is performed in moving 1 coulomb of positive charge from infinity to that point.

Similarly, for PD we have:

1 volt of PD exists between two points if 1 joule of work is performed in moving 1 coulomb of positive charge from one point to the other.

These definitions can be shown in the form of an equation:

$$\text{volts} = \frac{\text{joules}}{\text{coulombs}}$$ **Equation 5.7**

5.8.4   Electrical potential because of a point charge

Consider a point charge, Q, as shown in Fig. 5.4. A unit of positive charge has been moved from infinity to a distance r from Q. The nearer the charge comes to Q, the greater the force of repulsion (if Q is positive) or attraction (if Q is negative). Thus the potential is positive if Q is positive and negative if Q is negative because the potential is the work done on the unit positive charge. If we consider that the work done on all unit positive charges which are equidistant from Q will be the same, then it is logical to assume that equipotential surfaces will be concentric spheres with Q as the centre. It is also worth noting that the particular path chosen to bring a unit positive charge from infinity to the point r is of no

importance and so paths (1) and (2) give exactly the same electrical potential.

Electrical potential is usually given the symbol V and so we can produce the equation:

$$\text{work} = \text{force} \times \text{distance}$$
$$V = \frac{Q \times r}{4\pi\varepsilon_0 r^2}$$ **Equation 5.8**
$$V = \frac{Q}{4\pi\varepsilon_0 r}$$

where V is in volts, Q is in coulombs and r is in metres.

The electrical potential because of a point charge is given the term *coulomb potential* and the force between two charges is the *coulomb force* (see Section 5.4).

5.8.5   Electrical potential attributed to a conducting sphere

If we place a charge Q on a conducting sphere, then the charged particles will mutually repel each other and the charges will be evenly distributed on the outer surface of the sphere as shown in Fig. 5.5. This is true whether the sphere is hollow or solid. No PD exists between any points either on the surface or within the sphere (if a PD did exist, the charge would redistribute in such a way that the whole body was at a constant potential). When the potential exists outside the sphere, it may be shown mathematically that the sphere behaves as though all the charge Q is placed at its centre. This is shown in the graph in Fig. 5.5. Thus Eq. 5.8 can be used to calculate the potential of points outside the sphere where r is the distance from the centre of the sphere. This is important from a practical viewpoint in radiography in the design of components such as the X-ray tube shield where we wish to have the charge distributed evenly over the internal surfaces of the tube shield.

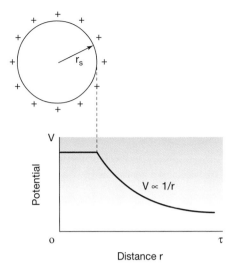

Fig. 5.5 Distribution of electrical potential on a conducting sphere of radius *r*. The potential is constant within the sphere and reduces outside it ($V \propto 1/r$).

5.9   DISTRIBUTION OF ELECTRICAL CHARGE ON AN IRREGULARLY SHAPED CONDUCTOR

Having considered the charge distribution on a sphere, it is now useful to consider the distribution of charge on a conducting body of irregular shape. Such a body is shown in Fig. 5.6. Again the charge is distributed so that no PD exists between any points *within the body*. This gives the charge distribution shown in Fig. 5.6. Note that there are large collections of charge at parts of the body that have a small radius of curvature. This is important in the design of the X-ray tube both in the prevention of coronal discharge (where electrons are forcibly removed from their orbits to create an electrical spark) from sharp corners and also in the use of a sharp-edged focusing cup for electron focusing (see Chapter 12).

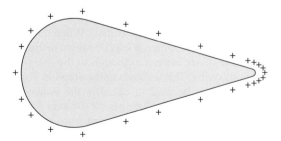

Fig. 5.6 Distribution of positive charge on an irregularly shaped conductor. Note the high intensity of charge at the area of low radius of curvature.

5.10   ELECTRICAL CAPACITY (CAPACITANCE)

The capacitor is a device for storing electrical charge. It has many applications in medical imaging equipment as it can be charged and discharged quickly, unlike a battery. The ability to store electrical charge on the plates of a capacitor has important practical consequences. Some of the practical uses of capacitors are the following:
- Capacitor discharge mobile X-ray units
- Voltage smoothing
- Phase splitting for alternating current (AC) induction motors
- Electronic timers.

We have previously shown that when a body has a net positive or negative charge it also possesses an electrical potential, because work must be done in moving a unit positive charge from infinity to the body. This potential is positive if the charge on the body is positive and negative if the charge on the body is negative.

The electrical capacity or capacitance of the body is the relationship between the charge put on the body and its potential:

$$\text{capacitance} = \frac{\text{charge}}{\text{potential}}$$

$$\text{or } C = \frac{Q}{V}$$

Equation 5.9

5.10.1   Definitions and unit of capacitance (farad)

The definition of capacitance varies slightly depending on the type of body holding the charge. When a body consists of one surface only (e.g., a sphere) the following definition applies:

> **DEFINITION**
>
> The capacitance of a body is the ratio of the total charge on the body to its potential.

If the body consists of two surfaces close together, we must consider the potential differences between the surfaces rather than the potential on each. This leads to the following alternative definition of capacitance:

> **DEFINITION**
>
> The capacitance of a body is the ratio of the total charge of one sign (such as positive or negative) on the body to the potential difference between its surfaces.

Remember that capacitance involves both charge and potential and so it is not correct to think of capacitance as the 'amount of charge a body can hold' unless we add the phrase 'per unit PD'. The SI unit of capacitance is the farad and may be defined as:

> **DEFINITION**
>
> An electrical system has a capacitance of 1 *farad* if a charge of 1 coulomb held by the body results in a potential (or potential difference) of 1 volt.

Thus, Equation 5.9 may be expressed as:

$$\text{farads} = \frac{\text{coulombs}}{\text{volts}} \qquad \textbf{Equation 5.10}$$

> **DEFINITION**
>
> An alternative definition of capacitance, and one that is often more useful in medical imaging, is to consider capacitance in terms of the *change* of charge divided by the corresponding change in potential.

If a capacitor starts with a charge Q and a PD V, then by definition:

$$C = \frac{Q}{V} \qquad \textbf{Equation 5.10A}$$

If an extra charge, ΔQ, is added to the plates and an extra PD, ΔV, results, then:

$$C = \frac{(Q + \Delta Q)}{(V + \Delta V)}$$

that is, capacitance is the total charge divided by the total PD.

By cross-multiplying the above equation, we get:

$$CV + C\Delta V = Q + \Delta Q \qquad \textbf{Equation 5.10B}$$

However, we can say from Equation A that:

$$CV = Q$$

Thus, Equation B can be rewritten:

$$C\Delta V = \Delta Q$$
$$\therefore \ C = \frac{\Delta Q}{\Delta V}$$

This gives the alternative definition of capacitance, which can be used in imaging equipment for calculations involving capacitor discharge circuits, and so on.

For practical purposes, the farad (F) is a rather large unit in which to measure capacitance and so it is more commonly expressed in units of microfarads (µF) or picofarads (pF), where:

$$1\mu F = 10^{-6} F$$

and

$$1pF = 10^{-12} F$$

5.11 CAPACITANCE OF A PARALLEL-PLATE CAPACITOR

Fig. 5.7 shows a parallel-plate capacitor with two plates of equal area, separated by a distance, d. The plates are made of electrical conductors so that charge may flow in and out of each plate. If the capacitor is charged, for example, by connecting it across a battery as shown, then a charge of $+Q$ will exist on one plate and a charge of $-Q$ on the other. If the battery is disconnected, the charge will continue to be stored on the plates of the capacitor as the positive charge on one plate attracts the negative charge on the other. This is why a capacitor is often described as a device for storing charge. (A large capacitor will retain this charge for a long period of time after it has been disconnected from the source of electromotive force (EMF). For this reason, it should be treated with extreme care because severe electric shock may result from touching the plates or the electrical connections to the capacitor.)

When the capacitor is fully charged, a PD equal to that of the battery exists across the plates. Thus, the capacitance of the parallel-plate capacitor is given by the equation $C = Q/V$ where Q is the charge of one sign on one of the plates and V is the PD between the plates.

Certain characteristics of the capacitor will affect its capacitance, and these will now be considered.

5.11.1 Area of the plates

If the area of the plates (A) is increased, then more charge will be able to flow onto the plates from the battery until

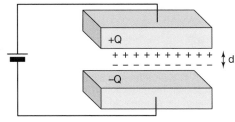

Fig. 5.7 A parallel-plate capacitor charged by a battery.

the charge per unit area is the same as before. It can be seen that if the area of the plates is doubled then the amount of charge which they will hold, to give the same charge per unit area, will also be doubled. In this situation, V remains unaltered, as it is the same as the PD from the battery and $Q \propto A$. Because $C = Q/V$, we can say that:

$$C \propto A$$

Note that if the plates are not directly opposite each other, then the area taken for this calculation of capacitance is the effective area, that is, the area of the plates which are in direct opposition to each other.

5.11.2   Separation of the plates

If the rest of the capacitor remains unaltered but the plates are brought closer together, then the charges on opposite plates will experience a greater force of attraction so that the battery will be able to 'push' more charge onto the plates. Once again, V is constant, but $Q \propto 1/d$. Because $C = Q/V$ we can then say that:

$$C = \frac{1}{d}$$

5.11.3   Dielectric constant of material between the plates

A material with a high dielectric constant is an insulator where it is relatively easy to induce a charge on its surface. The effect of placing such a material between the plates of a charged capacitor is shown in Fig. 5.8. The close proximity of the charges on the plates and on the dielectric results in some 'cancellation' of charges (as shown ringed in Fig. 5.8B). If this capacitor is now reconnected to the battery, it will be seen that more charge will flow onto the capacitor. Thus, once again, V is the same value but Q has

increased and so the capacitance of the capacitor increases with the dielectric constant (K), so we can say:

$$C \propto K$$

This leads to the definition of the dielectric constant.

> **DEFINITION**
>
> The dielectric constant of a material is the ratio of the capacitance of the capacitor with the dielectric to the capacitance without the dielectric (i.e., with a vacuum between the plates of the capacitor).

From this, it can be seen that the dielectric constant of a vacuum is unity (1). If we take the above three components together we get:

$$C \propto \frac{KA}{d}$$

By the addition of a constant of proportionality (ε_0), this now becomes:

$$C = \frac{\varepsilon_0 KA}{d} \qquad \textbf{Equation 5.11}$$

5.12   DISCHARGING A CAPACITOR THROUGH A RESISTOR

In Fig. 5.9A, a charged capacitor with a potential V_C across its plates is allowed to discharge through the resistor R when the switch S_2 is closed. When this happens, electrons travel from the negative plate of the capacitor, through the resistor R and onto the positive plate and the charge on the plates and the potential between them (V_C) is reduced. The reduction in V_C means that there will be less 'push' on the electrons in the next time interval resulting in a smaller drop in V_C. This situation continues, as shown in Fig. 5.9B,

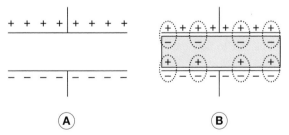

Fig. 5.8 (A) Parallel-plate capacitor with no dielectric between the plates. (B) Capacitor after a dielectric has been introduced between the plates. The induction of charge in the dielectric 'cancels' some of the charges stored on the plates (shown as ringed charges). This means that the battery can now place more charge on the plates of the capacitor.

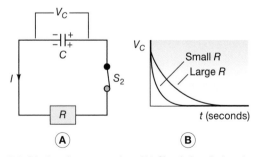

Fig. 5.9 Discharging a capacitor. (A) Circuit for discharging capacitor (C) through resistor (R). (B) Graph showing the effect of different resistors on the rate of discharge.

until the capacitor is discharged and the potential difference is zero. Again, the effect of R is to slow down the current and so the rate of fall of V_C.

5.13   THE TIME-CONSTANT FOR A CAPACITOR RESISTOR CIRCUIT

This is an example of an exponential law (see Section 10.11). The PD between the plates of a discharging capacitor can be calculated from the equation:

$$V_C = V_0 e^{-t/RC}$$ **Equation 5.12**

where V_0 is the PD between the plates before discharging the capacitor, t is the time of the discharge (in seconds), R is the resistance in ohms and C is the capacitance in farads. The quantity RC is called the *time-constant*. After a discharge time of 1 time-constant, the PD across a discharging capacitor has dropped to 1/e of its initial value, that is, 0.37 of its initial value. If the original PD is 6 V, the value after 1 time-constant is $0.37 \times 6 = 2.2$ V. After 2 time-constants, the value will be reduced to a further 0.37, that is, $0.37 \times 2.2 = 0.8$ V. Note that this is very similar to the concept of half-life discussed in Section 10.11 because both are examples of exponential decay, being instances of decay of charge and radioactivity respectively.

If we consider a capacitor being charged, then the equation for the potential across it is:

$$V_C = V_0(1 - e^{-t/RC})$$ **Equation 5.13**

V_0 is the charging source EMF. Again, RC is the time-constant. After 1 time-constant the potential across the capacitor will be $1 - 1/e$, which is 0.63. Thus for a charging capacitor, after 1 time-constant the potential across its plates will be 0.63 of its final value (the final value will be the same as the charging source EMF).

5.14   CAPACITORS IN MEDICAL IMAGING

There is insufficient space in this text to describe all these uses in detail and so only a brief overview of each will be given.

5.14.1   Capacitor discharge mobile X-ray units

Capacitor discharge mobile X-ray units have been important historically and possess the advantage of being independent of local mains electricity during an X-ray exposure but the disadvantage of suffering a fall in voltage during exposure during capacitor discharge. This can reduce the penetration of the X-ray beam because beam energy is

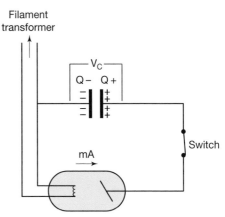

Fig. 5.10 Simplified diagram of the principles of a capacitor discharge X-ray circuit.

proportional to the voltage across an X-ray tube. Fig. 5.10 shows the basic principles of such a circuit. When an exposure is made on a mains-dependent mobile unit, a large current (around 30 A) is drawn from the mains during the exposure. This large current can cause large power losses in the mains cables (remember, $P = I^2R$). The capacitor discharge mobile works on the principle that a small current is drawn from the mains to charge a capacitor before the X-ray exposure, and this capacitor is allowed to discharge through the X-ray tube during the exposure. Because the electrical energy to the tube comes from the capacitor, no significant stress is applied to the mains supply during the exposure.

With the switch open, the capacitor is initially charged until the required potential (V_C is the same value as the kV which will be applied to the tube) is established across its plates. On closing the switch, electrons flow from the negative plate of the capacitor to the positive plate via the X-ray tube. This means that a PD (kV) is applied across the tube and charge (mAs) flows through it, comprising a radiographic exposure. At the end of the exposure, the switch is opened.

As a result of the exposure, the capacitor loses some of the charge on its plates and so the PD at the end of the exposure is less than the initial PD. However, when long exposures are made, there is a significant drop in the energy of the X-ray beam during the exposure as the energy stored in the capacitor falls. This must be considered when selecting exposure factors on such a unit.

5.14.2   Voltage smoothing

When an alternating voltage is full-wave rectified (see Chapter 7) and applied to a component, the voltage waveform will be as shown in Fig. 5.11A. Thus during each half-cycle a PD ranging from the peak voltage to 0 V is applied

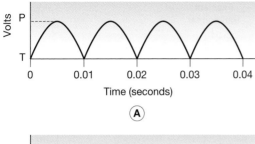

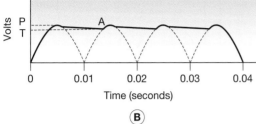

Fig. 5.11 (A) Voltage waveform from a single-phase transformer after it has been rectified. (B) The same waveform after capacitor smoothing, where *P* represents the peak and *T* the trough. The difference between the peak and the trough is known as the *ripple*. Note how capacitor smoothing reduces the voltage ripple.

across the component. This difference between the peak and the trough in the voltage is known as the *voltage ripple*. In this case, the ripple is 100%. There are some situations where it is beneficial to reduce this ripple. This is done by connecting a capacitor (or sometimes two capacitors) in parallel with the component so that the voltage supply is smoothed by the capacitor before it is applied to the component. The result of capacitor smoothing of the voltage is shown in Fig. 5.11B. The broken line shows the voltage waveform from the rectification circuit. Initially the capacitor charges so that the potential between its plates is the same as the peak potential from the rectification circuit. As this supply voltage drops, the capacitor discharges through the component so that the PD between its plates slowly drops. When this potential has dropped by a small amount, the potential from the supply 'catches up' with it (point A on the graph) and charge will once again flow on to the capacitor so that it reaches its peak PD at the same time as the supply voltage.

This application is important in medium-frequency rectification systems because, by using capacitors that are suitably matched to the components being supplied with electrical energy, the voltage ripple can be reduced to less than 1%.

5.14.3   Phase splitting for AC induction motors

When a capacitor is introduced into an AC supply, it causes a phase shift between the current and voltage. This is used in the AC induction motor. The role of the capacitor is to produce a current in one pair of coils that is 90 degrees out of phase with the current in the other pair. This produces a magnetic field, which appears to rotate at the same speed as the mains frequency and so produces rotation of the motor rotor.

5.15   BATTERIES

Batteries provide a source of electrical charge and hence of electrical current when connected to an electric circuit. Traditionally, batteries have consisted of a chemical solution or gel, termed an *electrolyte*, that provides a source of negative ions and positive ions which migrate to two electrodes, which are termed the *anode* and *cathode*, respectively. This charge difference results in an electrical PD across the electrodes. Rechargeable batteries such as lithium-ion or nickel-cadmium designs are able to reverse the chemical reactions during the charging process, so that the source of ions is replenished. Modern batteries may be solid state rather than incorporating an electrolyte, but still produce a source of charge. Batteries may be found powering mobile X-ray machines, both for providing voltage to an X-ray tube and for powering the drive motor.

5.16   ELECTRICITY

Electricity consists of a flow of electrons through a conductive circuit. The electrons may flow in a single direction, in the case of DC electricity, or back and forth in both directions over time, in the case of AC electricity. Capacitors and batteries provide a source of DC, whereas mains electricity is AC. In solid material such as an electrical conductor, atoms are bound to other atoms and so the flow of charge consists only of electrons, not of ions as might be the case in a liquid or gas. The electrical properties of a given solid are determined by the way in which the electrons surrounding the atom behave.

5.17   SIMPLE ELECTRON THEORY OF CONDUCTION

To explain why some materials readily allow a flow of electrons (i.e., are good electrical conductors) and other materials will only allow electron flow in extreme conditions (i.e., are good insulators), we need to look more closely at the structure of the atom. The nucleus of the atom contains protons (+ve charge) and neutrons (no charge) and around this in orbitals are electrons (−ve charge). We can appreciate that electrons near the nucleus experience a high level of attraction (because unlike charges attract) and are thus said to be tightly bound. Electrons in the more remote orbitals experience less force of attraction from the nucleus (remember $F \propto 1/d^2$) and are also repelled by other electrons which lie between them and the nucleus and so are said to be more loosely bound. Because the electrons in a given single atom are influenced by only that atom, the electrons lie at discrete energy levels, as shown in Fig. 5.12A.

When electrons are brought closer together, as in a solid, the orbitals of the electrons are strongly influenced by the proximity of neighbouring atoms. This means that electrons are no longer at discrete energy levels but that they are now within a band of energies. This situation is shown in Fig. 5.12B.

For the purpose of this discussion, only the outer two energy bands are of interest to us: the valence band and the conduction band. The valence band is that band which contains the outermost electrons of the atom and may be partially or completely full of its permitted maximum number of electrons. The configuration of electrons in the valence band determines the chemical properties of the atom, that is, its ability to form chemical bonds with other atoms. If electrons exist further away from the nucleus than the valence band, then their energies lie in the conduction band. This band is populated with electrons that have, for some reason, become free from their original atoms. Because of this, once an electron is in the conduction band of a solid, it is able to move relatively freely and may take part in electrical conduction through the material. A material with a large number of electrons in the conduction band is a good electrical conductor whereas a material with no electrons in the conduction band is a perfect electrical insulator. Whether or not a material is a conductor, an insulator or a semiconductor is determined by the number of electrons in the conduction band. This number is in turn determined by the size of the forbidden energy gap (E) which exists between the top energy of the valence band and the bottom energy of the conduction band. The arrangement of the valence and conduction bands for conductors, semiconductors and insulators is shown in Fig. 5.13. Each of these will now be considered individually.

5.17.1 Electron arrangements in a conductor

As can be seen from Fig. 5.13A, the conduction band and the valence band of energies overlap in a conductor. As a result, a large number of electrons always exist in the conduction band and because of this there is a ready exchange of electrons between the valence and conduction bands. This means that these electrons can be moved through the solid with little resistance to their flow. The main opposition to their flow arises from collisions with other electrons or atoms. If the temperature of the conductor is increased, there is an increase in the vibration of the atoms and a corresponding increase in the likelihood of collision with moving electrons. From this we can see that the opposition (or resistance) to the flow of electrons in a conductor will increase with an increase in its temperature.

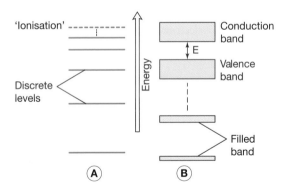

Fig. 5.12 (A) Electron energy levels in a solitary atom. (B) Electron energy bands in an atom of a solid.

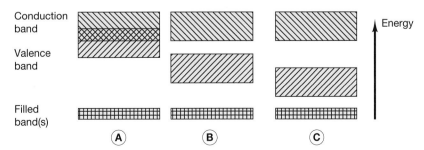

Fig. 5.13 Energy bands for (A) a conductor, (B) a semiconductor and (C) an insulator.

5.17.2   Electron arrangements in a semiconductor

In a semiconductor, there is a gap between the maximum energy of the valence band and the minimum energy of the conduction band (Fig. 5.13B) and so electrons need to be given energy to bridge this gap and flow through the material. Thus, semiconductors have a greater resistance to the flow of electrons than conductors. If we increase the temperature of the semiconductor, we will increase the energy of the electrons in the valence band and so make it easier for them to transfer to the conduction band and move through the solid. Thus increasing the temperature of a semiconductor will reduce its resistance to the flow of electrons.

5.17.3   Electron arrangements in an insulator

In an insulator, there is a significant gap between the maximum energy of the valence band and the minimum energy of the conduction band (Fig. 5.13C). This means that electrons cannot readily bridge this energy gap, and so the conduction band contains no electrons, making conduction impossible. If the material is heated, then the electrons in the valence band gain energy, and so the gap between the valence and the conduction bands is narrowed, making it more likely that electrons can jump the gap. Thus, increasing the temperature of an insulator reduces its resistance.

The effect on the resistance to the flow of electrons of increasing the temperature is shown in Fig. 5.14.

5.18   ELECTRIC CURRENT

Electricity is the flow of electrons in a material. The rate of flow of electrons is a measure of the electric current. To produce a current, the following conditions must be satisfied:
- There must be a source of electric *PD*.
- There must be a complete circuit around which the electrons are able to travel.

These two points are illustrated in Fig. 5.15. The battery (B) is a source of PD, but if the switch (S) is open (as in Fig. 5.15A), no electric current flows and the bulb does not light up. When the switch is closed (Fig. 5.15B), a complete circuit exists around which electrons are able to flow and so the bulb lights up. The *PD* may be thought of as the driving force that causes electrons to flow, whereas the current is the rate of flow of electrons, that is, the number of electrons passing a given point in unit time.

DEFINITION

An electric current of 1 ampere (A) flows at a point if a charge of 1 coulomb (C) flows past that point *per second*.

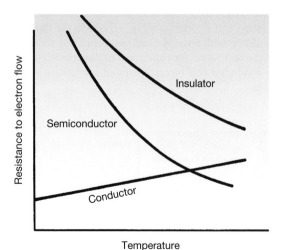

Fig. 5.14 Effect of temperature on the electrical resistance of a conductor, a semiconductor and an insulator.

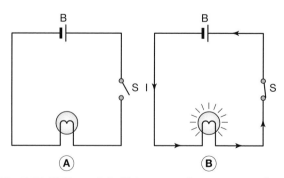

Fig. 5.15 (A) The switch (S) is open and so no current flows through the circuit. (B) When the switch is closed, current will flow through the circuit and the bulb will light. This shows that a continuous circuit is necessary for electrical current to flow.

Thus we can say mathematically:

$$\text{amperes} = \frac{\text{coulombs}}{\text{seconds}} \quad \textbf{Equation 5.14}$$

From Section 5.4, we know that a charge of 1 coulomb is equivalent to approximately 6×10^{18} electrons, so 1 ampere is simply this number of electrons passing a point in 1 second.

> **INSIGHT**
>
> We are accustomed to an instant response when we close an electrical switch and so it is surprising to discover that the average velocity of electrons in a circuit is only in the order of 0.5 mm.s^{-1}. When the switch is closed, electrons start to flow through the whole circuit and so the bulb in Fig. 5.15 will light up even if the electrons from the battery have not yet reached it—this is similar to the situation where water enters a pipe from a reservoir when a tap is opened; water leaves the tap immediately, although it might be some time before the water from the reservoir reaches it.

5.19 mA, mAs AND MILLICOULOMBS

The electric current through an X-ray tube is a small one and so it is measured in milliamperes (mA) rather than in amps: 1 mA = 10^{-3} That is, a one thousandth of an amp. This relates to the rate of flow of electrons through the X-ray tube. If we wish to consider the total number of electrons that have travelled across the tube during a given radiographic exposure, then we need to multiply the rate of flow by the time of the exposure. This unit is in milliampere-seconds (mAs) where:

$$\text{mAs} = \text{mA} \times \text{seconds} \quad \textbf{Equation 5.15}$$

Now the total number of electrons, which have crossed the X-ray tube, is just a measure of the charge, measured in *coulombs*. From Equation 5.14:

$$\text{amps} = \frac{\text{coulombs}}{\text{seconds}}$$

By cross-multiplying (see Appendix A):

$$\text{coulombs} = \text{amps} \times \text{seconds}$$

so:

$$\text{millicoulombs} = \text{milliamps} \times \text{seconds} \quad \textbf{Equation 5.16}$$

So we can say that:

$$1\,\text{mAs} = 1\,\text{millicoulomb} \quad \textbf{Equation 5.17}$$

5.20 POTENTIAL DIFFERENCE AND ELECTROMOTIVE FORCE

We have already considered PD in Section 5.8.2 and defined the PD in volts:

> **DEFINITION**
>
> The potential difference in volts is the work done in moving 1 coulomb of positive charge from one point to another.

Thus:

$$\text{volts} = \frac{\text{joules}}{\text{coulombs}} \quad \textbf{Equation 5.18}$$

In electricity, we are concerned with moving charges and, as mentioned previously, we can regard the PD as the impetus which moves the electron along a conductor. The greater the PD (charge difference) between two parts of a circuit, the greater will be the force that makes electrons pass from the negative to the positive ends of that circuit.

EMF is also expressed in *volts* and is a measure of electrical potential energy developed across a source of electricity (e.g., a battery or a generator). The EMF is the 'driving force' behind the electron flow in the circuit.

It is therefore possible to speak about the PD across any part of the circuit including the source of electricity, whereas the term EMF is reserved solely for the latter. It would not be correct to use the term 'EMF across a resistor' as a resistor is not a source of electricity—the appropriate terminology would be 'the PD across a resistor'.

5.21 RESISTANCE

The elementary theory of conduction discussed earlier in this chapter refers to two mechanisms that impede electron flow:
1. Lack of 'free' electrons in the conduction band—as in an insulator.
2. Collisions between flowing electrons with other vibrating electrons in the material.

This impedance to the flow of electrons is given the term *electrical resistance* or simply *resistance* and is measured in ohms. From the earlier discussion, insulators have much higher resistance than conductors of the same shape and size. The resistance of a conductor can vary depending on a number of factors, which will be discussed later.

5.21.1   Factors affecting resistance

The resistance of a substance will be affected by:
- the dimensions of the substance
- the type of the substance
- the temperature of the substance.

Note that the resistance of the substance is not affected by either the PD across it or by the current flowing through it.

5.21.1.1   Dimensions

The shape of a body is capable of infinite variation, so for simplicity we shall consider circular conductors of constant cross-sectional area.

Fig. 5.16 illustrates such a body and the effect on the resistance R of altering its length l and its cross-sectional area A.

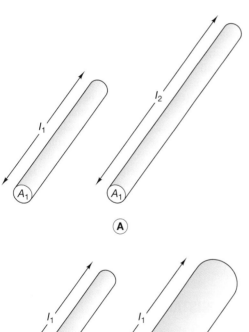

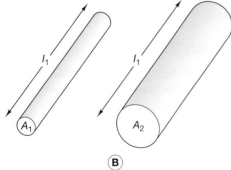

Fig. 5.16 Factors affecting resistance of a conductor. In (A) the conductors are of different lengths and the resistance increases with the length. In (B) the conductors have differing cross-sectional areas and the resistance is inversely proportional to the cross-sectional area.

The resistance is proportional to the length of the conductor ($R \propto l$). If we consider a situation where the length of the conductor is doubled, then electrons travelling along the conductor have twice as many vibrating atoms to get past, so the resistance to their flow will be doubled.

The resistance is inversely proportional to the cross-sectional area ($R \propto l/A$). If the area is doubled, there are twice as many electrons capable of conducting charge. The number of atoms each electron must get past for the length of the conductor remains the same and so doubling the area will halve the resistance.

5.21.1.2   Type of substance

By definition, good electrical conductors will have a lower resistance than insulators. Different metals also have different values of resistance. As we have just seen, the shape of the substance also affects its resistance, so that a standard shape and size must be used when comparing the resistance of different materials. The standard used is a cube of side 1 metre and the resistance is measured when a current is passed between opposing faces of the cube. The value of the resistance so obtained is called the *resistivity* or the *specific resistance* of the material and is measured in ohm-metres. Resistivity is given the symbol ρ (Greek rho) and it is clear that the resistance of the material will be directly proportional to its resistivity: $R \propto \rho$.

If we now consider all the factors discussed, we have:

$$R \propto \frac{\sigma l}{A} \qquad \textbf{Equation 5.19}$$

In the SI system, ρ is defined so that the constant of proportionality in the above equation is unity and we can say:

$$R = \frac{\sigma l}{A} \qquad \textbf{Equation 5.20}$$

The resistivity of insulators is about 1 million times greater than those of semiconductors, which in turn are about 1 million times greater than those of metallic conductors.

5.21.1.3   Temperature

As described at the beginning of this chapter, a change in temperature affects the resistance of a body. This effect is different for conductors, semiconductors and insulators, as shown in Fig. 5.14. Because of these variations, resistance is usually quoted at a particular temperature (e.g., 20° C). The temperature coefficient of resistance, α, is defined as the fractional change in resistance (or resistivity) per unit temperature change:

$$\alpha = \frac{\text{change in resistivity}}{\text{original resistivity}} / \text{temperature change}$$

Note: α is different for different conductors.

5.22 OHM'S LAW

Ohm's law applies to metallic conductors and combines, in a simple way, the relationship between current, PD and resistance. It is found experimentally that the current flowing through a conductor is proportional to the PD applied across it—as the driving force on the electrons is increased, so the number of electrons passing a point in unit time increases by a proportional amount. If a PD of 2 volts causes a current of 1 amp to flow through a conductor, then a PD of 4 volts will cause a current of 2 amps to flow. Ohm's law may be formally stated as follows:

> **The current flowing through a metallic conductor is proportional to the PD that exists across it provided that all physical conditions remain constant.**

The main physical condition, which must remain constant, is the temperature of the conductor, as an alteration in the temperature will cause an alteration in the resistance (see Section 5.20).

Ohm's law may be stated mathematically thus:

$$I \propto V \qquad \textbf{Equation 5.21}$$

where I and V are the magnitude of the current and the PD respectively.

Note that Ohm's law does not mention the word resistance. The resistance of the body (R) is introduced into Equation 7.8 as a constant of proportionality (see Appendix A) and so the equation may now be rewritten:

$$\begin{aligned} V &\propto I \\ \therefore V &= R \times I \\ \therefore V &= I \times R \end{aligned} \qquad \textbf{Equation 5.22}$$

As we have already established, R is a constant for a given conductor at a given temperature and *does not* depend on V or I.

R is measured in ohms (Ω) and we can see from Equation 5.22 that when $V = 1$ volt and $I = 1$ amp, then R will be 1 ohm. The ohm may be defined as follows:

> **DEFINITION**
>
> A body is said to have an electrical resistance of 1 ohm if a potential difference of 1 volt across it produces an electrical current through it of 1 ampere.

Note that a PD always occurs across a body, never through it. Likewise, an electrical current always flows through a body and does not exist across it.

Although Ohm's law is simple in its formulation, it has far-reaching implications which can be applied to radiological physics.

5.23 ELECTRICAL ENERGY AND POWER

To get an electric current to flow through a conductor, the electrons must be driven by a PD. As the electrons move through the conductor they are involved in collisions with the atoms of the conductor and so work must be done to keep all the electrons moving in the same direction. The electrons dissipate energy to the atoms of the material, which they pass through, and so heat is produced in the material—this is the mechanism by which the filament of the X-ray tube is heated to produce electrons by thermionic emission (see Chapter 12).

5.23.1 The joule

As already discussed (see Chapter 3), the joule is the SI unit of energy. The key to the method of calculating electrical energy lies in the definition of PD. As we discovered in Section 5.8.3, the PD between two points is 1 volt when 1 joule of work is done in moving 1 coulomb of positive charge from one point to the other. Thus, we can say:

$$\text{volts} = \frac{\text{joules}}{\text{coulombs}} \qquad \textbf{Equation 5.23}$$

or:

$$\text{joules} = \text{volts} \times \text{coulombs} \qquad \textbf{Equation 5.24}$$

Because the ampere is a rate of flow of charge of 1 coulomb per second, then we can say:

$$\text{joules} = \text{volts} \times \text{amperes} \times \text{seconds} \qquad \textbf{Equation 5.25}$$

5.23.2 The watt

We also saw in Section 4.3 that the SI unit of power is the watt, where 1 watt = 1 joule per second. Thus, we can say that:

$$\frac{\text{joules}}{\text{seconds}} = \frac{\text{volts} \times \text{amperes} \times \text{seconds}}{\text{seconds}}$$

or:

$$\text{watts} = \text{volts} \times \text{amperes} \qquad \textbf{Equation 5.26}$$

This is a general equation used in the calculation of electrical power, which applies to any electrical system. It is, however, particularly useful to apply this formula to a metallic conductor which obeys Ohm's law.

5.23.3   Power in a resistor

Consider a current I passing through a metallic resistor of resistance R when a PD V is applied across its ends. As previously discussed:

$$W = V \times I$$

However, we can apply Ohm's law to the resistor:

$$V = I \times R$$

so

$$W = I \times I \times R$$

or

$$W = I^2 R$$

By similar manipulations of Ohm's law, we can get two possible equations for the electrical power in a resistor:

$$W = VI$$
$$W = I^2 R$$ **Equation 5.27**

The second equation is probably the most useful one in radiography.

5.24   POWER LOSS IN CABLES

If we consider electricity in the form of a current I passing through a cable with a resistance R, it becomes apparent that some of the available electrical power will be 'lost' in the cable. The term lost does not imply that there is a breach of the law of conservation of energy but that the power is not available for the user at the far end of the cable—the lost energy is in fact converted into heat.

It is obviously desirable that the power which is lost in the cables be kept to a minimum as this is not available to the user. If we consider that the power loss is given by the equation $P = I^2 R$, then it can be seen that the power loss can be kept to a minimum in one of two ways:
1. Reducing the current flowing within the cable.
2. Reducing the resistance of the cables.

5.24.1   Reducing the current flowing within the cable

Electrical power (P) is a combination of the PD (V) across the cables and the current (I) flowing through them, that is, $P = VI$. If we wish to transmit a given amount of electrical power with the minimum loss in the cables, this can be done by using a high voltage and a low current. This is

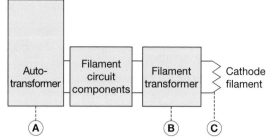

Fig. 5.17 Transmission of electrical power from the voltage selector to the X-ray tube filament. Between points A and B power is in the optimum form for transmission with minimum power loss—high voltage and low current. Thus 100 watts of power would be transmitted in the form of 100 volts and 1 ampere. Between points B and C power is in the optimum form for heat generation at the filament. Thus 100 watts of power would be transmitted in the form of 10 volts and 10 amperes.

shown in Fig. 5.17 where a power of approximately 100 watts is required to heat the filament of the X-ray tube. This power is transmitted from the voltage selector to the filament transformer (see Section 12.7.3) in the form of a relatively high voltage and low current. At the filament we wish to use this power to generate heat, so it is converted to a relatively low voltage and high current at the filament transformer. Similar techniques are used in transmitting power from the generating stations to our homes.

5.24.2   Reducing the resistance of the cables

This is achieved in two ways: making the cables of a material with a low resistivity (usually copper) and making the cables as thick (large cross-sectional area) as possible. Because the cables are required to transmit power from one point to another, there is little scope for the third possibility—reducing the length of the cables.

5.24.3   Mains cable resistance and X-ray exposures

As we have previously discussed, there is a PD across any resistor which is related to the current through the resistor ($V = IR$). This volt drop is removed from the EMF available when a current flows to an X-ray unit. This can be seen in Equation 5.28:

$$V = EMF - IR_c$$ **Equation 5.28**

where R_c is the resistance of the mains cables and V is the PD available at the mains supply when the unit is 'on load'. It is also worth noting that this volt drop is related to the resistance of the cables and the current to the X-ray unit.

In practice, with static X-ray units, the resistance of the mains cables is fairly constant so it is possible to compensate for this volt drop using a static mains resistance compensator. For mains-dependent mobile units the volt drop can vary for different parts of the hospital—obviously, the mains cables that reach the 10th floor are longer than the cables to the ground floor. This means that this type of mobile unit has an adjustable mains resistance compensator. Usually, the plug for the unit in the ward is coded in some way so that we know the correct setting for the compensator.

INSIGHT

Many modern mobile X-ray units overcome this problem by being 'mains independent'. Such units remove power from the mains in small amounts between exposures (they require to be plugged into the mains when not in use) and then release this power through the X-ray tube during the exposure. The electrical power may be stored in special batteries or in capacitors.

5.25 ALTERNATING CURRENT

DC electricity is representative of a flow of electrons in one direction only. AC is the situation where electrons flow through a circuit first in one direction and then in the other (because of the changing polarity of the ends of the circuit)—this is known as an *AC flow*.

5.26 TYPES OF DC AND AC

Fig. 5.18 shows different types of DC and AC in graphical form—the magnitude of the current (the dependent variable) is plotted on the vertical axis against time on the horizontal axis.

Fig. 5.18A is a case where the number of electrons passing a point per second in the circuit is constant producing a horizontal straight line. This is an example of DC. Fig. 5.18B is a case where the electrons always move in the same direction but the number of electrons passing a point varies with time—the electrons move as a series of pulses and this is known as *pulsating DC*. In Fig. 5.18C there is no discernable pattern in the flow of electrons,

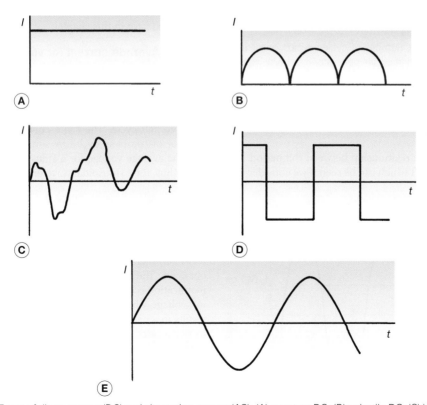

Fig. 5.18 Types of direct current (DC) and alternating current (AC): (A) constant DC; (B) pulsatile DC; (C) irregular AC; (D) square waveform AC; (E) sinusoidal AC.

except to say that they flow in both directions at different times. This is an example of an irregular AC waveform. Fig. 5.18D shows a situation where the number of electrons travelling in one direction is constant for a short period of time and then the same number of electrons travel in the opposite direction for the same period of time. This is an example of a square waveform. Fig. 5.18E shows an example of a sinusoidal AC wave form. This is the most common AC waveform and will be discussed in detail later.

5.27   SINUSOIDAL AC

The sinusoidal AC waveform is shown in more detail in Fig. 5.19, together with some of the quantities used to measure it.

DEFINITIONS

One cycle: One complete waveform starting at a point and continuing until the same point on the pattern is reached. This is usually measured from zero to zero (ABCDE) or from peak to peak (BCDEF).

Period (T): The time taken to complete one cycle, measured in seconds.

Frequency (f): The number of cycles which occur in 1 second, measured in cycles per second or hertz (Hz).

Amplitude: The maximum value of positive or negative current (or voltage) on the waveform. This may be referred to as the *peak value*.

There is a simple relationship between the period (T) and the frequency (f) which can be seen if we consider the following situation. Suppose we have a frequency of 10 Hz (10 cycles per second). Because the waveform is regular, each cycle must last for 0.1 second. Thus, we can say:

$$f = \frac{1}{T} \qquad \textbf{Equation 5.29}$$

For a sinusoidal current, this equation may be rewritten as:

$$I_t = I_p \sin 2\pi\, ft \qquad \textbf{Equation 5.30}$$

where I_t is the current at a time t and I_p is the amplitude or the peak value of the current. A similar equation can be produced for the voltage.

5.27.1   Peak current (or voltage)

The peak current is the same as the amplitude, that is, it is the maximum positive or negative value of the current. Similarly, the peak voltage is the maximum value of the voltage. In radiography, the peak voltage across the tube, when the anode is positive and the cathode is negative, is usually quoted. If an X-ray tube is operating at 75 kVp then the peak PD between the anode and the cathode is 75 kV. The reasons for quoting the tube voltage as kVp will be considered later in this chapter.

5.27.2   Average current (or voltage)

As we can see from Fig. 5.19, the average current flowing in one cycle of a sinusoidal waveform is zero, as the current flowing in one direction during the positive half-cycle has the same overall value (but of the opposite sign) during the negative half-cycle. The same conclusion applies to any number of complete cycles. A similar argument suggests that the average voltage for a sinusoidal waveform is also zero. Thus, for a sinusoidal waveform:

$$\begin{aligned} I_{AV} &= 0 \\ V_{AV} &= 0 \end{aligned} \qquad \textbf{Equation 5.31}$$

However, if the waveform is rectified (or made unidirectional) then a value of the average current (or voltage) is obtained. The voltage waveform produced for half-wave rectification is shown in Fig. 5.20A. This results in a pulsating voltage which (assuming a complete external circuit) results in a net electron flow in one direction—this allows us to consider average values of voltage and current which are not zero.

The voltage waveform for a full-wave rectified circuit is shown on the same scale in Fig. 5.20B. Again, a pulsating voltage is produced where the average value is twice that for the half-wave rectified circuit as there are twice as many peaks in unit time.

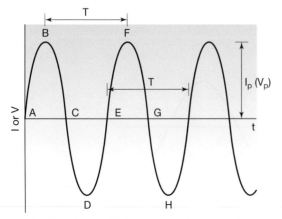

Fig. 5.19 A sinusoidal current or voltage waveform.

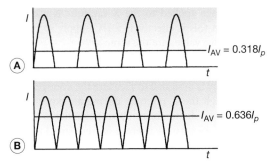

Fig. 5.20 Forms of rectified sinusoidal alternating current: (A) half-wave rectification; (B) full-wave rectification.

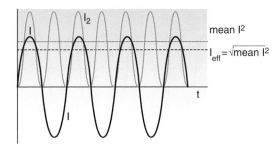

Fig. 5.21 Graphic representation of an effective (root mean square [RMS]) value of current.

Thus, we can say for half-wave rectification:

$$I_{AV} = 0.318I_p$$
$$V_{AV} = 0.318V_p$$

Equation 5.32

and for full-wave rectification:

$$I_{AV} = 0.636I_p$$
$$V_{AV} = 0.636V_p$$

Equation 5.33

5.27.3   Effective (or root mean square) current or voltage

If an AC supply is connected across a resistor, then electrons will flow in one direction during the first half-cycle and in the opposite direction during the second half-cycle. As there is no net movement of electrons for any given number of complete cycles, the average current is zero.

This does not mean that the net heating effect is zero. Electrons will produce heat within a resistor irrespective of their direction of travel. The average current is therefore a quantity, which is not suitable for determining the energy or power expended in a circuit which is connected to an AC supply. The quantity of importance is the effective or root mean square (RMS) value of the current and may be defined as Fig. 5.21:

> **DEFINITION**
>
> The effective current is that value of constant current which, flowing for the same time, would produce the same expenditure of electrical energy in a circuit as the AC.

The effective value of the current is also known as the *RMS value*, for reasons which we will consider below. The effective or RMS voltage is defined in a very similar manner:

> **DEFINITION**
>
> The effective voltage is that voltage which, being present for the same time, would produce the same expenditure of energy in a circuit as the alternating voltage.

5.28   AC AND THE X-RAY TUBE

To produce X-rays, the X-ray tube requires a high PD (voltage) across it and a current flowing through it. The voltage available from the mains supply is far too low for use directly across the X-ray tube so a means of increasing it to the high values of thousands of volts is required. This is relatively easy to accomplish using an AC transformer (Chapter 12). Because this transformer increases the voltage, it is known as a *step-up transformer*. The filament of the X-ray tube requires a low voltage supply so that it can produce the electrons that form the mA through the tube, and so the mains voltage passes through a step-down transformer before being applied to the filament. Thus an alternating voltage may be either increased using a step-up transformer or decreased using a step-down transformer.

In AC circuits, the voltages or currents are usually expressed in terms of their effective values unless otherwise stated. When considering the X-ray circuit, the following conventions apply:

- The voltage across the tube (kV) is expressed in terms of the peak voltage, that is, kVp.
- The current flowing through the tube (mA) is expressed in terms of the average current.
- The mains voltage and current to the X-ray generator are expressed as effective or RMS values.

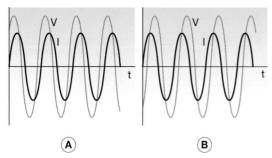

Fig. 5.22 Phase differences between current and voltage waveforms: (A) *I* lags behind *V*; (B) *I* leads *V*.

5.28.1   Voltage across the X-ray tube (kVp)

The PD across the X-ray tube is expressed in terms of the peak value for the following reasons Fig. 5.22:

- The maximum energy of X-ray photons emitted by the anode is the same value in keV, that is, an X-ray tube operated at 100 kVp will emit X-ray photons with a maximum energy of 100 keV.
- The voltage rating of the high-tension cables must be able to withstand the maximum voltage applied to them. This occurs during the peak value of the voltage.

If the voltage applied to the X-ray tube is a constant potential, then this is effectively a DC supply so the peak and the effective values are the same.

5.28.2   Current through the X-ray tube (mA)

The mA display is designed to measure the average current flowing through the X-ray tube during an exposure. The intensity of the radiation beam is proportional to the average current. If we take the average current (mA) and multiply this by the exposure time in seconds, we get the mAs for that exposure. This represents the total charge that has passed through the X-ray tube during the exposure. The quantity of X-rays produced during the exposure is proportional to the mAs.

FURTHER READING

Ball, J.L., Moore, A.D., & Turner, S. 2008. *Ball and Moore's Essential Physics for Radiographers*. 4th edn. London: Blackwell Scientific. (Chapters 5, 6, 7.)

Bushong, S. 2016. *Radiologic Science for Technologists: Physics, Biology, and Protection*. 11th edn. St. Louis: Mosby. (Chapter 4.)

Dobson, K., Grace, D., & Lovett, D. 2008. *Collins Advanced Science – Physics*. 3rd edn. London: Collins Educational.

Magnetism and electromagnetism

CHAPTER CONTENTS

6.1   AIM

In this chapter the key principles of magnetism and electromagnetism are considered. Magnetism plays a vital role in the scanning technique called *magnetic resonance imaging* (MRI), which uses powerful magnetic fields to portray human tissues (see Chapter 25). These scanners are normally specialised electromagnets which produce powerful magnetic fields by having their conducting coils cooled to very low temperatures, at which point there is zero electrical resistance. Permanent magnets are sometimes used in MRI but have a lower field strength. Electromagnets are found in other imaging applications too, such as in the case of motors used in the rotating anode X-ray tube (see Chapter 12).

6.2   MAGNETIC FIELDS

As long ago as the 11th century, the Chinese were employing magnetic compasses. These consisted of a length of permanently magnetised iron which will tend to align itself in the direction of the Earth's magnetic field when free to pivot. The phenomenon that two like magnetic poles (such as two north poles) repel and two unlike magnetic poles (such as a north and a south pole) attract was demonstrated by Peter Peregrinus in the 13th century.

Whenever an electrical charge is in motion, a magnetic field is produced. This takes place when electrons flow in a conductor such as a metal wire. There are also electron orbital motions and spins in atoms, which produce tiny magnetic fields.

Whenever a field is produced in a volume of space, an energy gradient exists. In other words there is a change of energy within that volume. The energy gradient means that force may be exerted on a charge present within the field. For example, force may be exerted on a current-carrying wire, on a compass needle which experiences a twisting force, or on the magnetic spins of nuclei within the field of an MRI magnet. Materials which are capable of being temporarily magnetised experience a force when placed in a magnetic field. A vivid demonstration of this effect (not to be attempted!) is the sight of an object such as a pair of scissors accelerating through the air towards the bore of an MRI magnet. This is an example of the 'projectile effect' in which a magnetic field exerts a 'torque' (or twisting force) on a ferromagnetic object such as iron, tending to align it with the field and bring it closer to the strongest point in the field.

A magnetic north and magnetic south pole separated by a distance is known as a *magnetic dipole*. A dipole can comprise the two poles of a permanent magnet or the two ends of a current-carrying loop of conductor. If two magnetic

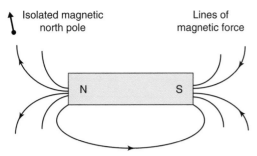

Fig. 6.1 Lines of magnetic field surrounding a permanent bar magnet.

poles of strength p are separated by a distance l, then the *magnetic dipole moment* of the system, $m = p \times l$.

The force F between two magnetic poles is equal to the product of their individual strengths divided by the square of the distance between them.

F is proportional to $(p_1 \times p_2)$ divided by d^2, where p_1 and p_2 are the individual magnetic pole strengths and d^2 is the square of the distance between them. Thus it can be seen that the force on an object entering a magnetic scanner room increases greatly as the distance to the scanner decreases. This is an example of an 'inverse square law'. A further example of the law, which is particularly important in radiography, can be found in the case of X-ray emission.

The direction of a magnetic field is taken as the direction in which a hypothetical isolated magnetic north pole would move if placed in the field. Hence lines of magnetic field pass from the north to the south pole of a permanent magnet, as shown in Fig. 6.1.

> ## INSIGHT
>
> It is not correct to talk about the north and south poles of a magnetic resonance imaging (MRI) scanner. Such scanners produce a very powerful magnetic field in the z-axis (or long axis) of a patient lying within the scanner, and we can talk about a 'spin-up' orientation parallel to the field and a 'spin-down' orientation antiparallel to it. But the concept of an MRI scanner as a large bar magnet is misleading.

The field around a bar magnet is nonuniform, that is it varies in strength and direction with location. In contrast, the Earth's magnetic field is relatively uniform and the magnetic field lines run fairly parallel to each other. Although this is generally true, there may be small local variations caused by the presence of iron-containing rock. The Earth's magnetic flux density is typically about 0.5 gauss

(G) or 0.5×10^{-4} tesla. A tesla equals 10,000 gauss. The gauss is an old centimetre gram second (cgs) unit but is still in common use as it is sometimes easier to use. For example, it is easier to talk about a '5-gauss exclusion zone' surrounding an MRI scanner than a 0.0005 tesla zone! The larger and more current SI unit of tesla (T) for magnetic flux density and magnetic inductance is used a lot to describe the 'field strength' of MRI scanners, where 0.2 T would be regarded as a 'low field' magnet and 3 T as a 'high field' magnet. A 3-T magnet provides a magnetic field about 60,000 times more powerful than that of the Earth.

Note that although the tesla is commonly used to describe the 'strength' of the magnetic field B in radiography, strictly the tesla is a unit of magnetic flux density or inductance.

The static (or constant) magnetic field produced by an MRI magnet needs to be as uniform as possible within the bore itself, to maximise image quality. Magnetic field homogeneity needs to be achieved, with a maximum permissible variation of 1 part in 100,000 for clinical MR imaging and to about 1 part in 10 million for in-vivo (living) magnetic resonance spectroscopy, which produces spectral signatures of chemicals present in the body. In practice, small inhomogeneities (nonuniformities) arise when an object such as a patient is present within the magnetic field.

> ## INSIGHT
>
> There are two contributions to the magnetic moment of an electron, namely an orbital magnetic moment caused by angular momentum around the nucleus, and a spin magnetic moment caused by spin about the electron's own axis. The permitted spins of an electron are +1/2 and −1/2. Paired electrons within full orbitals have opposing spins and cancel out each other's magnetic moments. Likewise, the net magnetic moment of a filled electron shell is zero, because all the orbitals within it are full. Only the unfilled electron shell needs to be considered when examining magnetic properties. Contributions to the spin and angular momentum for each individual outer shell electron need to be added vectorially.

Paramagnetic materials have a small positive magnetic susceptibility, symbol χ, of the order of $+10^{-3}$ to $+10^{-5}$. The magnetic susceptibility of a material refers to the extent to which it can become temporarily magnetised in a magnetic field. Materials with positive susceptibility reinforce the effect of a magnetic field. The magnetisation of paramagnets is weak but parallel to the direction of the applied magnetic field. These materials usually have unpaired electrons. They include atoms and ions of transition elements, rare Earth elements, some metals, oxygen and free radicals. Examples are aluminium, platinum, manganese and the gadolinium ion Gd^{3+}, which is used within MRI contrast agents to reduce MRI T1 relaxation times and hence brighten the signal. Ferrous Fe^{2+} ions in the liver, bound to organic molecules, also reduce T1 times. See Chapter 25 for an explanation of the T1 process.

Diamagnetic materials have a small negative magnetic susceptibility, of the order of 10^{-5}. Their magnetic response is in opposition to the applied magnetic field. These materials, such as copper, silver, gold, bismuth and beryllium, have filled electron shells and no net magnetic moment. Their induced magnetisation opposes the magnetic field, in a manner predicted by Lenz's law. The applications of Lenz's law are covered later in this chapter.

Ferromagnetic materials have a very high positive magnetic susceptibility of the order of +50 to +10,000. Ferromagnetic materials retain their magnetisation once exposed to a magnetic field. They are used within permanent MRI magnets. The disadvantage of such magnets is their low maximum field strength. The property of ferromagnetism is because of the bulk effects of many electrons within the material, rather than to the magnetic effects of the electrons within individual atoms. Examples are iron, cobalt and nickel.

Superparamagnetic materials exhibit a large positive magnetic susceptibility. They differ from ferromagnetic materials in consisting of small size particles which do not display the bulk properties of ferromagnetic materials. They become transiently magnetised within a magnetic field. An example is coated particles of iron oxide, used as a negative contrast agent which reduces MRI T2 times and reduces signal intensity.

> **INSIGHT**
>
> The magnetic susceptibility properties of body tissues can be used in magnetic resonance imaging (MRI) to provide useful signal information. For example, the magnetic susceptibility of liver and haemorrhage is altered by their iron content. Metallic implants often produce a large magnetic susceptibility artefact in MRI, by distorting the local magnetic field. The magnetic susceptibilities of oxygenated and deoxygenated blood differ, and this can be used in functional MRI of tissue blood supply.

So far we have only considered the magnetic effects attributed to electrons. However, there is a small contribution to the total angular momentum of the atom from the nucleus because of its spin. This contribution is about one-thousandth of that of an electron but is a very important property in MRI.

> **INSIGHT**
>
> Nuclei, like electrons, possess ground energy levels and excited energy levels. Protons and neutrons, the constituents of nuclei, have a spin quantum number of +1/2 or −1/2. They also have orbital angular momentum by virtue of their motion in the nucleus. Both the proton and the neutron possess a magnetic moment (the latter despite not having an overall electrical charge, for reasons which need not concern us here). The sum total of the spin and orbital angular moments of the nucleons in the nucleus is referred to as the *nuclear spin*. Because an odd number of spin 1/2 particles always combine to give a half integer total spin, it follows that nuclei with an odd mass number have nuclear spins of values 1/2, 3/2, 5/2, etc. It is these nuclei that concern us in magnetic resonance imaging (MRI) and have useful magnetic spins. The most important one is the hydrogen-1 nucleus, which is just a single proton and has a 1/2 spin. Phosphorus-31 is used in magnetic resonance spectroscopy. Note that the individual nucleon spins are cancelled out in nuclei with even mass numbers and thus these nuclei are of no use to us in MRI.

MRI used to be termed *nuclear magnetic resonance*, because it depends upon the magnetisation of the atomic nucleus. The name was changed because the public tended to confuse it with the nuclear reactions, involving the fission of atomic nuclei, that occur in power stations and atom bombs.

We commented earlier that the magnetic moment of an electron is much greater than that of a nucleus. Indeed, electron spin resonance has been studied to examine its potential for imaging. However, electron spin resonance occurs on the gigahertz or GHz frequency range and leads to considerable heating of tissues. In addition, these frequencies are absorbed superficially in the body, leading to poor deep imaging.

6.3 BULK MAGNETIC PROPERTIES AND PERMANENT MAGNETS

We saw earlier that some elements and materials like iron are highly magnetic (ferromagnetic) whereas others like gold, plastics and most body tissues have almost no magnetisation. A ferromagnetic material like a block of iron in fact consists of many tiny crystals, not just one slab of homogeneous material. These small crystals can be considered

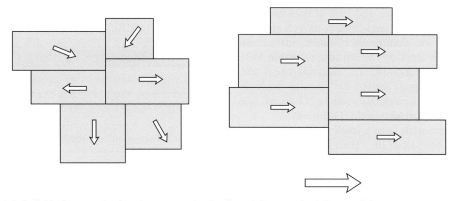

Fig. 6.2 Individual magnetic domains are randomly aligned (but can be influenced) in nonpermanent magnetic materials (*left*) whereas permanent magnets (*right*) have their domains in fixed alignment, giving an overall magnetisation.

as individual domains, each with an overall magnetisation in a particular direction. If the domains are aligned randomly, very little overall magnetisation will result, although the domains may become more aligned in the presence of a strong magnetic field, producing temporary magnetisation. This is the case when a pair of scissors hurtles into an MRI magnet!

In permanent magnets, the domains tend to align in a particular direction and are fixed in this direction, giving a permanent overall magnetisation, as shown in Fig. 6.2.

A small number of MRI scanners employ permanent magnets to produce a magnetic field. These magnets have the disadvantages of being bulky and producing a relatively low magnetic field strength. More will be said about the types of available MRI scanners in Chapter 25. There have been improvements in the technology of permanent magnets, and a range of materials, such as neodymium iron, ceramics, ferrites and rare Earth elements, can be employed in their construction.

6.4   ELECTROMAGNETISM

An electric current in a wire (for example) can also produce a magnetic field, because an electric current is just the flow of electrons in a conductor. This is found to be so in practice and the term *electromagnetism* is used to describe this effect (i.e., electricity producing magnetism).

6.5   ELECTRON FLOW AND 'CONVENTIONAL' CURRENT

When electricity was first discovered, it was assumed that it was the positive charges that flow in a conductor, and not the negative charges. This concept is now known as the

'*conventional*' current. It is now known that the positive charges in a solid material do not have any net movement (although they vibrate with heat energy) because they form the protons in the nuclei of atoms. Thus it is the electrons that move in a solid, as explained by the elementary electron theory of conduction.

In gas or liquid, any positive and negative charges present may take part in current flow, because the positive charges are free to move, unlike in a solid. In radiography and many other subjects, it is the electron flow in conductors which is most frequently under consideration, and herein lies a difficulty, for many rules (or conventions) in electromagnetism and electromagnetic induction are based upon the totally false assumption of the 'conventional' current, which in a mathematical sense is supposed to flow in the opposite direction to that of the electrons.

This and further chapters will therefore discuss both electromagnetism and electromagnetic induction on the basis of electron flow only, in an attempt to eliminate much of the confusion that undoubtedly exists at present in many people's minds. Some caution is therefore required when studying these subjects from other books, as they may invoke the 'conventional' current for their rules. Differences in the two approaches are explained in the Insights where appropriate.

6.6   MAGNETIC FIELD RESULTING FROM A STRAIGHT WIRE

The presence of a magnetic field around a current-carrying conductor was first discovered by Oersted when passing a current through a straight wire placed near a magnetic compass, as illustrated in Fig. 6.3.

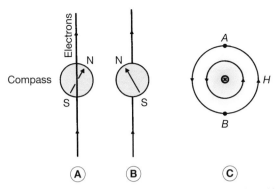

Fig. 6.3 (A and B) The effect of the magnetic field produced by the electrons flowing in the wire upon a magnetic compass. (C) If we look along the wire in the direction of electron flow, then the field is an anticlockwise direction (⊗ means that the electrons are flowing away from the eye of the observer).

If the wire is aligned in a north–south direction (i.e., along the direction of the compass needle), then an electric current through the wire causes deflections of the compass, as shown in Fig. 6.3: clockwise when the wire is above the compass (A) and anticlockwise when the wire is below the compass (B). This is only possible if the lines of magnetic force are circular and in an anticlockwise direction when viewed along the same direction as the movement of the flowing electrons. We may therefore use the following convention.

> **CONVENTION**
>
> Each moving electron produces an anticlockwise magnetic field about itself when viewed along the direction of its motion.

This convention is illustrated in Fig. 6.3C, where the symbol ⊗ means that electron flow is away from the eye (and ⊙ is towards the eye). The arrows on the lines of force are in an anticlockwise direction, in accordance with our convention, and give the direction in which a north pole would move if placed in that position. Thus, a weightless north pole would, if released, travel round and round the wire indefinitely in an anticlockwise circle.

6.7 MAGNETIC FIELD RESULTING FROM A CIRCULAR COIL OF WIRE

Fig. 6.4A shows a circular coil of wire in which an electric current is made to flow. Now, each individual moving electron produces anticlockwise magnetic lines of force about itself, as illustrated in Fig. 6.4A. The closeness of the lines

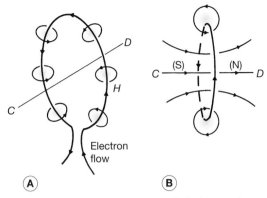

Fig. 6.4 The magnetic field around a coil of wire carrying a current. Note the similarity to the field around a small bar magnet.

of force to each other represents the total magnetic effect (i.e., the magnetic flux density). The addition at a point of all the magnetic flux densities represented by the lines of force produces the total magnetic flux density at that point. Note that, within the coil, the lines of force all tend to be in the direction C to D, whereas outside the coil, they are from D to C. A top view of the coil (Fig. 6.4B) shows the pattern of the overall lines of force so obtained. It is interesting to note the similarity of these lines of force to those of a short bar magnet (see Fig. 6.1), where they emerge from the north pole end and travel around the magnet to the south pole end and back again.

6.8 MAGNETIC FIELD RESULTING FROM A SOLENOID

A solenoid consists of several coils joined together, and so produces magnetic lines of force, as shown in Fig. 6.5A, similar to a bar magnet.

The effect of a piece of soft iron within the solenoid is to increase the magnetic flux density many times because of the induced magnetism within the soft iron. This effect is reflected by an increase in the number of lines of force in Fig. 6.5B compared with Fig. 6.5A. The combination of solenoid and soft iron in this manner is known as an *electromagnet*. The coils in an alternating current (AC) transformer act as a solenoid inducing a magmatic flux in the core of the transformer.

6.9 ELECTROMAGNETIC INDUCTION

Electromagnetic induction is the production of electricity by the interlinking of a conductor with a changing magnetic field or moving a conductor relative to a stationary magnetic field (also known as the *generator effect*).

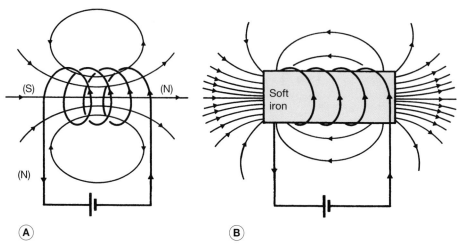

Fig. 6.5 (A) The magnetic field produced by a current-carrying solenoid. (B) The large increase in the magnetic field produced when using a soft iron bore in the solenoid.

6.10   CONDITIONS NECESSARY FOR ELECTROMAGNETIC INDUCTION

Consider the simple experiment depicted in Fig. 6.6. A solenoid L is joined to a meter that can measure both the magnitude and the direction of the current flowing through the solenoid. The following effects are observed:

- No current flow is observed on the meter if the magnet is stationary with respect to the solenoid (Fig. 6.6A and C).
- A current flows through the meter whenever the magnet is moved towards or away from the solenoid (Fig. 6.6B and D).
- The magnitude of the induced current is greater if the magnet is moved faster.
- Reversing the direction of the movement of the magnet reverses the direction of the induced current (Fig. 6.6B and D).
- Reversing the pole of the magnet, which is closer to the solenoid, reverses the direction of the induced current for a given movement.

From this simple experiment, we can conclude that only a changing magnetic field relative to the conductor is able to induce electricity in the conductor. We can also see that the amount of electricity produced is in some way related to the rate of change of the magnetic field relative to the conductor. Finally, we can conclude that the direction of movement of the magnetic field influences the direction of the induced current. These concepts will be discussed in more detail in the following sections of this chapter.

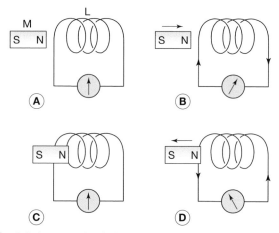

Fig. 6.6 An example of electromagnetic induction. A current flows only when there is relative movement between the bar magnet (*M*) and the solenoid (*L*).

6.11   FARADAY'S LAWS OF ELECTROMAGNETIC INDUCTION

Faraday produced two laws of electromagnetic induction that cover some of the observations we made in the previous section. These may be defined as follows:

1. A change in the magnetic flux linked with a conductor induces an electromotive force (EMF) in the conductor.
2. The magnitude of the induced EMF is proportional to the rate of change of the magnetic flux linkage.

To understand Faraday's laws, we need to have a clear understanding of EMF and magnetic flux linkage.

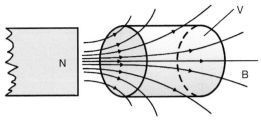

Fig. 6.7 The magnetic flux linkage associated with a volume *V*.

EMF was considered in Chapter 5 and can be considered as the force which is capable of causing electrons to flow (i.e., EMF will cause a current to flow in a complete circuit). Note that Faraday's laws do not specify whether or not the conductor is connected to an external circuit but, in either case, an EMF will be induced in it.

Magnetic flux and magnetic flux density were discussed earlier in this chapter. The magnetic flux through a volume *V* can be visualised as being proportional to the number of lines of flux passing through that volume (Fig. 6.7). Thus, if a magnetic flux of 10 weber passes through *V*, then the magnetic flux linkage with *V* is also said to be 10 weber. If the magnet in Fig. 6.7 is moved to the left of the page, then the number of lines of flux (or the flux linkage) in the volume *V* will be reduced.

We now see that moving the magnet relative to the solenoid will alter the flux linkage between the magnet and the solenoid and so an EMF will be induced—Faraday's first law. Also, a rapid movement of the magnet increases the rate of change of flux linkage and so increases the size of the induced EMF—Faraday's second law.

Changing the magnetic flux linkage associated with a particular conductor may be achieved in two ways:
1. By moving the conductor relative to a stationary magnet—this principle is used in the AC generator or dynamo.
2. By varying the magnitude of the magnetic *flux* while the conductor is stationary—this principle is used in the AC transformer.

6.12 LENZ'S LAW

In our initial observations regarding the induced current we noted the direction as well as the size of the current. Faraday's laws apply to open or closed circuits, but because Lenz's law concerns the direction of the induced current, it can only be applied to closed circuits. The law can be stated as follows:

The direction of the induced current in a conductor caused by a changing magnetic flux is such that its own magnetic field opposes the changing magnetic flux.

When the north pole of a bar magnet is moved towards a solenoid (Fig. 6.6B), the current will flow in the solenoid in such a direction that it produces a north pole at the end closest to the magnet. This has the effect of producing a force of repulsion between the bar magnet and the solenoid and so work must be done against this force to keep the magnet moving towards the solenoid. Thus mechanical energy is transformed to electrical energy and the law of conservation of energy is maintained. The reverse occurs when the magnet is withdrawn.

6.13 SIGN CONVENTION FOR THE INDUCED CURRENT

When current flow was considered as the flow of positive charge, this was determined using Fleming's right-hand rule. As we now know that current flow *is* a flow of electrons, Fleming's hand rules are liable to cause confusion and so the direction of current flow will be determined using the convention shown in Fig. 6.8.

CONVENTION

Consider a situation similar to that shown in Fig. 6.8A. Here a conductor is moved at right angles to a magnetic field (Fig. 6.8B)—the direction of the movement and the direction of the magnetic field are as shown in the diagram. We wish to determine whether the induced electron flow along the conductor will be either into the page or out of the page. This can be determined as follows:
1. Mark the position of the conductor and draw a line to indicate the direction of movement.
2. Draw a second line (*B*) to represent the permanent magnetic field direction to intersect the first line at the point *P* (Fig. 6.8B).
3. Now, draw a circle with the conductor at its centre such that its circumference passes through the point *P*.

4. This circle represents the magnetic field that will be caused by the current induced in the conductor. The direction of this magnetic field is the same as the direction of the permanent magnetic field at the point P—the field is in a clockwise direction.

5. As we learnt earlier, the magnetic field around a current-carrying conductor is anticlockwise when the electrons are travelling away from us. Thus because of the clockwise magnetic field, we can conclude that the electrons (of the induced current) are travelling towards us.

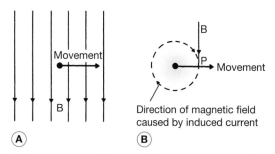

Fig. 6.8 An example of the use of the convention described in the text for establishing the direction of the induced current.

6.14   MUTUAL INDUCTION

If a changing current is passed through one conductor, then this will produce a changing magnetic field around this conductor. If a second conductor is placed within this changing magnetic field, then (by Faraday's laws) an EMF will be generated in the conductor and a current will flow in it if the conducting loop is complete (Fig. 6.9).

By Lenz's law, this current will be in the opposite direction to the original current. The size of this secondary current will vary with the magnetic field; it will be a current of changing magnitude because there is a changing magnetic field. This changing secondary current will produce its own changing magnetic field, which will induce an EMF and current in the first conductor. Thus each conductor induces electricity in the other and the effect is known as *mutual induction*.

Consider Fig. 6.9. When the switch, SW, is closed, electrons will flow from the negative pole of the battery to its positive pole via the coil P. During the time while the rate of flow of electrons builds up, there is a changing magnetic field around P. This is linked to S via the iron core (the iron core greatly enhances the flux linkage) and so an EMF and current flow will occur in S. The direction of the pointer on the ammeter, M, indicates that this flow of electrons in S is

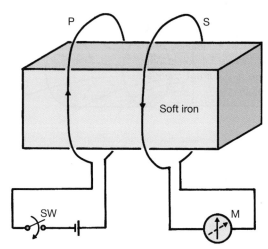

Fig. 6.9 Principles of mutual induction. A changing current in coil P (the primary coil) induces a current in coil S (the secondary coil) and vice versa. The soft iron core magnifies the effect by improving the magnetic flux linkage between the coils. M, Ammeter; SW, switch.

in the opposite direction to that in P, verifying Lenz's law. After a short time, the current in P is constant and so S is no longer influenced by a changing magnetic field. As a result, no EMF is generated in S (Faraday's first law). If the switch, SW, is now opened, the magnetic field around P collapses and so an EMF is again generated in P, but this time it is in the opposite direction. If a more powerful battery is now used, this produces a greater current in P, thus a greater magnetic field and consequently a greater EMF in S (the magnitude of the induced EMF is proportional to the rate of change of the magnetic flux). Finally, if we undertake the experiment with the iron bar present, and then with the iron bar removed, we find that the EMF produced in the coil S is greatest when the iron bar is present. This is because of improved magnetic flux linkage (Faraday's second law).

From this experiment, we can show that the EMF induced in the secondary winding E_S is:
- proportional to the rate of change of the current in P (the primary)
- dependent on the detailed design of the two conductors and the flux linkage between them. This is called the *mutual inductance* (M).

Thus:

$$E_s = M \times \text{rate of change of primary current}$$

Equation 6.1

The greater the mutual inductance, M, the greater the mutual effect between the two conductors. M is measured in henrys, and may be defined as:

A mutual inductance of 1 henry exists between two conductors if 1 volt is induced in one conductor where there is a current change of 1 ampere per second in the other.

6.15 SELF-INDUCTION

Consider the solenoid in Fig. 6.10A. If the switch, SW, is closed, current flow starts to build up in the solenoid. As this current increases, each turn of the solenoid produces a changing magnetic flux, which is linked to the other turns of the solenoid (the flux from one turn is shown in Fig. 6.10A). Thus, from Faraday's and Lenz's laws, an EMF in the opposite direction to the EMF from the battery will be induced in the solenoid. This is known as a *back-EMF*. This effect is known as *self-induction* and, if the self-induction is large, the current in the coil will take an appreciable time to build up to its maximum value. The self-induction in an electrical system is defined in a very similar manner to the mutual induction and is given by the equation:

$$E_B = L \times \text{rate of change of current} \quad \textbf{Equation 6.2}$$

Here E_B is the back-EMF and L is the self-inductance, measured in henrys. Thus we can say that:

DEFINITION

A conductor has a self-inductance of 1 henry if a back-EMF of 1 volt is induced when the current flowing through it changes at 1 ampere per second.

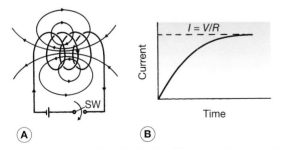

(A) **(B)**

Fig. 6.10 Principles of self-induction. The changing magnetic flux produced by the current flow through the solenoid when the switch, *SW*, is closed links with all the turns of the coil. This produces a back-electromotive force, which slows down the rate of growth of current in the coil.

A graph of the current flowing through the solenoid is shown in Fig. 6.10B. As can be seen, the induced back-EMF slows down the rate of growth of the current and so it takes an appreciable time to reach its maximum value, determined by Ohm's law. If the wire of the solenoid were unwound to become a straight conductor, then there would be no magnetic flux linkage and consequently no back-EMF. Thus, the current would rise to its maximum value very quickly.

As in the case of mutual induction, a soft iron bar placed in the solenoid will enhance the self-induction as the magnetic flux linkage between the coils is improved.

6.16 THE AC GENERATOR

Electric power is produced from an AC generator. This is an example of a situation where mechanical energy is converted to electrical energy. The basic components of such a generator are shown in Fig. 6.11A. A permanent magnetic field exists between the poles of the magnet, and coils of copper wire rotate through this field. For simplicity, only one coil is shown in the diagram. The EMF generated in the device is collected at brushes positioned at A and B.

Now consider the situation where the coil shown is rotated in a clockwise direction. Thus from the initial position, side X of the coil will move upwards through the magnetic field and side Y will move downwards (Fig. 6.11B). At this point in its movement, the coil is cutting the maximum number of lines of flux as it is moving at right angles to the flux lines, and so the maximum EMF will be generated. If we use the convention discussed earlier to establish the direction of electron flow, we can see that electrons will travel towards us on side X and away from us on side Y. Thus an excess of electrons will exist at brush A and a shortage of electrons will exist at brush B: brush A is negative and brush B is positive. This situation is shown as position 1 on the graph in Fig. 6.11C. Now consider the situation when the coil has turned in a clockwise direction from its initial position through 90 degrees: this is the second position of the coil shown in Fig. 6.11B. In this position, both side X and side Y of the coil are moving parallel with the lines of magnetic flux and so no current is generated; this is again shown as position 2 in Fig. 6.11C. In position 3, the coil has rotated through 180 degrees from its original position. Side X of the coil is now moving downwards through the magnetic field and side Y is moving upwards. As in position 1, a maximum number of lines of flux are being cut as the conductor is moving at right angles to the flux, and so, again, the maximum EMF will be generated. The polarity

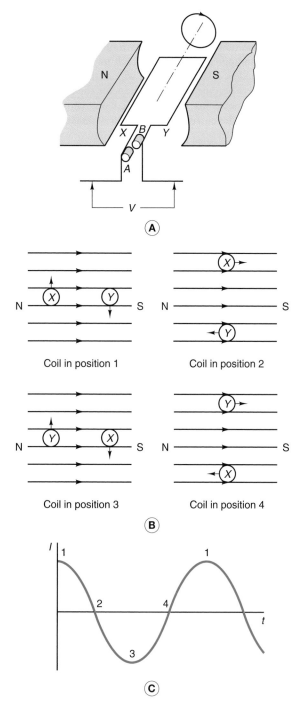

Fig. 6.11 (A) Simplified diagram of an alternating current generator; (B) four positions of the coil relative to the magnetic field; (C) the current waveform produced when the coil moves through positions 1, 2, 3, 4 and returns to 1. A complete turn of the coil will produce one cycle of current. See text for further details.

of A and B is now the reverse of position 1. In position 4, the conductor is again moving parallel to the lines of flux, so no EMF is generated. The conductor then returns to position 1 and so one cycle is complete. The process is then repeated. The type of current shown in Fig. 6.11C is known as *alternating current, AC*.

In cases where there is no external circuit connected, then no current is able to flow and only sufficient work to overcome the frictional resistance is necessary to keep the rotational movement at the same speed. As soon as an external circuit is connected, then a current is able to flow in the circuit and in the winding.

It should come as no surprise to discover that this current will flow in such a direction as to oppose the motion of the coil (remember Lenz's law). This means that mechanical work must be performed to overcome this resisting force, that is, mechanical energy is converted into electrical energy.

The effect of suddenly increasing the electrical load demanded from the generator (e.g., when making an X-ray exposure) is suddenly to increase the opposition to its rotation. Hence, as the generator slows down momentarily, the induced EMF (which depends on the speed of rotation) is reduced. We find that, in times of increased demand on the generators, there is a drop in the voltage they supply. In X-ray units, this is taken into account by the inclusion of a mains voltage compensator on the unit.

SUMMARY

In this chapter you should have learnt the following:
- Magnetic properties exist at the atomic level and also in whole materials at the macroscopic level.
- Magnetism may be temporary or permanent and many materials become magnetised within a magnetic field.
- There are many applications of these principles in MRI and general radiography.
- Circular magnetic fields exist around moving charges: anticlockwise around negative charges and clockwise around positive charges when viewed along the direction of motion.
- The magnetic flux density resulting from a current-carrying solenoid may be increased many times by inserting within it a material of high permeability (e.g., soft iron because $B = \mu$). The magnetic domains become aligned with the direction of H, so adding to the overall magnetic flux density.
- That an EMF is induced in a conductor if it is linked with a changing magnetic field.

- Faraday's first and second law of electromagnetic induction.
- Lenz's law, which determines the direction of the current flowing as the result of the induced EMF.
- The sign convention for the direction of the induced current.
- The meaning and a simple application of mutual induction and self-induction.
- The mode of operation of an AC generator.

FURTHER READING

Ball, J.L., Moore, A.D., & Turner, S. 2008. *Ball and Moore's Essential Physics for Radiographers*. 4th edn. London: Blackwell Scientific. (Chapters 8, 9, 10.)

Bushong, S. 2016. *Radiologic Science for Technologists: Physics, Biology, and Protection*. 11th edn. St. Louis: Mosby. (Chapter 4.)

Dobson, K., Grace, D., & Lovett, D. 2008. *Collins Advanced Science – Physics*. 3rd edn. Glasgow: Collins Education.

X-ray circuit components

CHAPTER CONTENTS

7.1 AIM

This chapter explains how circuit components are used to enable X-ray tubes (see Chapter 12) to be used as a source of X-rays. The functions of these components are as follows:

- To provide a high voltage (potential difference) across the X-ray tube to accelerate electrons across the vacuum of the X-ray tube insert, so that they have sufficient energy to produce X-rays (see Section 12.7.6). This is achieved using a generator.
- To provide an electric current through the X-ray tube filament, thereby heating the filament and causing the thermionic emission of electrons (see Section 12.7).
- To maintain current flow in a single direction across the X-ray tube (direct current) because electron flow must always be from the cathode to the anode. Mains supply is alternating current (AC) and thus this must be *rectified* to be converted to direct current (DC).
- To control and adjust the X-ray exposure factors such as kept, mA, mAs and exposure time.

7.2 GENERATORS – OBTAINING ENERGY FOR RADIATION PRODUCTION

As was seen in Chapter 3, energy cannot be created out of nothing, but may be converted from one form to another. This principle is called the *law of conservation of energy*. It is a bit like saying that we must have cash in our bank account before we can make a purchase, with no borrowing permitted! So we must have energy available before we can produce the X-rays that are used in diagnostic radiography. The production of X-rays in radiography involves a conversion of electrical energy into wave energy, via various stages.

The first step is to obtain electrical power from the mains (National Grid). There are two voltages available in the United Kingdom—a single-phase 240-volt supply for low-powered hospital devices such as dental X-ray tubes and domestic use, and a three-phase 415-volt supply where more power is needed, as in conventional static X-ray sets. The number of phases refers to how many voltage waveforms are combined within the electrical output.

To the world at large, the term 'generator' means a device for producing electricity. This might range from a huge apparatus at a power station to a mobile unit at a camp site. But in radiography, the term 'generator' normally refers to a device that increases (or 'steps-up') the mains voltage to values sufficient to produce X-rays. At one time the generator tank in an X-ray room was a bulky affair, containing a large transformer and various switches, surrounded by insulating oil. But modern generator tanks tend to be much more compact, because of the advent of more efficient 'medium-frequency' or 'high-frequency' voltage converters. An example of a modern generator tank can be seen in Fig. 7.1.

As mentioned previously, the 'driving force' for X-ray production at X-ray energies up to 150 keV (150 kiloelectron volts, or 150,000 electron volts) is a source of current electricity from the mains. This mains electricity is AC which means that the electrons in the circuit flow first in one direction and then another. Electricity is a flow of small negatively charged electrons drifting through a conducting material, as explained in more detail in Chapter 5.

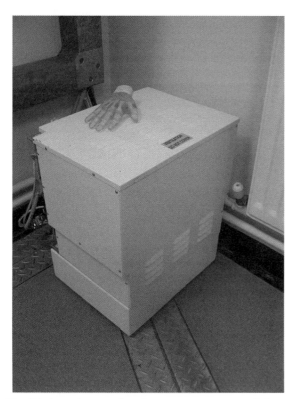

Fig. 7.1 A modern medium-frequency generator tank in an X-ray room. The compact size of the unit can be seen with reference to the hand phantom.

> ## INSIGHT
>
> Why is mains electricity produced as alternating current (AC)? The generators found in power stations consist of three large coils of wire, at 120 degrees to each other. Mechanical power makes the coils rotate through a magnetic field and this motion induces electrical current in the coils. The topic of electromagnetic induction is covered in Chapter 6. The changing motion of each coil relative to the magnetic field during each revolution produces an alternating positive and negative voltage in the coil. This alternating voltage drives an AC flow. There is also a big practical advantage to AC; an AC waveform generates a lot of magnetic field change (because there is a lot of changing current flow) and this is good news because devices called *transformers* (which increase or decrease voltages) work more efficiently within a rapidly changing magnetic field.

The voltage across the X-ray tube in kilovolts corresponds to the maximum possible X-ray energy in kiloelectron volts, as will be explained in Chapter 12. Another term which needs explaining is the 'kVp' or 'peak kilovoltage' applied to an X-ray tube. There is a peak value because there may be slight voltage fluctuations in the AC output of an X-ray generator.

Traditional X-ray generators included large 'step-up' transformers, designed to increase the mains voltage of 415 volts to the kilovoltage levels needed for X-ray production. The transformer consists of two coils of conducting wire, termed primary and secondary coils, mounted on an iron core. AC electrical current in the primary coil produces a time-varying magnetic field which in turn induces an alternating electrical current in the secondary coil. The relative size of the primary and secondary voltages depends on the relative number of loops of wire on the primary and secondary coils. AC is especially good at this process of electromagnetic induction, as it produces a lot of magnetic flux change.

Modern X-ray generators make use of 'high-frequency' devices, which are not only more compact and more efficient but also offer more precise control of electrical output. The term *high frequency* means a frequency higher than the 50 Hz (Hertz or cycles per second) supply obtained from the mains and is typically about 5000 Hz or more in radiographic generators. A key principle of working with voltages that vary with a high frequency is that they are very efficient at producing electromagnetic induction in a transformer. The transformer can be more compact as a result of this. The frequency of a wave is the number of wave cycles which will fit into a second. The modern generator assembly additionally first converts mains AC to DC. This DC is fed to a voltage inverter, which in turn provides a high-frequency AC supply for the primary coil of a step-up transformer.

7.3   TRADITIONAL TRANSFORMERS

A transformer is a device for changing the value of a voltage. If the voltage is increased, for example to the high values required across an X-ray tube, then the device is called a 'step-up transformer'. If the voltage is decreased, for example, to the low values required for the X-ray tube filament supply, then the device is called a 'step-down transformer'. Simple transformers consist of an iron core, with primary and secondary windings (loops of wire) wrapped around the core. They have been largely replaced by more modern devices in X-ray circuits but will be briefly discussed because they are still mentioned in many textbooks.

7.3.1   The ideal transformer

An *ideal transformer* is one whose output electrical power is equal to its input electrical power – there is no power 'lost' in the transformer itself.

There is, of course, no such thing as the ideal (or perfect) transformer, although real transformers with efficiencies of 98% or more are not uncommon. Consider an ideal transformer, shown in Fig. 7.2 where two isolated sets of windings share a common core; there are a number of other configurations of core and windings but the one shown in Fig. 7.2 is the simplest. The input or primary side of the transformer consists of n_p turns around the core and

has an alternating voltage V_P across it. The output or secondary side of the transformer consists of n_s turns and has a voltage V_s induced in it. This is a case of mutual induction, as discussed in Section 6.14. The sequence of events is as follows:

- The alternating voltage in the primary winding V_P causes an AC to flow through the winding.
- This AC, I_p, produces a changing magnetic flux density (B) in the soft iron core.
- The changing magnetic flux density is linked to the secondary winding so that an electromotive force (EMF), V_s, is induced in it according to Faraday's and Lenz's laws of electromagnetic induction.

An AC supply is essential for the operation of the transformer because no EMF will be generated in the secondary if the magnetic flux is constant (Faraday's first law).

The purpose of the soft iron core is to contain all the magnetic flux within it so that the magnetic flux linkage between the primary and the secondary is as near perfect as possible. The core can do this because of its strong induced magnetism, resulting from its high magnetic permeability.

The mathematics of the ideal transformer are relatively simple if we first consider the effect of the magnetic flux on a single turn of wire around the core. Because we are assuming that the transformer is ideal, there is no magnetic flux loss and the EMF induced is independent of the position of the wire. Thus, the same voltage will be induced in each turn of the primary and in each turn of the secondary. If we call this voltage v, then we can say that the total

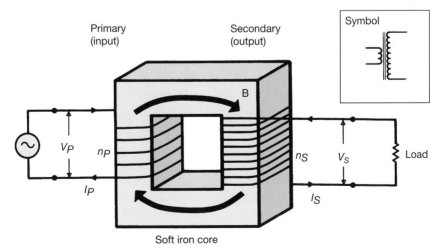

Fig. 7.2 An 'ideal' transformer showing the core and the primary and secondary windings. In practice, the core is laminated, as shown in Fig. 7.3. Because there are more turns on the secondary winding than on the primary winding, this is a step-up transformer. The symbol for a step-up transformer is also shown.

primary voltage is the voltage in each turn multiplied by the number of turns. Thus:

$$V_p = v \times n_p$$

$$\text{or } \frac{V_p}{n_p} = v$$

Similarly, for the secondary:

$$V_s = v \times n_s$$

$$\text{or } \frac{V_s}{n_s} = v$$

Thus, we can combine the two equations to get:

$$\frac{V_p}{n_p} = \frac{V_s}{n_s}$$

By cross-multiplying this equation, we get the formula:

$$\frac{V_s}{V_p} = \frac{n_s}{n_p} \qquad \textbf{Equation 7.1}$$

The ratio V_s/V_p is known as the *voltage gain* of the transformer. This is greater than unity for a step-up transformer and less than unity for a step-down transformer.

The ratio n_s/n_p is known as the *turns ratio* of the transformer. Again, if this is greater than unity, we have a step-up transformer, and if it is less than unity, we have a step-down transformer.

If we have a transformer with a turns ratio of 200:1, we know that there are 200 times as many turns on the secondary as on the primary and that the voltage across the secondary is 200 times that of the primary.

The current flowing in the secondary of the transformer may be calculated from the power in the primary winding and secondary winding (for simplicity, in the following discussion, RMS values are assumed). In the ideal transformer, the power in the primary and the power in the secondary are equal. Thus:

$$V_p \times I_p = V_s \times I_s$$

$$\therefore \frac{I_p}{I_s} = \frac{V_s}{V_p}$$

From Equation 7.1 we know:

$$\frac{V_s}{V_p} = \frac{n_s}{n_p}$$

Thus, for an ideal transformer, we can say:

$$\frac{I_p}{I_s} = \frac{n_s}{n_p} \qquad \textbf{Equation 7.2}$$

> **DEFINITION**
>
> The efficiency of a transformer is the ratio of the output power to the input power.

Note that it is often convenient to express the transformer efficiency as a percentage. For example, if a transformer is 95% efficient and 100 watts of power is supplied to the primary of that transformer, then 95 watts is produced in the secondary. In this case, 5% of the power is 'lost' because of power loss in the windings and core, that is, this 5% is not available as useful electrical power.

7.3.2 Transformer losses

Various factors contribute to the fact that real world transformers are not ideal because they experience power losses as a result of the following causes.

7.3.2.1 Copper losses

The term *copper* refers to the copper wire of the windings of the transformer, which has a small but finite resistance. If we consider a current I_{RMS} flowing through a resistance R, then there is a power of $(I_{RMS})^2 R$ watts produced within the resistor. (The copper loss is often referred to as the I^2R loss of the transformer.) The copper loss produces a small heating effect within the coils of the transformer.

We wish to keep the copper loss as low as possible and, as it is related to I^2R, it makes sense to keep R low when I is large. As we saw in Chapter 5, the resistance of a conductor is inversely proportional to its cross-sectional area. For this reason, the winding of the transformer, which carries the larger current, is made of the thicker wire. In the step-up transformer, this is the primary winding whereas in the step-down transformer it is the secondary winding.

7.3.2.2 Iron losses

The term *iron losses* refer to the losses that occur in the soft iron core of the transformer. These take three forms, as outlined.

7.3.2.3 Magnetic flux losses

If the iron core is magnetically saturated, then all the magnetic flux will not be contained within the core. This means that magnetic flux will be produced by the primary, which is not linked with the secondary. The EMF induced in the secondary and the output electrical power will be lower than if the flux linkage were perfect. By the appropriate design of the transformer core, in practice this loss is made very small indeed and so can be neglected for most practical purposes. The losses are as a result of eddy currents and hysteresis.

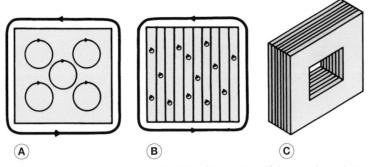

Fig. 7.3 (A) Flow of eddy currents in an unlaminated transformer core. If the core is laminated, as shown in (B) and (C), then the eddy current flow is restricted and so the eddy current losses are limited.

Eddy currents occur in the iron core of a transformer. Because the core is an electrical conductor, it will experience currents induced in it in response to changing magnetic flux. These induced currents will in turn produce a magnetic field which opposes the applied magnetic field.

This principle is shown in Fig. 7.3A where the direction of the eddy currents in the core is in the opposite direction to the current in the winding. The effect of these currents is twofold:

1. The flow of electrical current through the core causes heating of the core attributed to the electrical resistance of the core.
2. The magnetic flux associated with the eddy currents is in the opposite direction to the flux from the winding and so there is a reduction in the flux interlinking with the secondary; flux which interlinks with the secondary is the flux produced at the primary minus the eddy current flux. This constitutes a power loss within the transformer core.

Eddy currents may be reduced but not entirely eliminated by lamination of the core, as shown in Fig. 7.3B and C. The laminated sheets of soft iron are bolted together to produce the required cross-sectional area. Each lamination is insulated from its neighbours by the application of a thin layer of insulation (e.g., polyester varnish) to its surface. This means that the eddy currents produced in the core are now confined to the small cross-sectional area of each lamination. As resistance is inversely proportional to cross-sectional area, lamination produces an increase in resistance and a consequent reduction in the size of the eddy current. There is, however, some eddy current present and this causes heating of the transformer core. Because of this, the transformer core requires to be cooled either by air or by immersing the transformer in oil, the latter acting as both a coolant and an insulator.

Hysteresis is the lagging-behind of the induced magnetism in a ferromagnetic material when the applied magnetic field changes. Consider the changes which will occur in a transformer core during 1½ cycles of AC. The magnetising force H changes with the current (see Fig. 7.4A). This produces changes in the magnetic intensity I as shown in Fig. 7.4B. This graph is referred to as a *hysteresis loop* and the shape and size of this loop are important in the function of the transformer. The shape of this loop is explained as follows.

Consider a situation where the core is initially unmagnetised. Because the magnetic domains are in randomised directions, there is no magnetic intensity within the core. This represents the origin O on both of the graphs. The current increases until it reaches its peak value at point A. The magnetising force increases with the current and so initially does the magnetic intensity. This, however, flattens as magnetic saturation of the sample occurs so that the line is horizontal at point A on the hysteresis graph. The current now follows the curve AB and, as the magnetising force decreases, so the magnetic intensity reduces along the curve AB on the hysteresis graph. Note that at point B, the magnetising force is zero but there is still some magnetic intensity left in the ferromagnetic core sample. This magnetic intensity is known as the *remanence* in the core. To get rid of this remanence—so completely demagnetising the core—a coercive force, represented by OC, must be used. Because the current has been reversed, the magnetising force is also reversed and this continues until magnetic saturation is again produced at D. This occurs at the negative peak value of the current. As the current is reduced, the magnetising force is again reduced and it is zero when the current is at point E on the graph of current. At this point on the hysteresis graph, there is again a remanence represented by OE (equal and opposite to OB) and this must be destroyed by the coercive force OF. The magnetising force now continues to its positive peak, A, and the magnetic intensity follows the curve FA. The hysteresis loop is now complete.

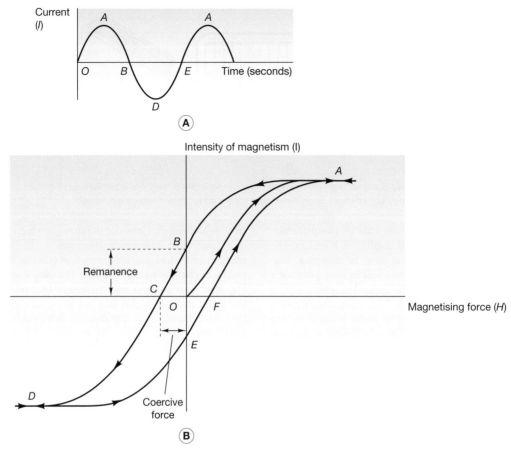

Fig. 7.4 (A) Typical alternating current supply for a transformer winding; (B) hysteresis loop for a ferromagnetic sample. For an explanation of the connection between the two, see the text.

The area of the hysteresis loop is important because it represents the work done in taking the sample through a complete hysteresis cycle. In considering the transformer core, the smaller the amount of work done, the smaller the iron loss from hysteresis. This should become clearer if we consider the hysteresis loops for soft iron and for steel.

The material usually selected for transformer cores is stalloy or permalloy because their small hysteresis loops limit the hysteresis 'loss'. The power loss resulting from hysteresis in the core increases the kinetic energy of the atoms of the core and so manifests itself in the form of heat.

7.4 THE AUTOTRANSFORMER

The autotransformer permitted the operator to manually select a range of output voltages values not very different from those of the input voltage (usually differing by a factor of between 0.5 and 2.0). Its principle function was to compensate for these slight variations, providing stable operating conditions for the other circuits of the X-ray generator. For this reason, it is more commonly known as the *mains compensator*. The autotransformer consisted of several turns forming a single winding connected to the incoming mains supply. The changing magnetic flux of the AC supply produces an EMF in the winding which is evenly distributed over every turn of the winding. In accordance with Lenz's law (see Chapter 6) a back EMF is also produced. The position of S_2 in Fig. 7.5 permits the operator to select a limited number of turns on the winding tapping the back EMF which has been produced in accordance with Lenz's law, thus producing a secondary voltage Vs and secondary current I_s.

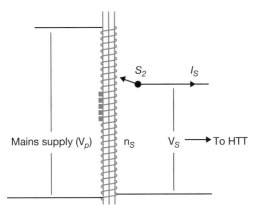

Fig. 7.5 A circuit diagram for an autotransformer. It operates on the principle of self-induction. The number of secondary turns of the transformer can be varied at S_2. Thus the output from transformer to the X-ray generator and high-tension transformer can be varied.

7.5 THE CONSTANT-VOLTAGE TRANSFORMER

Because it was manually operated the autotransformer was replaced by the constant-voltage transformer. This will now be discussed in more detail.

The constant-voltage transformer is designed in such a way that there can be considerable variation in the input voltage to the transformer, but the output voltage remains relatively constant. For reasons which will be discussed in Chapter 12, the output from the X-ray tube is sensitive to the temperature of the tube filament and so some units use a constant voltage transformer to ensure a well-stabilised voltage supply to the filament. Fig. 7.6A gives a diagrammatic representation of the construction of such a transformer. Fig. 7.6B shows a graph of the input and output voltages.

This transformer operates on the principle that the secondary limb of the core, B, is magnetically saturated during normal operation. The magnetic flux produced at the primary core, A, passes through two other magnetic circuits, the much thinner secondary core, B, and a central path of high magnetic resistance in core C. This high magnetic resistance is caused by an air gap between one end of C and the rest of the core (remember, air is less permeable than iron). The thinner core, B, is rapidly brought to magnetic saturation and the excess magnetic flux then passes through C. As can be seen from the graph, once B is saturated then an increase in input voltage does not produce any more magnetic flux in B and so the output voltage from the transformer remains fairly constant. Magnetic saturation occurs at an input voltage of X, and Y on the graph repre-

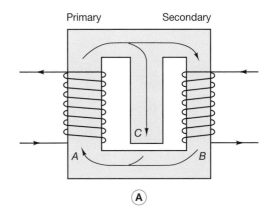

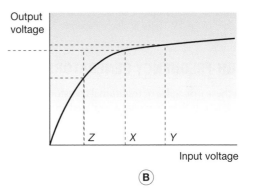

Fig. 7.6 (A) Construction of a typical constant voltage transformer; (B) graph of the input and the output voltage for such a transformer.

sents the normal operating input voltage of the transformer. Note that a large fall in the input voltage (say to Z on the graph) can result in the limb B becoming unsaturated with a resultant fall in the output voltage.

7.6 TRANSFORMER RATING

For transformer rating, the term 'rating' means the maximum combination of factors that a system can withstand without damage. If the rating is exceeded for a transformer, this may cause damage to the electrical insulation of the windings because of overheating or it may cause electrical breakdown.

The transformers in an X-ray unit are energised when the X-ray exposure is made. There are basically two types of exposure in radiography:
1. Fluoroscopy—this uses a low amount of power for a relatively long time.
2. Radiographic exposures—these use a relatively large amount of power for a short time.

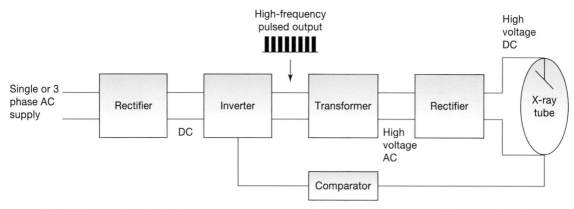

Fig. 7.7 An overview of a high-frequency generator circuit. The inverter produces a rapidly pulsing high-frequency voltage output, which is applied to a transformer. The comparator part of the circuit is designed to control the kV. There is also a separate X-ray tube filament circuit (not shown).

7.7   HIGH-FREQUENCY GENERATORS

Although these principles of traditional transformers are of historical interest, they have been replaced in all modern X-rays circuits by high-frequency generators. Such designs have the following advantages:
- Compactness, such that the circuit can even be fitted within an X-ray tube head
- Precise and instant control of voltage and mA output, via microprocessor control
- Linear output, in contrast to the nonlinearity that may affect traditional transformers
- Reduced cooling demands
- Unaffected by type of power supply (single phase or three phase).

There are several stages in the process for creating the high-voltage supply to the X-ray tube, as shown by Fig. 7.7.
1. The mains supply is rectified, which means that AC is converted to DC.
2. This DC is then fed into an inverter. The function of the inverter is to produce a very rapidly fluctuating AC output, consisting of many short pulses. Typically the frequency is 5000 Hz or more.
3. The high-frequency output is fed into a transformer (see earlier) to obtain a high voltage.
4. The output from the transformer is rectified to produce the direct current required across an X-ray tube.
5. Capacitors are used to 'smooth' the voltage and achieve a constant potential, which is important for maintaining the energy of the X-ray beam.

The key principle explaining the efficiency of the high-frequency generator can be explained in terms of Faraday's laws of electromagnetic induction (see Section 6.11) which are that:

- A change in the magnetic flux linked with a conductor induces an EMF in the conductor.
- The magnitude of the induced EMF is proportional to the rate of change of the magnetic flux linkage.

This means that if a rapidly fluctuating (high-frequency) electrical waveform is applied to a transformer, a very rapidly varying magnetic field will be induced in the transformer core. Because the rate of change of magnetic flux is high, a high induced EMF will result. The efficiency of the arrangement means that the size of the transformer core and number of transformer windings can be greatly reduced, producing a compact design with less cooling demands.

7.8   CONTROL OF EXPOSURE FACTORS

In modern high-frequency generator circuits, solid-state electronic devices detect the actual voltage across the X-ray tube and compare this with the voltage set by the operator. If there is any variation from the set value, the pulse frequency arising from the inverter is automatically compensated to adjust the voltage. Similarly the voltage can be manually adjusted by varying the inverter pulse frequency. Note that autotransformers were used to adjust voltage in older X-ray circuit designs.

A separate inverter is used to adjust the mA across the X-ray tube, by controlling the voltage that supplies the filament circuit. The filament circuit is distinct from the high-voltage circuit, because the filament requires a high current (and low-voltage) supply to generate the heat that is needed for thermionic emission (see Chapter 12).

7.8.1   Automatic exposure devices

Automatic exposure devices (AEDs) or automatic exposure controls (AECs) are designed to terminate an X-ray exposure when sufficient X-radiation has been received in an ionisation chamber. This helps to prevent exposure errors. Normally there are groups of three chambers in the X-ray table and upright bucky unit, one central and two side. Chambers can be selected depending on the body area under examination, for example, central for a spine or side for a chest. The ionisation timer makes use of the fact that X-radiation will cause ionisation in air. A radiolucent chamber is placed between the patient and the image recording device and as radiation passes through this chamber it ionises the air within it. The ionised air molecules are attracted to the electrodes in the chamber by a potential difference between them, and as a result, a small electrical current directly proportional to the amount of X-radiation flows between the electrodes. This small current is then amplified and used to charge a capacitor. The amount of charge which the capacitor receives is controlled by a variable resistor, R. An amplified voltage is received in an ionisation chamber which can measure the amount of radiation that has passed through the patient. Assuming that the amount of charge from the ionisation chamber is determined by the position of the variable resistor, then the remainder of the charge required to raise the potential of the capacitor to the trigger voltage of the switching device must be from the amplified voltage. Because this is directly related to the amount of radiation passing through the patient to the imaging device, this will be constant irrespective of the amount of radiation absorbed by the patient. The timer, in this case, terminates the exposure when the correct amount of radiation has passed through the ionisation chamber. If the ionisation chamber or photocell is positioned under the correct part of the patient, the radiograph will always receive the correct exposure. The resistance of the variable resistor controls the amount of charge required from the ionisation chamber, allowing imaging receptors of differing sensitivities (speeds) to be used.

With the AED, the operator has control over the selection of the exposure variables such as the kV, focus used, the image recording medium and, with some units, the mA used.

7.8.2 Anatomically programmed timers

With anatomically programmed timers, the operator selects the exposure by body part and projection from a number of preinstalled options. These options will determine the kV, mA, type of image recording medium, focus to film distance and the ionisation chamber to be used to detect the radiation that has passed through the patient.

This range of exposures, which is stored in the memory of a microprocessor, is programmed into the X-ray unit by the manufacturer of the X-ray generator. On installation of the unit, a senior operator programs the final selection of exposure factors for each permitted exposure in the range into the computer memory, which is then 'locked' to prevent unauthorised access. A simplified diagram of this type of device is shown in Fig. 7.8.

On exposure, interlocks are used to check that the X-ray tube is at the correct focus to film distance and the recording medium is in place. The radiation detection device is then selected and exposure commences. When sufficient radiation has passed through the detector, the microprocessor terminates the exposure through the exposure switching circuit.

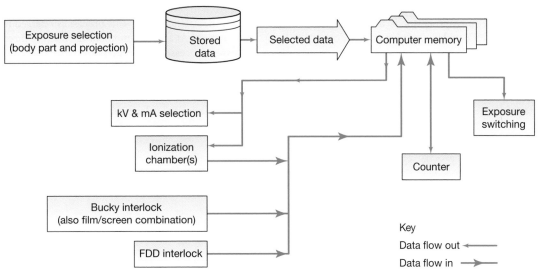

Fig. 7.8 Simplified diagram showing the principles of an anatomically programmed exposure device. *FDD,* Focus to detector distance.

Because the radiation dose received by the patient and the amount of scattered radiation produced are dependent on the quality and amount of radiation delivered during the exposure, this type of device ensures that the optimum quantity of radiation is delivered and kV is used for each exposure, minimising both the dose to the patient and the amount of scattered radiation produced.

7.9   RECTIFICATION

Rectification means that AC is converted to DC, both for the supply to the inverter circuit and then subsequently for the supply across the X-ray tube. This is achieved via solid-state semiconductor devices termed rectifiers, which permit a flow of current in one direction only. To understand how they work, the science of semiconductors will now be considered.

7.10   SEMICONDUCTORS

The use of semiconductor materials and the associated technology play an increasingly important part in our everyday lives as well as in radiographic science. Today it is possible to produce millions of electronic circuits on a small silicon chip using ultra-large-scale integration (ULSI) techniques. This has enabled the production of microprocessors that are capable of being programmed to perform specific tasks. Such devices are cheap and easy to program. They can perform a wide range of functions and are very reliable. Because of this, microprocessors are found in devices from wristwatches to aircraft flight systems and it is not surprising to learn that they are used in many devices in diagnostic imaging and radiotherapy departments.

However, the microprocessor is a complicated solid-state device, and a detailed description of its operation is beyond the scope of this text.

Other, simpler, solid-state devices are widely used in X-ray circuitry and are suitable for inclusion in this chapter after a general description of the properties of semiconductor materials.

7.11   INTRINSIC SEMICONDUCTORS

An intrinsic semiconductor is a chemically pure semiconductor, which is also assumed to have perfect regularity of atoms within its crystalline structure or lattice. The concept of semiconducting materials was briefly introduced in Section 5.16 where the properties of conductors, insulators and semiconductors were compared in terms of the energy band model for the orbiting electrons. This was illustrated in Fig. 5.13 and this diagram is reproduced here as Fig. 7.9. As shown in Fig. 7.9B, one of the characteristics of semiconductors is that there is a small energy gap (up to a few eV) between the top of the valence band and the bottom of the conduction band. At very low temperatures, all the outer electrons have energies near the bottom of the valence band, and no electrons are able to take part in electrical conduction, as there are no free electrons in the conduction band. As mentioned in Chapter 5, increasing the temperature of a semiconductor increases its conductivity. At normal room temperatures, many electrons can gain sufficient energy (because of the increased kinetic energy of the atoms) to jump up to the conduction band and so take part in electrical conduction.

7.11.1   Positive holes

Associated with each electron that can jump up to the conduction band is a 'vacancy' in the valence band, referred to as a positive hole or just hole. This hole may be filled by an electron from the valence band of a neighbouring atom, but in doing so the electron leaves a hole in the valence band of that atom. In this way, a hole may appear to move around the crystal lattice of a semiconductor (behaving like a positive charge) until eventually an electron drops down from the conduction band to fill the hole and remove it from the valence band. This process is referred to as recombination. At any one moment in time, all three of the discussed processes are occurring:
1. Electrons are being excited into the conduction band creating holes in the valence band.
2. There is movement of electrons in the conduction band and holes in the valence band.

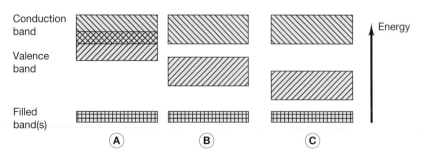

Fig. 7.9 Energy level bands for (A) a conductor, (B) a semiconductor and (C) an insulator.

3. There is a recombination of electrons in the conduction band with holes in the valence band.

The overall conductivity of such an intrinsic semiconductor is the sum of the effects of the movements of the electrons in the conduction band and the holes in the valence band.

INSIGHT

Consider the situation depicted in part A of the diagram, where there is a row of ball bearings at the base of a box, with no available space between them for sideways movement to take place. If we now lift ball bearing C onto the lid of the box, it is possible for ball bearing D to move to the left to fill the space once occupied by C. In doing so, D has now created a space to its right, that is, the hole may be considered as moving in the opposite direction to the ball.

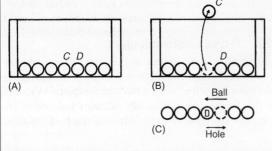

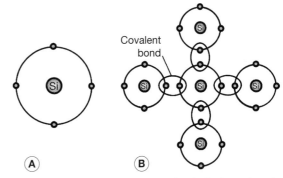

Fig. 7.10 Pure silicon as an example of an intrinsic semiconductor. (A) A silicon atom showing the four electrons in its valence shell; (B) the covalent bonds formed in a pure silicon crystal by each silicon atom sharing electrons with four neighbouring silicon atoms.

Now consider this situation as it refers to the valence and conduction bands of a semiconductor. No net movement is initially possible in the valence band because it is full of electrons. When an electron is raised to the conduction band, movement within the valence band is possible. Thus if an electron moves from right to left within the band, it leaves a hole in its starting position, that is, the hole appears to move from left to right. If an electron is removed from the valence band of an atom, then the atom is positively charged because the protons in the nucleus now outnumber the orbiting electrons; the hole is referred to as a positive hole. If a semiconductor is passing a current such that the electron flow in the conduction band is from left to right, there will also be an effective flow of positive charge associated with the movement of positive holes in the valence band in the opposite direction.

7.11.2 Silicon

Silicon is currently the most widely used general semiconductor material. It has an atomic number of 14 and has 14 protons in its nucleus and 14 electrons orbiting that nucleus This means that the two inner shells (K- and L-shells) are completely full and contain two and eight electrons, respectively. The next shell out from the nucleus is the M-shell, and this also exhibits a stable configuration when it contains eight electrons. In this case, it contains four electrons and so may be regarded as an incomplete shell in the solitary silicon atom. However, in the silicon crystal there is a regular arrangement of atoms in which each silicon atom shares its outer electrons with four neighbouring atoms so that each atom appears to have eight electrons in its M-shell and thus stability (see Fig. 7.10). Such electron bonds are known as covalent bonds and the electrons are termed valence electrons and inhabit the valence energy band of the atom. The covalent bonds give the crystal its regularity by inhibiting the movement of any particular atom. At room temperature, these bonds are being continuously broken and reformed as some of the valence electrons are gaining sufficient energy to reach the conduction band (bond broken) and electrons from the conduction band fall back into the valence band (bond reformed). The eight-electron configuration of the M-shell behaves like a full shell and so the valence band is effectively full until an electron moves up to the conduction band. As previously explained, when this happens, electron flow in the conduction band and positive-hole flow in the valence band are both possible.

Intrinsic semiconductors, which we just considered, have very limited practical use because of their low conductivity. If small amounts of specific impurities are added to them (by a process called doping), they are then known as extrinsic semiconductors and have properties which allow us to use them as rectifiers and integrated circuits (ICs), all of which are found in most X-ray generators. Extrinsic semiconductors will now be discussed.

7.12   EXTRINSIC SEMICONDUCTORS

The addition of small amounts of specific impurities to silicon or germanium is the basis on which most extrinsic semiconductors are produced. The doping may be heavy or light, depending on the component being produced. A typical concentration is one part of impurity to 10 million parts of pure silicon. The electrical conductivity of the extrinsic semiconductor is much greater than that of an intrinsic semiconductor and the level of conductivity can be controlled by altering the ratio of doping material to pure material. The impurity atoms within the silicon crystal lattice are the source of this greatly increased electrical conductivity. This is because the type of impurity is chosen either to enhance electron flow in the conduction band (this gives an *N*-type semiconductor) or to enhance the flow of positive holes in the valence band (a *P*-type semiconductor). These two types of extrinsic semiconductor will now be considered.

7.12.1   *N*-type semiconductors

As we have seen, single atoms of intrinsic semiconductors have four valence electrons. To produce an *N*-type extrinsic semiconductor, a pentavalent impurity (one with five valence electrons) is used as the doping material. Arsenic, antimony and phosphorus are examples of pentavalent elements that are suitable. Fig. 7.11 illustrates the effect of introducing an atom of phosphorus into the crystalline

structure of silicon. Four of the valence electrons in the phosphorus form covalent bonds and the fifth electron is unbonded. This electron has an energy level which is just below the bottom of the conduction band (see Fig. 7.11B). At normal room temperatures, it is therefore virtually a free electron because it is easily lifted into the conduction band and can take part in electrical conduction if a potential difference is applied across the crystal.

Because such pentavalent atoms provide a 'spare' electron, they are known as *donor impurities*. It must be remembered that some electrons from the valence band will also be able to jump into the conduction band because of the normal vibrational energy within the atom at room temperature (this is similar to the intrinsic semiconductor). Positive holes will also be produced in the valence band and add to the conductivity. At normal room temperatures, this effect is much less than the effect produced by the donor atoms. In the case of an *N*-type semiconductor, the majority carriers are the electrons in the conduction band and the minority carriers are the holes in the valence band.

7.12.2   *P*-type semiconductors

As discussed in the previous section, the *N*-type semiconductor has enhanced conductivity because of the movement of electrons (negative, hence the *N*), so it is logical to assume that the *P*-type semiconductor functions because of the movement of positive holes. In the case of intrinsic

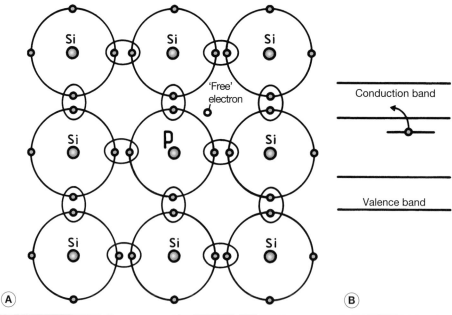

Fig. 7.11 An example of an *N*-type extrinsic semiconductor. (A) The introduction of a pentavalent impurity produces a 'free' electron which does not take part in the covalent bond formation; (B) the energy of such free electrons is close to the conduction band so that they can readily be enabled to take part in electrical conduction.

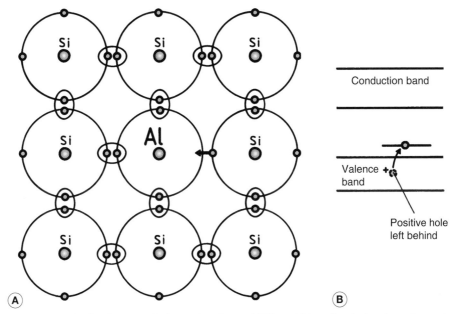

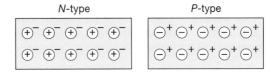

Fig. 7.12 An example of a *P*-type extrinsic semiconductor. (A) The addition of a trivalent impurity produces a 'hole' in the outside electron shell; (B) such acceptor atoms take an electron from the valence band, leaving a positive hole capable of flowing through this band.

semiconductors, we saw that holes were in the valence band, and that this allowed the movement of electrons within this band, giving the appearance of positive-hole movement (see previous Insight). In the *P*-type semiconductor, the movement of electrons within the valence band is encouraged by the creation of more positive holes within this band.

Fig. 7.12 illustrates the result of introducing a trivalent material (one with three valence electrons) into a silicon crystal lattice. The material used in this case is aluminium, and it results in a broken covalent bond between it and the silicon atoms as there are not sufficient electrons in its outer shell to form the four covalent bonds. The energy level of this broken bond is only just above the valence band (Fig. 7.12B) and so, at normal room temperatures, electrons have sufficient energy to leap this small gap. Thus the electrons that have left the valence band of the silicon leave positive holes behind them and so there is an increase in the number of positive holes in the valence band because of the trivalent impurity. This type of impurity is known as an *acceptor impurity* because it accepts electrons from the silicon atoms, creating holes in the valence band.

The majority carriers in the *P*-type material are positive holes in the valence band and the minority carriers are electrons that have sufficient energy to rise to the conduction band at room temperature, as in pure silicon.

Table 7.1 summarises the main points we have considered so far regarding intrinsic semiconductors and the *N*-type and *P*-type of extrinsic semiconductor. Note that an

increase in temperature does not affect the conductivity attributed to the majority carriers, but only that attributed to minority carriers. This is the result of the increased numbers of electrons able to reach the conduction band from the valence band as the temperature increases.

7.12.3 Diagrammatic representation of *N*- and *P*-types

When we discuss the *PN* junction in the next section, we need to form a mental picture of what occurs when an *N*-type and a *P*-type semiconductor are fused together. This is made easier if we have a simple symbolic representation of each, as shown in Fig. 7.13. In the *N*-type, the majority carriers are the free donor electrons, represented by the minus (−) sign. Each nucleus of the donor impurity

Fig. 7.13 A diagrammatic representation of *N*- and *P*-type semiconductors. In both illustrations the ringed charges represent the fixed charges whereas the unringed charges represent the free charges which form the majority carriers (electrons for the *N*-type and positive holes for the *P*-type).

TABLE 7.1   Summary of the properties of semiconductors

	Intrinsic Semiconductor	Extrinsic Semiconductor	
Typical material	Pure silicon or germanium	Silicon or germanium with added impurities	
Type of impurity	None	Pentavalent	Trivalent
Term for impurity	–	Donor	Acceptor
Conductivity	Low	High	High
Majority carrier	Electrons and positive holes in equal numbers	Electrons in conduction band	Positive holes in valence band
Minority carrier	–	Positive holes in valence band	Electrons in conduction band
Effect of temperature	Increases both the number of electrons and the number of positive holes	Increases number of minority carriers (positive holes) only	Increases number of minority carriers (electrons) only

has an excess positive charge because of the loss of its outer electron. These fixed positive charges are represented by the circles enclosing the + sign. In the *P*-type, the positive holes are free and so are shown as a plus (+) sign whereas the electrons captured by acceptor atoms give these an overall negative charge. Because these atoms form part of the crystal lattice, they are not free to move so the minus sign is shown enclosed in the circles. Thus in both diagrams the ringed charges are fixed and the unringed charges are free or mobile.

Note that in both diagrams there are minority carriers caused by the elevation of electrons from the valence band to the conduction band. Because these play little part in the electrical properties of the material, they have been omitted from the diagrams for simplicity.

Before considering the *PN* junction in the following section in which the *PN* junction is discussed as a rectifier, let us first remember that the term *diode* applies to any two-electrode electrical device. The X-ray tube is an example of a thermionic diode as it has two electrodes—an anode and a cathode. Other examples of solid-state diodes used in radiography are light-emitting diodes (LEDs), which have replaced bulbs as indicators. LEDs operate in a forward-bias mode (see Section 7.13.2), whereas the photodiode is a semiconductor diode which converts light into electrical current in a reverse-bias mode (see Section 7.13.3), and has replaced the photo-multiplier valve in many applications where its smaller size, low power consumption and high current output are important, (e.g., computed tomography [CT] scanners).

7.13   THE *PN* JUNCTION

When *P*- and *N*-types are heat-fused together to form *PN* junctions, interesting effects appear. Examples of the *PN* junction include the junction diode, the transistor and the

thyristor, which have one, two and three *PN* junctions, respectively.

If we use the diagrammatic representation that we have just discussed, then the *PN* junction may be shown as in Fig. 7.14. When *P*- and *N*-types are brought together and heat-fused in intimate contact, free electrons from the *N*-type and free positive holes from the *P*-type can penetrate across the boundary between them. This diffusion of

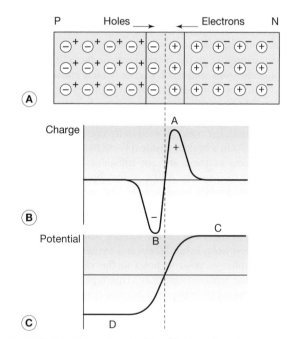

Fig. 7.14 The *PN* junction. (A) The diffusion of electrons across the *PN* junction in one direction and positive holes in the other forms a charge barrier, which prevents further flow. (B) Gain in charge across the junction and (C) potential difference established across the barrier.

charge across the barrier results in recombination of the positive holes and the free electrons (the free electrons drop into the positive holes so that their charges are cancelled). Thus for a short distance on either side of the *PN* junction (about 0.5×10^{-6} m), no free carriers exist; this is known as a *depletion layer*. However, a net charge exists on either side of the junction because the *N*-type has lost electrons and the *P*-type has lost positive holes (Fig. 7.14B), resulting in a negatively charged area just within the *P*-type region and a positively charged area just within the *N*-type region. The two peaks of charge shown in Fig. 7.14 increase in size until no further net flow of majority carriers takes place. For example, a free electron from the *N*-type will be able to pass over to the *P*-type only if it has sufficient energy to overcome the repulsion of the negative peak at the *PN* junction.

The charge distribution produces its own potential difference, as depicted in Fig. 7.14C. The height of *CD* is known as the *potential barrier* because it acts in opposition to the flow of majority carriers from either side of the barrier. For a silicon *PN* junction, this potential barrier is about 0.4 eV, so free carriers of energy lower than 0.4 eV cannot overcome this barrier.

7.13.1 Minority carriers at the *PN* junction

The earlier discussion concerned only the effect of the *PN* junction on the majority carriers. For majority carriers, a potential barrier is formed which prevents any further flow. However, this barrier actually aids the transport of minority carriers between the materials. Consider the potential gradient between *D* and *C* (Fig. 7.14). If a free electron (the minority carrier in a *P*-type material) is in position *D*, it is strongly attracted by the positive potential of the *N*-type material and rapidly moves to *C*. At equilibrium, of course, there are equal numbers of minority carriers moving in both directions.

Minority carriers are dependent on temperature, because an increase in temperature increases the number of electrons which can jump from the valence to the conduction band. Thus, the flow of minority carriers across a PN junction increases with temperature. This affects the behaviour of the *PN* junction under conditions of reverse bias, as will be explained later in this chapter.

7.13.2 Forward bias

If a source of potential difference (e.g., a battery) is connected across a *PN* junction, as shown in Fig. 7.15A, then a current will flow across the junction because the potential barrier is lowered. This is shown graphically in Fig. 7.15B. The negative side of the battery reduces the positive potential of the *N*-type and the positive side of the battery reduces the negative potential of the *P*-type.

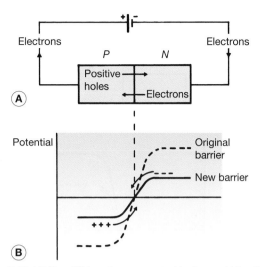

Fig. 7.15 (A) The *PN* junction connected in forward bias. The potential from the battery lowers the potential barrier and allows current to flow across the junction. (B) The position of the barrier before connection into the circuit and after the device is connected, as shown in (A).

The original height of the barrier is lowered and energetic free carriers from either side can surmount the barrier. A steady electrical current is set up as long as the battery is connected. This type of connection, which produces current flow across the *PN* junction, is called forward bias. The removal of the battery results in the full height of the barrier being reestablished and so no further current can flow.

7.13.3 Reverse bias

If the source of potential difference is now connected in the opposite orientation, as shown in Fig. 7.16A, then this is known as *reverse bias*. No current flows through this circuit because of the increase in the potential barrier at the *PN* junction. The graph in Fig. 7.16B shows that the negative side of the battery increases the negative potential of the *P*-type and the positive side of the battery increases the positive potential of the *N*-type. Thus no current flows because none of the majority carriers has sufficient energy to surmount this higher barrier. In fact, when a *PN* junction is connected in reverse bias, the depletion layer extends further into each semiconductor on either side of the *PN* junction.

The discussion so far has been regarding majority carriers. However, as discussed earlier, a small electrical current resulting from the thermally generated minority carriers can flow.

The *PN* junction can act as a one-way valve (a diode) which allows current only to *flow* in one direction. For this

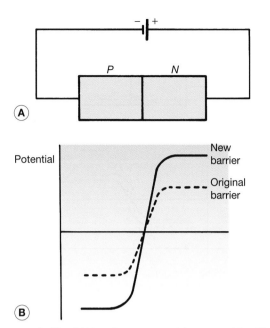

Fig. 7.16 (A) The *PN* junction connected in reverse bias. The potential from the battery raises the potential barrier, as shown in (B), and further prevents electrical conduction.

reason, *PN* junctions are used to create *solid-state rectifiers* or *PN junction diodes*. The symbol for such a device is shown later.

7.13.4   The *PN* junction as a rectifier

In our discussion in the last two sections we have shown that current will readily flow through a *PN* junction when it is forward biased, but very little current will flow through the junction when it is reverse biased. Thus the *PN* junction can act as a one-way valve allowing current to flow in only one direction. For this reason, *PN* junctions are used to create solid-state rectifiers or *PN* junction diodes. The symbol for such a device is:

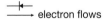

electron flows

Note that electrons may flow through the diode only against the direction of the arrow or bar of the symbol. Such devices have replaced old-fashioned thermionic diodes for the following reasons:

- They contain no filament and thus have a longer life, consume less power and produce less heat.
- They are smaller in size than thermionic diodes, thus enabling the production of a more compact X-ray unit.
- They have a smaller forward voltage drop than thermionic rectifiers and are more efficient rectifiers enabling a higher kVp to be applied to the X-ray tube.

7.13.5   *PN* junction characteristics

If the current flowing through a *PN* junction is plotted against the potential difference across it, then the graph produced is referred to as the characteristic curve for the device. Such a graph is shown in Fig. 7.17. As the potential difference across the diode is increased in a forward direction, so the current through it increases, as shown by *OA* on the figure. If we compare this with the forward-bias characteristic for the vacuum diode, we can note that, in this case, there is no saturation current. However, passing too high a current through a *PN* junction diode can cause irreparable damage.

A normal reverse bias produces only a very low reverse current because of the flow of minority carriers that happen to move into the vicinity of the *PN* junction and so get swept across it. As already discussed, this reverse current is very sensitive to temperature because this alters the production of minority carriers caused by thermal excitation. If the reverse bias is further increased, then the reverse current increases dramatically (see *BC* in Fig. 7.17). This is called the *zener voltage* or *breakdown voltage* and at this value of reverse bias the diode ceases to act effectively as a rectifier. At this negative bias, the minority carriers that cross the potential barrier gain enough energy to ionise atoms with which they collide. This results in the liberation of additional electrons and hence the large current. This phenomenon is also referred to as *solid-state multiplication* or *electron avalanching*.

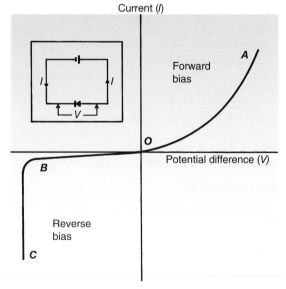

Fig. 7.17 The *PN* junction characteristic. For explanation, see text.

TABLE 7.2 Applications of semiconductor devices

Semiconductor Device	Applications
Solid-state diode	Rectification of the high-tension supply to the X-ray tube using multiple *PN* junctions connected in series to form stick rectifiers. Rectification of the supply to devices that require a unidirectional supply, e.g., solid-state 'chips'
Transistors	Electronic timing circuits Safety interlocks that avoid exceeding the rating of the X-ray tube
Triacs	Primary switching of the X-ray exposure, i.e., the triac switches the exposure on and off – following the signal from the timer
Integrated circuits (ICs)	ICs have replaced many semiconductor devices. These can check that a number of functions have taken place in sequence, e.g., they can check that the anode is rotating at the correct speed before an exposure is made
Microprocessors	These have many applications in more sophisticated measurement and controls, e.g., microprocessors can check a certain set of exposure factors to ensure that they are not outside the rating of the selected tube focus

7.14 SEMICONDUCTOR DEVICES IN RADIOGRAPHY

Semiconductor devices are used extensively in radiography. This chapter has given a brief overview of some of the types that are used. The development of ICs in the 1960s resulted in the production of complete miniaturised circuits which now perform many of the functions previously carried out by discrete solid-state devices or by ICs. ICs are produced on a single chip of silicon about 1 mm^2 and about 0.1 mm thick. This process, using ULSI, can produce circuits containing in excess of over 100 million transistors per chip. This technology offers components of very high reliability at very low production costs. There is also significant space saving over electromechanical devices. Both of the discussed devices have resulted in many of the circuits in modern X-ray generators containing significant amounts of 'chip technology'.

The microprocessor is another development based on silicon chip and ULSI technology. Using Boolean logic and inbuilt programs, microprocessors are used to monitor and control many pieces of equipment used in radiography.

The full description of the function of such ICs is the subject of a book in its own right and as such is beyond the short introduction in this text.

Table 7.2 outlines some of the applications of semiconductor technology in radiography.

SUMMARY

In this chapter you should have learnt that:

- X-ray circuits previously relied on traditional voltage transformers to provide the high voltage supply across an X-ray tube.
- These have now been replaced by high-frequency generators, which are more efficient.
- High frequency generators still include a transformer but apply a high-frequency pulsed-voltage waveform to it, via an inverter.
- Control of kV, mA and time is undertaken electronically, via circuits linked to the generator.
- Semiconductors are solid-state devices that will conduct electricity under certain conditions. Such devices that will conduct in one direction only are called rectifiers and permit a DC supply across the X-ray tube. Other semiconductor devices include switches.

FURTHER READING

Ball, J.L., Moore, A.D., & Turner, S. 2008. *Ball and Moore's Essential Physics for Radiographers.* 4th edn. London: Blackwell Scientific. (Chapter 13.)

Bushong, S. 2016. *Radiologic Science for Technologists: Physics, Biology, and Protection.* 11th edn. St. Louis: Mosby. (Chapter 5.)

Johnston, J., & Fauber, T. 2015. *Essentials of Radiographic Physics and Imaging.* 2nd edn. St. Louis: Mosby. (Chapter 4.)

8

The laws of modern physics

CHAPTER CONTENTS

8.1 AIM

The aim of this chapter is to introduce the reader to the laws of modern physics. In many cases these are refinements or extensions to the laws of classical physics which were discussed in Chapter 3, and in this chapter reference will be made to the laws outlined in Chapter 3. In other areas, there is disagreement between the classical and the modern laws, and these will be identified and discussed.

8.2 INTRODUCTION

The laws of classical physics were discussed in Chapter 3, and these have been sufficient to explain the phenomena outlined in previous chapters of this text. In the following chapters on atomic and radiation physics, some important aspects of modern physics must be introduced to explain many of the phenomena discussed. The purpose of this chapter is to describe the laws of modern physics which are relevant to our need in the rest of the text.

8.3 CLASSICAL VERSUS MODERN LAWS

What we might term 'modern' physics was developed at the turn of the 20th century with Planck's quantum hypothesis in 1900, in which he conjectured that radiation energy could be absorbed or emitted only by a body at discrete values of energy. Other dates of interest to the rest of this text include the mass–energy relationship postu-

lated by Einstein in 1905, the Bohr model of the atom which was suggested in 1913, and the de Broglie wavelength of particles which was introduced in 1924. Since these dates, there have been major technical and theoretical strides, but these form part of the firm experimental foundation upon which modern physics is built.

One of the essential differences between classical and modern physics is the way in which matter is regarded. In classical physics, matter and energy are completely separate entities and so we have the law of conservation of matter (see Section 3.2) and the law of conservation of energy (see Section 3.3) with no interconnection being produced between the two laws. In classical physics, matter is supposed to behave in one way—like solid particles—and waves are supposed to behave like waves, and one cannot behave like the other; classical physics does not allow for the existence of a particle with a wavelength. There are no such rigid boundaries in modern physics. In particular, the work of Einstein showed that matter can be thought of as being interchangeable with energy if the conditions are right. This principle is known as *mass–energy equivalence* and will be discussed in more detail later in this chapter (see Section 8.4.1). In addition, it is found in modern physics that particles of matter do behave like waves and vice versa, and this is known as the *wave–particle duality principle* (see Section 8.6). In this way, an X-ray beam may be considered as photons (particles) which have a specific energy and so can liberate electrons from atoms of the materials they pass through.

With these concepts in mind, we will now consider the laws of modern physics in more detail in the remainder of this chapter.

8.4   LAW OF CONSERVATION OF ENERGY

This law now states that the amount of energy in a system is constant. In the context of modern physics, this can be thought of as the sum of all the energies (rest energies + kinetic energies + potential energies) being a constant for any given system. The phrase 'a system' can be used to define either a very small or a very large area, provided the influence of other bodies outside the system is negligibly small. In the context of modern physics, the use of the term 'energy' in the above law embraces the contribution of matter to the total energy of a system under consideration. This concept of mass–energy equivalence will now be discussed.

8.4.1   Mass–energy equivalence

Einstein showed that the mass of a body, m, and its energy, E (excluding potential energy), are related by the formula:

$$E = mc^2 \qquad \textbf{Equation 8.1}$$

where c is the velocity of electromagnetic radiation (often referred to as the velocity of light, as light is probably the best-known form of electromagnetic radiation). Because c is a constant, the energy of a body is proportional to its mass (and vice versa). If we consider a stationary body with a rest mass, m_0, then the rest energy of this body is given by $E_0 = m_0c^2$. If we now consider this body travelling with a velocity, V, then its energy is now E_V and Einstein's equation is $E_V = m_Vc^2$. Because the energy of the body when moving, E_V, is greater than the energy of the body when at rest, E_0, and because c is a constant, then m_V must be greater than m_0: a body increases in mass as its velocity increases. This statement seems to contradict our common experiences (because of the small values of velocity which we can normally produce), but if we take particles and accelerate them until they travel with a velocity close to the velocity of light (3×10^8 m.s^{-1}) then there is a measurable increase in the mass of the particles. The mass which they then possess is known as the *relativistic mass* of the particles. Thus if we take a car which is travelling at 80 kilometres per hour, we can observe no measurable increase in its mass, but if we take electrons travelling at high speeds in a linear accelerator, at over 90% of the speed of light, then there is a measurable increase in their mass. This is a factor contributing to the very high-energy X-rays produced in radiotherapy because the kinetic energy of the speeding electrons increases with their mass and velocity. This relativistic mass increase is not such an important factor in conventional X-ray tubes, where electron are only accelerated to about 10% of the speed of light as they pass across the vacuum of the tube.

The law of conservation of energy, stated earlier, is sometimes referred to as the law of conservation of *mass–energy* because of the concept of equivalence between mass and energy. It is also not uncommon to quote the *rest mass* of subatomic particles, either in units of mass or in units of energy—the rest mass of the electron can be stated as 9.1×10^{-31} kg (mass) or 0.511 MeV (energy). As we can see from this discussion, energy and mass can be considered as two manifestations of the same thing, and may be changed from one form to the other in appropriate circumstances, as the following examples show:

- The forces which hold the atomic nucleus together are obtained because some of the mass of the nuclear particles is converted into energy. Because of this, the mass of the nucleus is less than the sum of the masses of the individual nuclear particles.
- In positron emission tomography (PET), as described in Chapter 23, artificially produced radionuclides emit positively charged electrons ('positrons') as they decay. The positron created in this interaction will interact with an ordinary negatively charged electron ('negatron') and their mass will be converted into two photons of radiation, each photon having an energy of 0.511 MeV. The positron and the negatron will now cease to exist, and the radiation is referred to as *annihilation radiation*. This is a real-world example of the conversion of mass into energy. The positron can thus be regarded as the antiparticle of the electron. This interaction shows that mass can be converted into energy. The reverse of this process, conversion of energy into mass, can occur in radiotherapy when X-rays of greater energy than 1.02 MeV encounter an atomic nucleus, resulting in the production of a positron-negatron pair.

8.5   LAW OF CONSERVATION OF MOMENTUM

This law may be stated as the total linear momentum in a system is constant. The word 'system' is used in the same context as for the law of conservation of energy. As we discussed in the section dealing with the laws of classical physics, the momentum of a body is the product of its mass and its velocity. Thus we can say:

$$\text{sum of all}\,(\text{mass} \times \text{velocity}) = \text{constant for a system}$$

Here, the mass referred to in the equation is the relativistic mass of the body, that is, its mass when it is moving with the velocity, V. An example of the law of conservation of momentum being applied to modern physics is in Compton scattering (see Chapter 13) when some of the momentum of the incoming photon is given to an electron—the combined momentum of the scattered photon and the ejected electron is the same as the momentum of the incident photon.

8.6 WAVE–PARTICLE DUALITY

Duality simply means two different features of the same thing. As we have just seen, modern physics regards mass and energy as being two manifestations of the same phenomenon. Similarly, modern physics blurs the distinction which exists in classical physics between a particle and a wave.

8.6.1 Waves as particles

Classical physics was very successful in explaining many of the phenomena associated with electromagnetic radiation (e.g., diffraction and interference) by assuming that such radiation was made up of waves travelling at the velocity of light, c. In this case $c = v\lambda$, where v is the frequency of vibration of the radiation and λ is its wavelength. However, phenomena such as the Compton effect and photoelectric absorption (both will be discussed in detail in Chapter 13) are not easy to explain using the wave theory. These effects are explained by considering that sometimes electromagnetic radiation behaves as 'packets' of energy which have an associated momentum. Such a packet of energy is called a *photon* or a *quantum*, and the quantum theory predicts that:

- the quantum will have an energy, E, given by:

$$E = hv \qquad \text{Equation 8.2}$$

where h is a constant known as *Planck's constant* and v is the frequency of vibration of the associated wave. We will frequently use this formula in the chapters which follow on atomic physics!

- The quantum will have a momentum, p, given by:

$$p = \frac{hv}{c} \qquad \text{Equation 8.3}$$

The electromagnetic wave may also behave like a particle, possessing energy and momentum.

8.6.2 Particles as waves

Moving particles of matter, whether these are large or very small, have both kinetic energy and momentum. Are there then occasions when they behave as waves? Perhaps the most dramatic example of particles behaving like waves is in the operation of the electron microscope. Here high-energy electrons are passed through or are scattered by a sample. A very highly magnified image of the sample is obtained so that individual large molecules may be seen in materials. The reason for the high degree of magnification is because of the very small wavelength of the electrons. Whether we consider an optical microscope or an electron microscope, the smaller the wavelength of the radiation used, the finer the detail it is possible to see.

De Broglie proposed that the following relationship exists between the momentum, p, of the particle and its associated wavelength, λ:

$$p = \frac{h}{\lambda} \qquad \text{Equation 8.4}$$

In such cases, λ is called the *de Broglie wavelength*, and the existence of particles behaving like waves can be verified by a number of experiments.

Note the inverse relationship between the momentum of the particle and its associated wavelength. The wavelength decreases as the momentum increases and vice versa. For example, the de Broglie wavelength associated with an electron moving at half the velocity of light is about 4×10^{-12} m which is less than the diameter of the hydrogen atom (100×10^{-12} m). When the velocity of the electron is one-hundredth of that of light then the de Broglie wavelength is at the larger value of 240×10^{-12} m, which is now in the X-ray range of wavelengths (see Chapter 9) and so such electrons can be used for X-ray crystallography.

Within the context of imaging science, it is more common to consider waves behaving as quanta rather than quanta behaving as waves. This is particularly true when we consider the production of X-rays (see Chapter 11) and the interactions of X-rays with matter (see Chapter 13).

8.7 HEISENBERG'S UNCERTAINTY PRINCIPLE

In classical physics it is possible in principle to measure exactly a number of quantities concerning the state of a body (e.g., the body's energy, position and momentum). Furthermore, if it were possible to build measuring apparatus which was infinitely precise, it would be possible to make simultaneous exact measurements of several of these quantities. For example we could say that at a particular point in time, an electron could be observed at a single discrete position in an atom.

According to modern physics, it is not possible to treat quantities like mass and energy or matter and waves as being totally independent of each other. Heisenberg's uncertainty principle is an extension of the principle of wave–particle duality and concerns the maximum possible precision which may be obtained in ideal circumstances when measuring two quantities simultaneously. The central point of the principle is that measuring one quantity affects another quantity so that it is never possible to measure both quantities simultaneously with complete accuracy—if we try to measure the momentum of a particle, this will automatically affect the position of the particle so that it is never possible to measure momentum and position simultaneously with complete accuracy. Effects resulting from this principle are too small to be observed in everyday life and concern atomic and nuclear systems. This principle is yet another difference between modern and classical physics—in classical physics, it is assumed that perfect instruments produce perfect results.

If we now apply Heisenberg's uncertainty principle to the duality theory, we can say that, although we can demonstrate that waves can behave like particles and that particles can behave like waves, it is not possible to set up a situation where both properties are demonstrated simultaneously. In practice, we may consider an electron's 'orbital' within an atom in terms of the probability of finding the electron within a given volume of space, with the electron being considered as a 'standing wave', held in position around the atomic nucleus. This is of relevance to the concept of 'electron density' which affects the Compton attenuation of X-rays (see Chapter 13). We also may considerv X-ray photons and electrons as discrete particles or 'packets' (quanta) of energy when thinking about the 'collisions' between them that occur in photoelectric absorption (see Chapter 13).

SUMMARY

In this chapter you should have learnt the following:
- The differences which exist between the laws of classical physics and the laws of modern physics.
- The law of conservation of energy as applied to modern physics.
- The concept of mass–energy equivalence.
- The law of conservation of momentum as applied to modern physics.
- The concept of wave–particle duality.
- The concept that waves may behave as particles and that particles may behave as waves, with examples of each situation.
- A brief outline of Heisenberg's uncertainty principle.

FURTHER READING

Ball, J.L., Moore, A.D., & Turner, S. 2008. *Ball and Moore's Essential Physics for Radiographers.* 4th edn. London: Blackwell Scientific. (Chapters 14 and 15.)

Dobson, K., Grace, D., & Lovett, D. 2008. *Collins Advanced Science – Physics.* 3rd edn. Glasgow: Collins. (Chapter 16.)

Morrison, J. 2015. *Modern Physics for Scientists and Engineers.* 2nd edn. New York: Academic Press.

Electromagnetic radiations

CHAPTER CONTENTS

9.1 AIM

This chapter discusses the properties of electromagnetic (e/m) radiations. These radiations, which are quite separate in nature from sound waves, all travel at the speed of light and can be considered to have both wave-like and particle-like properties. This is often termed *wave–particle duality*. Electromagnetic radiations range from those of very low energy, such as radio waves, to those of high energy, such as X-rays and gamma rays. Many have essential roles to play in medical imaging, such as radio waves (in magnetic resonance imaging), infra-red (heat emissions in X-ray tubes), visible light (produced in imaging plates), X-rays (from X-ray tubes) and gamma rays (in radionuclide imaging). In addition, X-rays and gamma rays have ionising properties which contribute to attenuation and radiation dose in body tissues.

9.2 INTRODUCTION

As can be seen from Fig. 9.3, the electromagnetic spectrum encompasses a wide range of wavelengths and we are able to directly perceive only a small window of these radiations. We can see the world around us because the retinas of our eyes are sensitive to a section of the electromagnetic spectrum which we know as visible light. Similarly, we can feel heat from the sun because our skin responds to the infrared part of the electromagnetic spectrum. Conversely, we can also accidentally walk through a beam of X-rays or handle an isotope that is producing gamma radiation because none of our sense organs are able to detect them. Remember, when we consider radiation protection, that although our sense organs are not able to detect the presence of ionising radiations (X or gamma), our body tissues can still be damaged by them.

9.3 PROPERTIES OF ELECTROMAGNETIC RADIATIONS

All electromagnetic radiations exhibit a set of general properties which are listed as follows:
- The waves are composed of transverse vibrations of electric and magnetic fields. (Transverse vibrations are ones which are oscillating at right angles to the direction of travel.)
- The vibrations have a wide range of wavelengths and frequencies.
- All electromagnetic radiations travel through a vacuum with the same velocity: 3×10^8 m.s^{-1}.
- All electromagnetic radiations travel in straight lines.
- The radiations are unaffected by electric or magnetic fields.
- The radiations may be polarised so that they vibrate in one plane only.
- The radiations are able to produce constructive or destructive interference.

TABLE 9.1   Interactions of different electromagnetic radiations with matter

Interaction	Notes
Emission	All bodies will emit electromagnetic radiation in certain circumstances, but the most efficient emission is from a 'black body'
Reflection	Reflection of electromagnetic radiation is not possible for the higher energy radiations (X and gamma radiation)
Refraction	Refraction of electromagnetic radiation is not possible for the higher energy radiations (X and gamma radiation)
Transmission	Different materials are transparent to different wavelengths or photon energies
Attenuation	Different attenuation processes are possible depending on the photon energy of the radiation but, if the photons all have the same energy, the attenuation is always exponential. Photoelectric absorption can occur from ultraviolet to gamma radiations. Compton scattering is produced by X and gamma radiations. Pair production is an attenuation process which is possible if the photon energies are higher than 1.02 MeV
Luminescence – fluorescence and phosphorescence	Electron transitions within the material being irradiated cause the emission of photons that have less energy than the incident radiation. A single photon of incident radiation can produce many fluorescent photons

- All the radiations obey the wave-particle duality principle (see Chapter 8) and so can be considered either as waves or as quanta with energy and momentum.

From this list it is obvious that electromagnetic radiations have a lot in common, so how can they be used for such widely differing purposes? The answer to this lies in the differences which they exhibit in their interactions with matter. These are outlined in Table 9.1.

Electromagnetic radiations are produced when particles lose energy. For example, radio waves are emitted when electrons moving in an electrical circuit are decelerated as the current oscillates. Light may be emitted as an electron drops in energy from an excited state to a 'ground state'. X-rays result when electrons are either braked in speed or move between atomic shell energy levels. Gamma rays may be ejected from unstable atomic nuclei when the nuclei lose energy.

As discussed in Chapter 8, there is a wave–particle duality which is exhibited when electromagnetic radiation interacts with matter. This will be discussed further in the following sections.

9.3.1   Wave-like properties

As the term *electromagnetic* suggests, electromagnetic radiation consists of both electric and magnetic fields. These fields are at right angles to each other and to the direction of propagation and are shown diagrammatically in Fig. 9.1. As shown in E and B of the figure, both the electric and the magnetic vectors vibrate transversely to the direction of propagation of the wave. In addition, the vectors vary in

a sinusoidal manner, as shown in the figure. Thus if we draw the variations of the electric vector (for example), a sine wave results, as shown in Fig. 9.2. These periodic variations of the vectors are the reason why electromagnetic radiations are often referred to as *electromagnetic waves*, and this was the sole method of explaining the behaviour of such radiations adopted by classical physics.

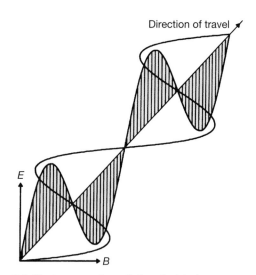

Fig. 9.1 Electromagnetic radiation depicted as a wave consisting of alternating electrical and magnetic vectors vibrating at right angles to each other and to the direction of motion of the wave.

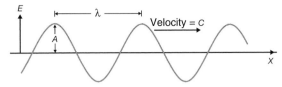

Fig. 9.2 An electromagnetic sine wave produced by plotting energy (E) against distance (X). The wave has amplitude of A and a wavelength λ and travels at the velocity of light, c (3×10^8 m.s^{-1}).

The same parameters can be used to describe this type of wave formation as can be used for any sinusoidal waves. These are:

- the cycle—one complete waveform (this can start from any point on the wave and end at the corresponding point on another wave)
- the wavelength—the distance travelled in completing one cycle (λ)
- the frequency—the number of cycles per second (Hz)
- the amplitude—the magnitude of the peak of the wave above the x-axis (A).

If we consider Fig. 9.2, it should be apparent that we can calculate the distance travelled by the radiation in 1 second by multiplying the wavelength (λ) by the frequency (v). However, the distance travelled in 1 second is simply the velocity of the radiation (c in a vacuum) and so we have:

$$c = v\lambda \qquad \textbf{Equation 9.1}$$

in a vacuum.

As mentioned earlier, one of the features of electromagnetic radiations is that they all travel with the same velocity (3×10^8 m.s^{-1}) in a vacuum. One ray is distinguished from another by the difference in wavelength and frequency—*blue light* has a wavelength of about 400 nm and a frequency of 7.5×10^{14} Hz whereas red light has a wavelength of about 800 nm and a frequency of 3.75×10^{14} Hz. From this, it can be seen that the greater the frequency, the smaller the wavelength and vice versa.

In an optically transparent medium, the light waves travel at a velocity V given by the equation $c = nV$, where n is a constant for a given medium and a given incident wavelength and is known as the *refractive index*. The frequency of the radiation is unaltered as it passes through a transparent medium, but the wavelength is reduced resulting from the reduction in the velocity of the wave. If the wavelength in the medium is λ', then Equation 9.1 becomes:

$$V = v\lambda'$$

Substituting the value of V for $c = nV$, we obtain:

$$c = nv\lambda' \qquad \textbf{Equation 9.2}$$

in a medium of refractive index, n.

> **INSIGHT**
>
> Chapter 6 showed that it is possible to produce both a magnetic field from moving electrical charges (electromagnetism) and an electric field from a changing magnetic flux (electromagnetic induction). It can be shown mathematically that a changing electric field can sustain a changing magnetic field, and vice versa, if they both travel at the velocity of light. This is the basis both for the linear propagation of electromagnetic radiations and for the fact that the wave does not gradually diminish in amplitude with time. Electromagnetic radiation can therefore be described as a self-sustaining interaction of electric and magnetic fields travelling with the velocity of light.

Two further properties of electromagnetic radiation which are a consequence of its wave-like nature are polarisation and interference.

9.3.1.1 Polarisation

A beam of light, from a bulb for instance, consists of many millions of waves whose electric vectors are pointing in random directions with respect to each other. If this light beam is passed through a polarising lens (similar to the one found in polarising sunglasses), then there is optimum transmission of the waves whose electric vectors are pointing in one direction and complete absorption of those at right angles to this direction (this is the mechanism by which polarising sunglasses limit the glare caused by light reflection from water). The emergent light is said to be plane-polarised—all its vibrations are in the one plane.

9.3.1.2 Interference

Further evidence of the wave-like properties of electromagnetic radiations comes from the phenomenon of interference where the amplitudes of two coherent beams (beams which are in phase with each other) can be added together. If the peaks of the waves coincide, we get constructive interference, and this produces bright areas. If the peak of the wave from one source coincides with the trough of the wave from the other source, we get destructive interference, and this produces a dark area. Such interference patterns are used in radiographic science to produce holograms, but further discussion on this topic is well outside the scope of this text.

9.3.2 Particle-like properties

In Chapter 8 we discussed how consideration of electromagnetic radiations as quanta or photons having energy and momentum enabled us to explain a number of properties which are not explained by the wave theory. The energy of such a quantum, E, is proportional to the frequency of the associated wave such that:

$$E = h\nu \qquad \textbf{Equation 9.3}$$

where h is a constant known as *Planck's constant* and ν is the frequency of vibration of the associated wave. Thus, because there is a direct relationship between frequency and the energy of the quantum, as the frequency increases so does the energy. The momentum, p, of the quantum is also proportional to the frequency, and is given by:

$$p = \frac{h\nu}{c} \qquad \textbf{Equation 9.4}$$

where c is the velocity of electromagnetic radiation in a vacuum.

The photon energy and its wavelength can now be related. If we take Equation 9.3 and substitute $\nu = c/\lambda$ from Equation 9.1, we get:

$$E = \frac{hc}{\lambda} \qquad \textbf{Equation 9.5}$$

In this equation, h is Planck's constant (6.62×10^{-34} J.s^{-1}), c is the velocity of electromagnetic radiation in a vacuum (3×10^8 m.s^{-1}), λ is the wavelength measured in metres and E is the photon energy measured in joules. For practical purposes, in radiography it is more convenient to measure the photon energy in keV (1 keV = 1.16×10^{-16} J) and the wavelength in nanometres (1 nm = 10^{-9} m). Because h and c are constants, Eq. 9.5 can now be rewritten:

$$E = \frac{1.24}{\lambda} \qquad \textbf{Equation 9.6}$$

This equation gives us an easy link between the energy of the photon in keV and the wavelength of the radiation in nanometres.

EXAMPLE

If the energy of the X-ray photon is 100 keV, what will be its wavelength in nanometres?
  Using Equation 9.6:

$$E = \frac{1.24}{\lambda}$$

$$\therefore \lambda = \frac{1.24}{E}$$

$$= 1.24\,/\,100\,\text{nm}$$

$$= 0.0124\,\text{nm}$$

Lengths as small as 0.0124 nm or 1.24×10^{-11} m are difficult to imagine. This is less than the diameter of an atom of body tissue (about 10^{-10} m) but is greater than the diameter of the atomic nucleus (about 10^{-14} m).

9.4   THE ELECTROMAGNETIC SPECTRUM

The previous sections of this chapter have shown that electromagnetic radiation may have a very large range of wavelengths, that is, a spectrum of wavelengths (and frequencies). It is convenient to split up such an electromagnetic spectrum into bands which are broadly categorised by their interaction with matter and hence the use to which the bands of radiation may be put. This is illustrated in Fig. 9.3, which also shows the wavelengths, frequencies and energies corresponding to the approximate boundaries between the various bands. As we have previously discussed, the table of the electromagnetic spectrum shows that the smaller the wavelength of the radiation, the higher the frequency and the energy.

The common factor which links the interactions between different types of electromagnetic radiations is that the value of the wavelength determines the size of object with which the radiation will directly interact. This is illustrated in Table 9.2.

INSIGHT

At the beginning of this chapter (see Table 9.1) are the types of interactions which are possible between electromagnetic radiations and matter, with brief comments. From this table you will note that refraction is associated with electromagnetic radiations which have wavelengths larger than X-rays. Refraction is a phenomenon associated with an interaction between a photon and the outer electron orbitals of atoms. It is therefore associated with wavelengths which are able to interact with these electrons—ultraviolet and longer wavelengths. Smaller wavelengths become progressively less affected by the outer electron orbitals, and so it is just possible to demonstrate refraction with very large wavelength X-rays but it is not possible to refract X-rays which have shorter wavelengths.

The interactions between X-rays and matter, which are of great relevance to medical imaging science, are discussed in detail in Chapter 13 of this book.

9.5   LIGHT AMPLIFICATION BY STIMULATED EMISSION OF RADIATION (LASER)

In the last few years, devices containing a laser source have increasingly become a part of our everyday life and are also increasingly used in radiographic imaging. For this reason,

TABLE 9.2   Common electromagnetic radiations and the type of body with which they will directly interact

Type of radiation	Body with which radiation directly interacts
Radio waves	Transmitted and received by large metallic conductors – aerials
Infrared radiation	Interacts with whole molecules or atoms giving them an increase in their kinetic energy in the form of heat
Visible light and ultraviolet radiation	Interacts with the outer electrons (more loosely bound) of the atom
X-rays and γ-rays	Interact with the inner electron shells or, if they have very high energy, with the nucleus of the atom

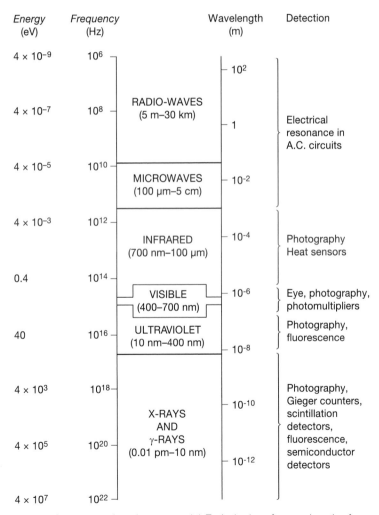

Fig. 9.3 The electromagnetic spectrum (not drawn to scale). Typical values for wavelengths, frequencies and photon energies for different bands of the spectrum are shown, together with some of the methods used for their detection. (Note: 1 Hz = 1 cycle per second.)

a short section is included here describing the basic physics of laser production and also a section indicating the hazards of lasers if used carelessly.

9.5.1   Basic physics of laser production

Laser is an acronym for light amplification by stimulated emission of radiation. The theory which was first proposed by Albert Einstein in 1917 was further developed in the 1950s and the first laser was produced in 1960. Lasers are used in medical imaging within computed radiography (CR) readers, as radiographic positioning devices and in interventional procedures. We already know from Section 2.6 that in an atom electrons can exist at various energy levels depending on their position relative to the nucleus. Electrons can be temporarily raised to a higher energy level by the absorption of photons of energy. In many cases, the electron remains in this excited state for only a few milliseconds and subsequently decays to its lower energy level by the emission of a photon of light (or other energy); this process is known as *fluorescence*. If the light emitted from an atom is incident on another atom which is in an excited state, then the first photon can stimulate the emission of a second photon from this atom. The two photons will be identical in wavelength, phase and direction. This is the basis of laser.

The basic components of a simple laser are shown in Fig. 9.4. The excitation of electrons to a higher energy level is achieved by illuminating the material with light of a frequency higher than that which the laser will emit. This light is produced from the flash lamp and is known as *optical pumping*. The two ends of the laser rod are polished flat and parallel. One end is coated with a completely silvered mirror and the other is coated with a semisilvered mirror. Pulsed light is flashed into the laser at high intensity from the flash lamp and this is reflected within the rods using the two mirrors, thus causing coherent photon emission from the atoms of the rod material. Eventually the high-intensity laser radiation will leave the rod through the semisilvered mirror. The wavelength of the light emitted depends on the design of the laser so the beam may not be visible to the eye.

9.5.2   Potential hazards of lasers

Laser light has several properties that are important when we consider its safe use:

- The light is monochromatic, with its wavelength determined by the design of the laser.
- The light is in the form of a tightly collimated parallel beam, often less than 1 mm in diameter.
- Because the light is in the form of a small, highly collimated area, even lasers of small power can deposit significant amounts of energy on a small area.

Assume that a 10-W laser beam is directed at a material. This does not sound much in terms of power in that many night lights are rated at 10 W. However, the laser beam is a parallel, very narrow beam. If this beam is 1 mm in diameter then the power deposited on the material is greater than 1000 $W.cm^{-2}$ —this can ignite paper or cause significant skin burns. If the laser beam enters the eye, the problem is further complicated by the fact that the lens of the eye focuses the beam onto a small area of the retina. Thus the power deposited on this small area of retina can be increased by a factor of up to 10^5 because of lens focusing. If we consider the original 10-W laser, this will mean a power deposited on a small area of the retina of 10^8 $W.cm^{-2}$ — compare this to power to the retina of about 10 $W.cm^{-2}$ if we stare at the midday sun, and it is easy to appreciate how damaging this can be to the eye.

As mentioned earlier, the wavelength of the light from the laser is determined by the laser design. The retina of the eye can detect from about 400 nm to just over 700 nm. Thus if a laser is operating at, say, 900 nm, we will not be able to see the beam from this laser. However, the beam can still penetrate the lens system of the eye and cause damage to the retina of the eye. For this reason it is important to wear eye protection whenever lasers are in use, for example, in an operating theatre, even if the laser beam is not visible.

9.6   ELECTROMAGNETIC RADIATIONS AND RADIOGRAPHY

The process of taking a radiograph (using a digital imaging system) results in the emission of radiations whose wavelengths and energies are from different parts of the electromagnetic spectrum, described in the previous section. These are summarised in Fig. 9.5. When the anode is bombarded by electrons, it emits both heat and light as well as X-rays. The X-ray spectrum is composed of a continuous

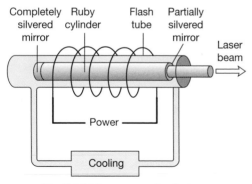

Fig. 9.4 Main components of a laser.

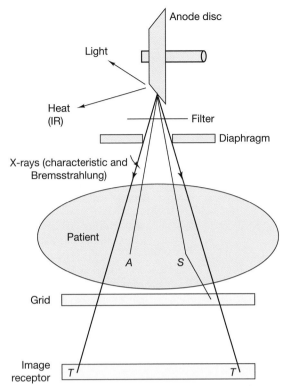

Fig. 9.5 The production of radiation from different parts of the electromagnetic spectrum used when a digital radiographic image is produced.

or Bremsstrahlung spectrum upon which is superimposed a characteristic or line spectrum from the tungsten target. The absorption processes within the aluminium filter and the lead collimators also produce characteristic radiation from these elements, although these are of fairly low intensity. When the radiation beam passes through the patient, some of the photons are absorbed (*A* in the diagram) and some are scattered (*S* in the diagram). The above processes produce a tiny amount of heat and other characteristic radiations from the elements which make up the body tissues. Some of the scattered radiation is absorbed by the grid. When the transmitted X-ray beam (*T*) strikes the digital imaging system, it produces changes in electron energies which can then be utilised to produce the digital image; this will be discussed in more detail in Chapter 15.

Further examples of electromagnetic radiation relevant to radiography include:

- the emission of light from thin film transistors (TFTs) to produce images on flat-screen imaging devices
- the emission of gamma rays from radioisotopes in radionuclide imaging (RNI)
- the production of radiofrequency (RF) pulses in magnetic resonance imaging (MRI)
- the emission of light from scintillators (in gamma cameras and computed tomography (CT) scanners) when bombarded with gamma rays or X-rays
- the emission of light from photostimulable CR plates when scanned using a laser beam
- the use of low-intensity lasers to aid positioning of the radiation beam.

SUMMARY

In this chapter, you should have learnt the following:
- The properties that are common to all electromagnetic radiations.
- The different ways in which electromagnetic radiations can react with matter.
- How electromagnetic radiation can be described as having wave-like properties and how these properties can be used to explain polarisation and interference.
- How electromagnetic radiation can be described as having particle-like properties and the equation which links the photon energy and the wavelength of the radiation.
- The various components of the electromagnetic spectrum and the principal interactions of the radiations with matter.
- A brief description of the physics of laser production and a note of its potential dangers.
- The electromagnetic radiations which are of importance to radiography.

FURTHER READING

Ball, J.L., Moore, A.D., & Turner, S. 2008. *Ball and Moore's Essential Physics for Radiographers*. 4th edn. London: Blackwell Scientific. (Chapters 14 and 15.)

Bushong, S. 2016. *Radiologic Science for Technologists: Physics, Biology, and Protection*. 11th edn. St. Louis: Mosby. (Chapter 3.)

Dobson, K., Grace, D., & Lovett, D. 2008. *Collins Advanced Science – Physics*. 3d edn. Glasgow: Collins Education. (Chapter 15.)

Radioactivity

CHAPTER CONTENTS

10.1 AIM

The aim of this chapter is to discuss the various types of radioactive decay which can occur. Within the chapter the relevance of these processes to nuclear medicine will be considered.

10.2 INTRODUCTION

Section 2.3 refers to various terms which may be used to define nuclear structure. This chapter will examine the changes that may take place in the nucleus during radioactive decay.

The term *radioactive* is applied to nuclei which are unstable. In these nuclei, the forces disrupting the nucleus are stronger than the forces that hold the nucleus together. The instability of the nucleus is demonstrated by the fact that it changes its internal structure to a more stable form, often (but not always) ejecting a charged particle from the nucleus in the process. Each time a nucleus changes its structure it is called a *radioactive disintegration* or a *nuclear transformation* and may result in a change in the atomic number—number of protons in the nucleus (and therefore element), or a change in the mass number—number of protons and neutrons in the nucleus, or a change of both the atomic number and the mass number.

A pictorial representation of the decay process (see Fig. 10.1) is called a *decay scheme*. In addition to this, it is possible for a nucleus to undergo more than one type of transformation (see Fig. 10.12), and this type of decay is called a *branching scheme*.

It is impossible to determine the exact time when a particular nucleus will transform, but the laws of probability may be used to determine the behaviour of a large number of nuclei (see Section 10.11 for a discussion of radioactive decay and the exponential law).

The unit of radioactivity is the becquerel (Bq) where 1 becquerel is 1 nuclear disintegration per second.

> ### INSIGHT
>
> Before the introduction of International System of Units, radioactivity was measured in curie (Ci). One curie was equal to 3.7×10^{10} nuclear disintegrations per second. Thus, an activity of 1 Ci is the same as an activity of 3.7×10^{10} Bq or 37 GBq. From this it can be seen that the curie was a much larger unit than the becquerel.
>
> It is often useful to know the specific activity of a sample. This is the activity of radionuclide per unit mass of the sample and so is measured in Bq.kg^{-1} or submultiples thereof.

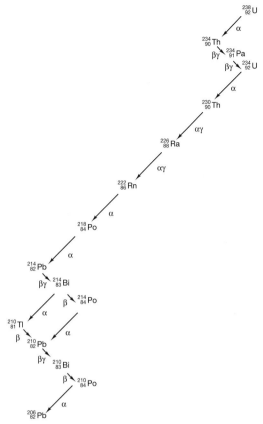

Fig. 10.1 The uranium decay series. Note that arrows to the right indicate an increase in the atomic number whereas arrows to the left indicate a decrease. The downward direction of the arrows indicates that the nucleus loses energy with each transformation (downward direction not drawn to scale).

10.3   NUCLIDE CHART

It is often useful to draw a graph, plotting the number of neutrons in a nucleus against the number of protons because all nuclides may be included in this nuclide chart. Such a chart is shown in simplified form in Fig. 10.2. Note that isotopes (lines of equal atomic number) are given by any vertical line on the figure. In such a graph, an angle of 45 degrees to the x-axis represents a situation where the nucleus contains equal numbers of protons and neutrons ($Z = N$).

It is found on such a graph that there is a broad band of nuclides with low atomic numbers at about 45 degrees to the x-axis and these are all stable or only weakly radioactive. Thus for the lighter elements, nuclear stability can be produced with equal numbers of protons and neutrons. From the graph it can be seen that, as the atomic number increases, a proportionately larger number of neutrons is

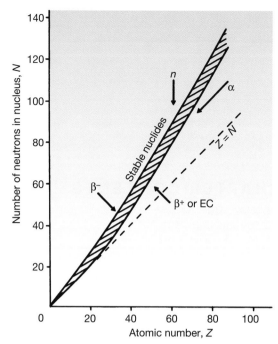

Fig. 10.2 A graph of the neutron number (N) plotted against the atomic number (Z) showing the position of the stable nuclides as a shaded band. Note that, as the atomic number increases, a higher proportion of neutrons to protons is required to achieve stability. Also shown are the directions which a nucleus takes for various forms of radioactive decay (these movements are not to scale). *EC,* Electron capture.

necessary to produce nuclear stability. Thus we can say that as the Coulomb repulsion (see Section 5.4) between the protons increases, then more neutrons are required to produce the short-range nuclear forces (see Section 2.3.1), thus producing the cohesive forces required for a stable nucleus. Nuclei which have atomic numbers greater than 83 (bismuth) are so large that it is impossible to produce a stable nuclear configuration.

Nuclides whose combination of neutrons and protons means that they land outside the band of stability shown in Fig. 10.2 have nuclei possessing higher energies than those within the band. Consequently, such a nucleus is unstable and tends, on decay, to produce a new nucleus of lower energy which is closer to, or within, the stable band. The energy difference between the nucleus before and after decay is emitted either as a charged particle or as a quantum (or quanta) of electromagnetic radiation. The decay scheme towards stability may be in the form of a single step (e.g., $^{14}_{6}$C decays to stable $^{14}_{7}$N[1] by the emission of a beta-particle, see Fig. 10.4) or it may be in the form of a multistage route involving many nuclear transformations (e.g., the decay of

$^{238}_{92}$U to $^{206}_{82}$Pb involves at least 14 steps, as shown in Fig. 10.1). As a rule, the greater the mass number of the nuclide, the more complicated the decay path to eventual stability.

The effect of different decay modes is illustrated using arrows on Fig. 10.2. The direction of the arrow shows the direction of change of position on the chart before and after the decay process. You may find it helpful to refer back to this chart while studying the decay processes in more detail in the following sections of this chapter.

10.4   ALPHA DECAY OR ALPHA-PARTICLE EMISSION

For the spontaneous emission of an alpha-particle from a nucleus, the nuclide must have an atomic mass number greater than 150. The nucleus must also have too few neutrons for the number of protons; a higher neutron-to-proton ratio would be required to produce nuclear stability. The alpha-particle consists of two protons and two neutrons tightly bound together (a helium nucleus). It may be considered as a free particle having high kinetic energy that is trapped in the parent nucleus. Thus the daughter nucleus has two protons and two neutrons fewer than the parent nucleus (see Equation 10.1).

The mechanism of production of the alpha-particle is quite complex. As we have already identified (see Section 2.3.1), the nucleus depends on a balance of disruptive electrostatic (Coulomb) forces and attractive forces between the nucleons caused by the short-range nuclear forces. In very large nuclei there is a large amount of electrostatic repulsion between the protons which extends across the whole nucleus. This is balanced by the short-range nuclear force which exists between adjacent nucleons. Thus if the nucleus becomes elongated, the electrostatic forces dominate, and the nucleus becomes even more elongated. This process continues until the nucleus divides into two fragments, the daughter nuclide and the alpha-particle.

An example of alpha decay is the decay of bismuth-212 to thallium-208 with the emission of alpha-particles. This process is shown in the following equation:

$$^{212}_{83}\text{Bi} \rightarrow {}^{208}_{81}\text{Tl} + {}^4_2\alpha \qquad \textbf{Equation 10.1}$$

Note that there is a reduction of four in the atomic mass number and two in the atomic number between parent and daughter product.

This reaction can also be written as shown in Fig. 10.3 (the decay of $^{212}_{83}$Bi also includes the emission of a beta-particle and is discussed later as an example of a branching programme; for simplicity, only the alpha-particle reaction is shown in Fig. 10.3 and the percentages shown refer only

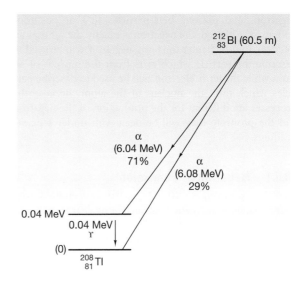

Fig. 10.3 An example of alpha-particle emission. The nucleus decreases its atomic number and energy as shown.

to the alpha-particles). Because the daughter product is to the left of the parent nuclide, this shows that there is a reduction in the atomic number. The reaction also shows that the difference in energy between the parent nuclide and the daughter nuclide is 6.08 MeV. If we consider only the alpha-particles emitted, we find that approximately 71% of these have an energy of 6.04 MeV and 29% have an energy of 6.08 MeV. In the case of the first group of alpha-particles, the nucleus is left in an excited state with excess energy of 0.04 MeV which it emits as a gamma ray.

The ejection of an alpha-particle means that, to preserve momentum, the nucleus must also recoil with an equal and opposite momentum to that of the alpha-particle. The energy of the recoiling nucleus is typically about 2% of that of the emitted alpha-particle. (Recoil also exists for beta decay but is much smaller because of the tiny mass of the beta-particle.)

Alpha-particles are intensely ionising but have a very short range in tissue so have little practical application in radiology.

10.5   BETA DECAY OR BETA-PARTICLE EMISSION

In the process of beta decay, a particle, having a mass equal to that of an electron, is ejected from the nucleus. The ejected particles, however, may have either a positive or negative charge and so, although they are known collectively as beta-particles, negative beta-particles (β^-) or negatrons and positive beta-particles (β^+) or positrons both exist. Although the negatron is exactly the same as an electron, in this chapter the term 'negatron' will be used to describe the particle which exits from the nucleus of an atom while the term 'electron' will be used to describe particles which orbit the nucleus of the atom. Because the processes are different for the production of the negatron and the positron, they will be dealt with under separate headings.

10.5.1   Negatron (β^-) emission

As we can see from Fig. 10.2, β^--particles are emitted from nuclei that have too many neutrons for nuclear stability. As we saw in Section 2.3.1, nucleons are being constantly changed from proton to neutron and back within the atomic nucleus. A neutron may be thought of as consisting of a proton and a negatron:

$$n \rightarrow p^+ + \beta^- \qquad \textbf{Equation 10.2}$$

It appears that in nuclei that have too many neutrons, there is a finite possibility that a neutron becomes isolated within the nucleus and then decays to form a proton and a negatron. The proton rejoins the nucleus and the negatron is ejected. This transformation results in the atomic mass number remaining unchanged (the combined number of protons and neutrons is still the same), but the atomic number will increase by one because one extra proton has been added to the nucleus (this results in the formation of a different element with the consequent rearrangement of electron orbitals to suit the new element).

An example of β^--particle decay is shown later, where carbon-14 decays to form nitrogen with the emission of a β^--particle:

$$^{14}_{6}C \rightarrow {}^{14}_{7}N + \beta^- \qquad \textbf{Equation 10.3}$$

This can also be illustrated using the methods discussed for alpha-particle emission to show the transformation from parent to daughter product. Such a diagram is shown in Fig. 10.4. Note that this time there is an increase in the atomic number so the line is down and to the right. This simple decay process is an example of pure beta emission because no other transformations are involved.

Fig. 10.5 shows a more complex emission pattern where the parent and daughter nuclei are separated by an energy difference of 2.81 MeV. The β^--particle has an energy of 0.31 MeV and so the nucleus is left in an excited state—2.50 MeV above its ground state. The nucleus emits this energy in the form of two gamma rays, one of energy 1.17 MeV and the other of energy 1.33 MeV. (This will be

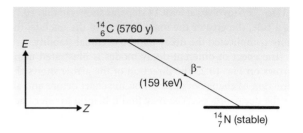

Fig. 10.4 An example of pure beta-particle (negatron) emission. The nucleus increases in atomic number and loses energy as shown.

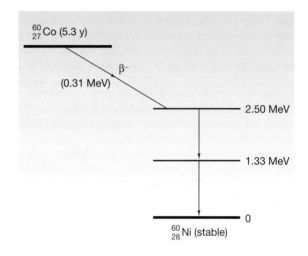

Fig. 10.5 The decay of cobalt-60 as an example of beta decay followed by a gamma decay of the daughter nucleus.

discussed further when we consider gamma-ray emission in Section 6.6.)

10.5.2   Positron (β^+) emission

As mentioned earlier, protons are continuously changing into neutrons and back. In these reactions we can consider a proton as consisting of a neutron and a positron.

$$p^+ \rightarrow n + \beta^+ \qquad \textbf{Equation 10.4}$$

If we consider Fig. 10.2, we see that positron emission takes place from nuclei that have too many protons to achieve stability. In such cases, protons appear to become isolated within the nucleus and then to decay to form a neutron which rejoins the nucleus and a positron that is ejected from the nucleus. In this reaction, the atomic mass

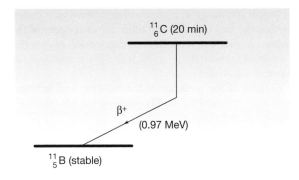

Fig. 10.6 An example of positron decay. The nucleus experiences a decrease in the atomic number and loses energy, as shown.

number will remain the same, but the atomic number will decrease by one (the total number of protons and neutrons is unchanged, but one proton has been converted into a neutron).

An example of such a reaction is the decay of carbon-11 to boron:

$$^{11}_{6}C \rightarrow {}^{11}_{5}B + \beta^{+} \qquad \textbf{Equation 10.5}$$

If we consider the energy changes which take place within the nucleus, as shown in Fig. 10.6, we see that the situation regarding energy of the β^{+}-particle is not as simple as it is for the β^{-}-particle. The energy difference between the parent and daughter nucleus in this case is 1.99 MeV. An energy loss of $2mc^{2}$ is required to create the positron and allow it to escape from the nucleus—where m is the mass of the positron and c is the velocity of electromagnetic radiation. As the mass of the positron is the same as the mass of the electron, then 1.02 MeV is required to create the positron and eject it from the nucleus, and any remaining energy (in this case 0.97 MeV) is given to the positron as kinetic energy.

INSIGHT

A negatron or a positron is influenced by the electrostatic forces which exist between it and the nucleus until it can escape from the atom. As a result, the kinetic energy of the β^{-}-particle is reduced by the force of attraction which exists between it and the nucleus, whereas the kinetic energy of the β^{+}-particle is increased by electrostatic repulsion. Energy and momentum are conserved in this process.

10.5.3   The fate of the positron

An energetic positron emitted by a nucleus will move through the surrounding atoms and will lose kinetic energy because of collisions with them. As its momentum decreases, it is more likely to interact with a free electron in the material. The positron is the antiparticle of the electron, and when they meet, they completely annihilate each other to form two gamma rays of annihilation radiation. This process is shown diagrammatically in Fig. 10.7, where the annihilation radiation consists of two photons, each of energy 0.511 MeV, ejected at 180 degrees to each other. In this way, both energy and momentum are conserved. The mutual annihilation of the electron and the positron is an example of the principle of mass–energy equivalence (see Section 8.4.1) as given by Einstein's equation $E = mc^{2}$, and shows that each particle has a mass–energy of 0.511 MeV, in agreement with Table 2.1.

The annihilation radiation produced by the reaction may now interact with neighbouring atoms by the processes of Compton scattering and photoelectric absorption (see Chapter 13) and may produce characteristic radiation and Auger electrons (see Section 10.6.3) by processes which will be discussed later in this chapter.

INSIGHT

The positron and the electron may annihilate each other when the positron still has considerable kinetic energy. In this case, the two quanta are not emitted at 180 degrees to each other and each has an energy higher than 0.511 MeV. The excess of energy of the positron is divided equally between each quantum. In each case, energy and momentum are conserved. A diagrammatic representation of the process is shown in the figure.

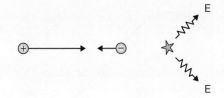

(A) collision between a positron and an electron where the positron has significant kinetic energy; (B) the direction of propagation of the annihilation radiation where the photons have energy in excess of 0.511 MeV each.

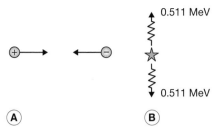

0.511 MeV

0.511 MeV

(A)   (B)

Fig. 10.7 (A) A collision between a positron and an electron where both have a minimal kinetic energy. (B) The annihilation radiation where two photons, each of 0.511 MeV, are produced at 180 degrees to each other.

10.5.4   The neutrino

Consider the carbon-14 reaction which we discussed earlier. Here the carbon-14 decayed to nitrogen where the difference in energy between the parent and the daughter nucleus was 159 keV. Because only beta decay takes place, we could confidently expect that all the β⁻-particles should have an energy of 159 keV. If we plot a graph of the energy of the beta-particles against the numbers emitted, we get a graph similar to the β⁻ graph shown in Fig. 10.8. The maximum or end-point energy of the β⁻-particles in this case is 159 keV. The graph means that, although only beta decay takes place and although the difference between the parent and the daughter nucleus is 159 keV, some of the β⁻-particles have energies less than 159 keV. Such a situation would appear to suggest that this does not obey the law of conservation of energy (see Section 8.4). This difficulty was overcome by Wolfgang Pauli in 1933 when he postulated that another particle—the neutrino—is always ejected with a beta-particle. He suggested that a neutrino (symbol ν) is ejected at the same time as a positron and that an antineutrino (symbol ν⁻) at the same time as a negatron. The total energy of the emitted negatron and antineutrino corresponds to the energy difference between the parent and daughter nucleus. How this energy is shared between the two particles will differ for each decay of the nucleus. In this way, a continuous distribution of energies is obtained for both the β⁻-particle and the antineutrino as shown in Fig. 10.8.

Because of the presence of the neutrino and antineutrino, we now need to modify some of the equations we considered earlier:

$$^{14}_{6}C \rightarrow {}^{14}_{7}N + \beta^- + \nu^-$$
$$^{11}_{6}C \rightarrow {}^{11}_{5}B + \beta^+ + \nu$$

Equation 10.6

INSIGHT

Although Pauli postulated the existence of neutrinos and antineutrinos in 1933, the presence of these particles proved difficult to detect until much later. There is now conclusive proof of their existence because of experiments performed using nuclear reactors and particle accelerators. The neutrino and the antineutrino differ in their direction of spin relative to their direction of motion—the neutrino spins anticlockwise and the antineutrino spins clockwise. They are antiparticles and if they are made to collide will produce electromagnetic radiation in the form of annihilation radiation. The reason the particles are so difficult to detect can be seen by considering their three major properties:
1. zero rest mass
2. zero charge
3. extremely small interaction with matter.

Because of these properties, it is extremely difficult to detect the presence of neutrinos (or antineutrinos) —they have a half-value thickness (see Section 14.3) of many miles in lead!

10.6   GAMMA DECAY OR GAMMA-RAY EMISSION

Gamma rays are part of the electromagnetic spectrum and are similar in many ways to X-rays. Gamma rays are emitted from a nucleus which has excess energy whereas X-rays are from electrons as they lose energy (this will be further discussed in Chapter 11). It is possible for gamma rays to have lower energies than X-rays and vice versa. However, the maximum energy possible from gamma rays exceeds that of X-rays.

We discussed in this chapter (see Section 10.5.1) the fact that cobalt-60 decayed with the emission of a β-particle but the daughter nucleus was left in an excited state. The situation for this daughter nucleus is depicted in Fig. 10.9A. The

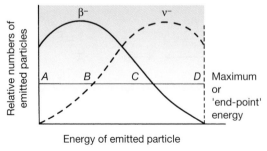

Fig. 10.8 The sharing of energy between the beta-particle and the neutrino in beta decay. The case shown is for negatron emission.

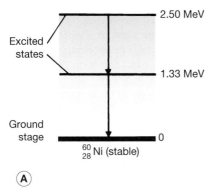

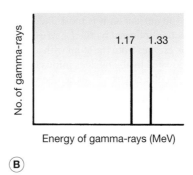

Fig. 10.9 (A) The excited states of a nickel-60 nucleus, which is left in an excited state as the result of the previous decay of a cobalt-60 nucleus. This decays to its ground state by the emission of two gamma photons, each representing the difference in energy between the excited states. (B) The line spectrum produced by the gamma radiation.

figure illustrates the energy states of the daughter nucleus by means of horizontal lines above the thick line representing the ground state of the nucleus. In this case, the $^{60}_{28}$Ni, nucleus is left at an energy 2.5 MeV above its ground state. It immediately decays to its ground state in two jumps:
1. It decays to 1.33 MeV above its ground state by the emission of a 1.17 MeV gamma ray.
2. It then drops to its ground state by the emission of a second gamma ray of energy 1.33 MeV.

Fig. 10.9B shows the line spectra of the gamma radiation emitted by the nucleus where each gamma ray has a precise energy corresponding to the discrete energy transformations within the nucleus.

10.6.1   Metastable states and isomeric transitions

In the case of $^{60}_{27}$Co decaying to $^{60}_{28}$Ni, the nucleus remains in an excited state before the emission of the gamma rays for a time so short that it is incapable of accurate measurement. However, this is not always the case, and those excited states which last sufficiently long for their durations to be measured are known as *metastable states*. The transition from a metastable state to a more stable state is known as an *isomeric transition*. Such metastable radionuclides prove to be useful in nuclear medicine because of the low dose which they deliver to the patient; the patient gets no dose from β⁻-particles emitted before metastability. Technetium-99m (usually written $^{99}_{43}$Tc^m or, less commonly, $^{99m}_{43}$Tc) is a radionuclide widely used in nuclear medicine. A simplified decay scheme for it is shown in Fig. 10.10 and it will be discussed in more detail in Chapter 22 which deals with radionuclide imaging. The half-life of $^{99}_{43}$Tc^m is 6 hours and it emits a gamma ray of energy 140 keV when it decays to $^{99}_{43}$Tc. The half-life of $^{99}_{43}$Tc is so long (2.1×10^5 years) that it can be considered stable for all practical purposes.

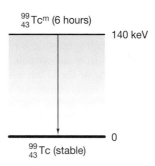

Fig. 10.10 An example of the decay of technetium from a metastable to a stable state with the emission of a 140 keV gamma photon.

The reaction can be written as:

$$^{99}_{43}\text{Tc}^m \rightarrow \,^{99}_{43}\text{Tc} + \gamma \qquad \textbf{Equation 10.7}$$

The next section of this chapter considers the possible effects of gamma emission from the nucleus on the whole atom rather than on the nucleus only.

10.6.2   Internal conversion

When a nuclide is decaying by gamma emission, there is a competing process within the atom called *internal conversion*. This process results in electrons with discrete energies (unlike the continuous spectrum of energies of negatrons) being emitted from the atom. The process is a result of a direct interaction between the nucleus and an orbiting electron, such that the nucleus can drop to its ground state by giving all of its excess energy to the electron.

The innermost electrons of the atom have orbitals which pass close to or even through the nucleus. Thus it is a matter of statistical probability whether the excess energy of the nucleus will result in a gamma-ray emission from the nucleus or electron emission from the inner shells. The K-shell is situated closest to the nucleus so it is most likely to participate in such a reaction followed by the L-, M-shells, etc. The *converted electron* escapes from the atom with an energy equal to the energy donated by the nucleus minus the binding energy of that particular electron. This can be stated:

$$\begin{aligned} \text{KE of converted electron} = \\ \text{nuclear energy transition} - \text{BE} \end{aligned} \quad \textbf{Equation 10.8}$$

where KE is kinetic energy and BE is binding energy of the electron.

The internal conversion coefficient, α, is defined as the ratio of the number of nuclear transformations resulting in internal conversion to the number resulting in gamma-ray emission. Thus α may take a value between 0, resulting in no internal conversions, and infinity, corresponding to complete internal conversion. This can be illustrated by considering the figures for the decay of $^{99}_{43}\text{Tc}^\text{m}$ to $^{99}_{43}\text{Tc}$. Approximately 9% of the nuclear transitions result in internal conversions of electrons from the K-shell, 1.1% from the L-shell and 0.3% from the M-shell. This means that 10.4% of the nuclear transitions result in internal conversions and 89.6% result in gamma-ray emission. This gives an internal conversion coefficient (α) for $^{99}_{43}\text{Tc}^\text{m}$ of 0.116.

10.6.3   X-rays and Auger electrons

If a radioactive decay results in a vacancy occurring within one of the inner electron shells of the atom, then electrons from orbitals further away from the nucleus will perform quantum jumps inwards until there are no inner-shell vacancies. Each such quantum jump will result in the emission of electromagnetic radiation from the atom equal to the energy difference between the two shells. For inner-shell transitions, the energy of this electromagnetic radiation may be in the X-ray part of the spectrum. Such radiation is known as *fluorescent radiation* and its energy is characteristic of the atom concerned. If we consider the internal conversion process which we have just described and take a situation where a K-shell electron is removed from the atom, the vacancy thus created in the K-shell may be filled from the L-shell (a $K\alpha$ transition) or from the M-shell (a $K\beta$ transition). Such a quantum jump would be accompanied by the emission of a photon of electromagnetic radiation equivalent to the energy difference between the two shells. If it was a $K\alpha$ transition, there would now be a vacancy in the L-shell and this might be filled from the M-shell, etc. This would again be accompanied by the emission of a photon of electromagnetic radiation equal to the energy difference between the L- and M-shells. This process continues until the atom is able to capture a free electron to fill the vacancy—usually in one of its outermost shells. Until this occurs the atom contains more protons than electrons and so is regarded as a *positive ion*.

This already rather complex situation is further complicated by the fact that some of the photons emitted by such transitions may have sufficient energy to interact with other electrons in the atom and to remove them from their orbitals and eject them from the atom; this process is called the *photoelectric effect* and may occur if the photon energy is greater than the binding energy of the electron (see Chapter 13 for a more detailed description). The electrons thus ejected are called *Auger electrons* and have discrete energies equal to the photon energy minus the binding energy of the electron. The ejection of an Auger electron from a shell leaves a vacancy in that shell which will be filled by electrons jumping down from orbitals even further away from the nucleus, with the release of more fluorescent radiation and perhaps the release of even more Auger electrons.

From this we can see that the ejection of an electron from one of the orbitals by internal conversion may result in a complicated sequence of orbital quantum jumps accompanied by the release of photons of electromagnetic radiation and the ejection of Auger electrons from the atom. The term *fluorescent yield* is used to describe the fraction of the electron transitions that result in the production of fluorescent radiation.

If we consider $^{99}_{43}\text{Tc}^\text{m}$ from the previous discussion, you may remember that 11.6% of the energy from the nucleus results in internal conversion ($\alpha = 0.116$). Of the resulting electron quantum jumps, 80% of the transitions result in fluorescent radiation and 20% result in the production of Auger electrons. Thus the fluorescent yield for technetium is 0.8. Some typical fluorescent radiation energies for $^{99}_{43}\text{Tc}^\text{m}$ are:

$$K_\alpha = 18.4\,\text{keV},\ L_\alpha = 2.4\,\text{keV},\ M_\alpha = 0.2\,\text{keV}$$

Note that the electrons emitted by this process carry discrete amounts of energy, which makes it easy to distinguish them from negatron emission where there is a continuous spectrum of energies.

INSIGHT

For each decay, the total energies for all the fluorescent radiation and of all the electrons emitted from the shells of the atom equal the energy lost by the nucleus in the nuclear transition. This is because the binding energy of each ejected electron is recovered in the fluorescent radiation emitted in the subsequent cascade of orbital jumps. Thus the whole process obeys the law of conservation of energy.

10.7 ELECTRON CAPTURE

If a nucleus of low mass number has too few neutrons for stability but has insufficient excess energy (<1.02 MeV) to eject a positron, then an alternative way by which the nucleus may undergo an isobaric transformation and lose energy is electron capture (shown in Fig. 10.11). In this process, the nucleus captures one of the orbiting electrons, the most likely being a capture of a K-shell electron. Sometimes the terms 'K capture' and 'L capture' are used to denote the shell from which the electron was captured. A situation where electron capture is the only process involved is shown in Fig. 10.11A where $^{131}_{55}$Cs decays to $^{131}_{54}$Xe.

In the diagram, the atomic number is reduced by one because the capture of an electron by the nucleus results in one of the protons in the nucleus changing into a neutron. Also note that during the process of electron capture, a neutrino is emitted by the nucleus. The processes involved in electron capture may be shown by Equation 10.9:

$$p^+ + e^+ \rightarrow n + \nu \qquad \textbf{Equation 10.9}$$

In situations where a low-mass nucleus has too few neutrons and an excess energy greater than 1.02 MeV, then the process of electron capture may compete with the process of positron emission. An example of such a competing process is shown in the decay of $^{58}_{27}$Co into stable $^{58}_{26}$Fe in Fig. 10.11B.

Note that both the process of electron capture and the process of positron emission involve the conversion of a proton to a neutron. Thus the atomic mass number remains unaltered but the atomic number is reduced by one.

As we mentioned earlier in this chapter (Section 10.6.2), creating a vacancy in an inner electron shell will result in the emission of characteristic fluorescent radiation from the atom. It is interesting to note that in the case of electron capture this is characteristic of the daughter product. This means that the electron orbitals of the daughter product are established before the consequent electron transitions occur.

10.8 BRANCHING DECAY PROGRAMMES

If the nucleus is very large, it is possible that it may disintegrate in more than one way. We have already encountered this (although it was not described in detail) in the uranium series in Fig. 10.2. In this case, $^{214}_{83}$Bi can either decay to $^{214}_{84}$Po by β⁻-particle emission or it can decay to $^{210}_{81}$Tl by alpha-particle emission.

Another isotope of bismuth, $^{212}_{83}$Bi, decays in a similar branching programme. The decay process for this isotope involves the emission of alpha-particles of energies 6.04 and 6.08 MeV, gamma rays of energy 0.04 MeV and β⁻-particles of maximum energy 2.25 MeV. The initial decay scheme for the $^{212}_{83}$Bi nuclide is shown in Fig. 10.12. Note that, for simplicity, only the first disintegrations are shown. As can be seen from the diagram, both $^{208}_{81}$Tl and $^{212}_{84}$Po have short half-lives and so are also radioactive.

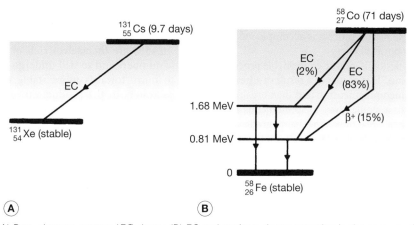

Fig. 10.11 (A) Pure electron capture (*EC*) decay. (B) EC and positron decay occurring in the same nuclide (85% EC and 15% positron decay). Also emitted are the X-rays from the iron-58 atoms and the 0.511 MeV annihilation radiations from the positron–electron annihilations.

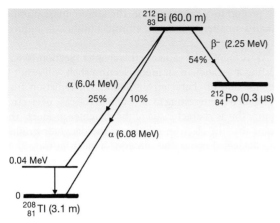

Fig. 10.12 A branching decay programme where alpha and beta decay processes compete in the decay of bismuth-212.

a chain reaction can be set up. Such a process is accompanied by the release of large amounts of energy (see Insight).

INSIGHT

On average, a uranium-238 nucleus will release an energy of 200 MeV on fission. If we consider the complete fission of a 1-kg mass of uranium (this is about the size of a golf ball), we need to consider the energy released by all the uranium atoms in a 1-kg mass. By applying Avogadro's equation (see Section 3.6) to this we can calculate that 1 kg of uranium-238 contains 2.5×10^{24} atoms. If each of these atoms releases 200 MeV of energy, th total energy released will be 5.1×10^{27} MeV. This is the same as 8.1×10^{13} joules of energy.

10.9   FISSION

As we mentioned in our discussion of alpha decay (see Section 10.4), the short-range forces holding the nucleus together exist between adjacent nucleons, whereas the Coulomb forces act across the whole of the nucleus. This fact becomes increasingly important as the size of the nucleus increases. A very large nucleus may be pictured as being rather like a liquid drop in which the nucleons are moving about with very high energy and continuously deforming the shape of the nucleus. During this process, it is possible for the nucleus to become very elongated and then to break into two fragments—usually of fairly similar sizes. Such a phenomenon is known as *spontaneous fission* and can occur for very large nuclei (e.g., thorium-232 is capable of spontaneous fission). As well as the fission fragments from such a reaction, one or more neutrons are usually liberated and the whole fission process is accompanied by the release of large amounts of energy.

Neutron-activated fission is a more controllable process than spontaneous fission. This occurs as a result of a heavy nucleus capturing an incoming neutron and then breaking into large fragments in a similar way to spontaneous fission. An example of such a reaction is the disintegration of $^{238}_{92}$U into two fission fragments of $^{145}_{56}$Ba and $^{94}_{36}$Kr if the uranium-238 nucleus is made to absorb a neutron. The fission of the nucleus is normally accompanied by the release of gamma rays and neutrons. Both of the fissile fragments are extremely rich in neutrons and so each will usually release a neutron. The neutrons from both of the discussed processes can now react with two $^{238}_{92}$U nuclei, resulting in the release of four fissile fragments and four neutrons, and so

A pictorial representation of the neutron-activated fission process is shown in Fig. 10.13. The incoming neutron is captured in Fig. 10.13A and delivers sufficient energy to the nucleus (Fig. 10.13B) to elongate its shape into an ellipsoid. As mentioned earlier, the Coulomb forces across the nucleus are now at an advantage over the short-range nuclear forces and the nucleus further distorts to form a 'peanut' shape (Fig. 10.13C) and eventually breaks to form two fragments because of the electrostatic repulsion between the two main nuclear masses. The two fragments fly apart (their kinetic energy accounts for about 80% of the total disintegration energy) and several neutrons and gamma-ray photons are usually emitted (Fig. 10.13D). The neutrons emitted by this reaction may now interact with other atoms to cause fission and the release of further neutrons and so a chain reaction is set up, with the consequent liberation of large amounts of energy. The fissile fragments (Fig. 10.13E) are themselves rich in neutrons for their atomic numbers and so will undergo further disintegration to move towards more stable nuclei. This initial process results in the production of β⁻-particles (with associated gamma rays) which produces a more stable proton/neutron configuration or, if the nucleus is very excited, the ejection of a neutron from the nucleus. These neutrons are known as *delayed neutrons* to distinguish them from the *prompt neutrons* which are emitted at the moment of fission.

Fission products from any type of nucleus are not always the same and may have different relative sizes on each disintegration. Thus a great range of other decay chains is possible from other fissile fragments.

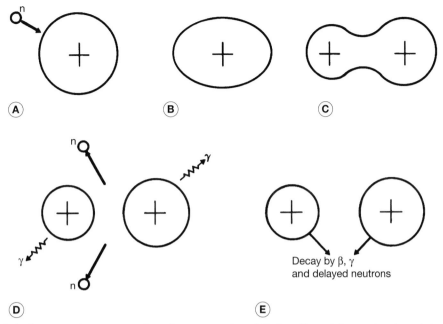

Fig. 10.13 A diagrammatic representation of neutron-activated fission. For a fuller explanation of the process, see the text.

> **INSIGHT**
>
> It is also possible to initiate fission in the nucleus by bombarding it with protons (or with alpha-particles) or by striking it with high-energy photons. Examples of these are:
>
> - Copper ($^{63}_{29}$Cu), if bombarded with protons, can be made to undergo fission to produce sodium ($^{24}_{11}$Na) and potassium ($^{39}_{19}$K). This process is accompanied by neutron emission.
> - Uranium-238 ($^{238}_{32}$U), if it is bombarded by photons of energy equal to or greater than 5.1 MeV, will undergo fission. This latter process is known as *photofission*.

10.10 SUMMARY OF RADIOACTIVE NUCLEAR TRANSFORMATIONS

Table 10.1 is a summary of the types of radioactive decay discussed so far in this chapter. You may find it useful to refer to this table when considering the production of artificial radionuclides and also in considering the use of radionuclides in medicine in Chapter 22.

10.11 EXPONENTIAL RADIOACTIVE DECAY PROCESSES

Provided that there are sufficient radioactive atoms in a sample, which is always the case because even a tiny weight of material will contain billions of atoms, radioactive decay is described as an exponential process. This is a mathematical relationship which simply means that equal time increments will result in equal fractional decreases in radioactivity. For example, if we take the commonly used isotope $^{99}_{43}$Tc^{m}, the activity will halve every 6 hours. So the number of remaining radioactive nuclei will be a half after 6 hours, a quarter after 12 hours, an eighth after 18 hours and so on. Eventually the activity will decay to almost nothing. The time taken for half of the radioactivity in a sample to decay is referred to as the half-life. The law of radioactive decay states that the rate of decay of a particular nuclide (i.e. the number of nuclei decaying per second) is proportional to the number of such nuclei left in the sample (i.e. it is a fixed fraction of the number of nuclei left in the sample). An example of radioactive decay is illustrated by Fig. 10.14.

TABLE 10.1   Summary of the effects of radioactive decay

Type of decay	Symbol	Effect on nucleus			Effect on atom	Comments
		Z	N	A		
Alpha	α	Z − 2	N − 2	A − 4	Electron orbits change to that of daughter nucleus.	Occurs in elements with a mass number greater than 150. Daughter products may undergo further decay by a variety of the processes mentioned later.
Negatron emission	β⁻	Z + 1	N − 1	–	Electron orbits change to that of daughter nucleus	Neutron changes to proton in nucleus. Negatron emitted from the nucleus with a spread of energies but the energy of the negatron plus the energy of the antineutrino is constant for a given nuclide. Daughter nucleus may further decay by prompt or delayed gamma-ray emission competing with internal conversion (IC).
Positron emission	β⁺	Z − 1	N + 1	–	Electron orbits change to that of daughter nucleus.	Proton changes to neutron in nucleus. The positron is emitted with a neutrino and the sum of their energies is constant for a given nuclide. The process only occurs if the energy loss by the parent nucleus can be greater than 1.02 MeV. Positron is annihilated by collision with electron and two photons of annihilation radiation, each of energy 0.511 MeV are produced. Daughter nucleus may decay by gamma radiation and/or IC.
Gamma radiation	γ	–	–	–	No effect on the number of nucleons in the nucleus but the process may compete with IC.	Produced by the quantum jump from excited state of the nucleus to a lower energy. Excited states of measurable half-life are defined as *metastable* and the transition is *isomeric*.
Internal conversion	IC	–	–	–	Characteristic radiation and Auger electrons emitted.	An inner orbital electron of the atom interacts with the nucleus and is ejected from the atom. The electron is given the excess nuclear energy. This creates a vacancy in the shell and results in the emission of characteristic radiation and Auger electrons.

TABLE 10.1 summary of the effects of radioactive decay **(Continued)**

Type of decay	Symbol	Effect on nucleus			Effect on atom	Comments
		Z	N	A		
Electron capture	EC	Z − 1	N + 1	–	Characteristic radiation and Auger electrons of the daughter nucleus are emitted.	An inner orbital electron is captured by the nucleus and changes a proton to a neutron. A neutrino is emitted, carrying energy changes of the nucleus. The nucleus may decay spontaneously by gamma-ray emission. The vacancy left in the electron orbit results in the emission of characteristic radiation and Auger electrons.
Fission	f	Size and structure of the fragments may vary.			Bonds may be broken or ionisation caused by fragment.	Fission may be spontaneous or neutron activated. The nucleus splits, producing two or more fragments, gamma rays and neutrons. Controlled fission is used in nuclear reactors and the neutrons can be used to produce artificial radionuclides.

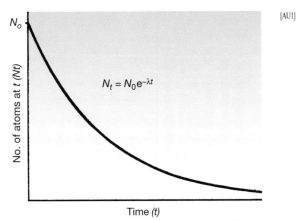

Fig. 10.14 An example of an exponential process, as illustrated by radioactive decay. Note that the number of remaining radioactive atoms decreases exponentially with time.

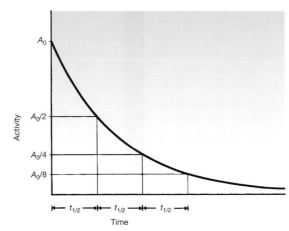

Fig. 10.15 Half-life ($t_{1/2}$) and radioactive decay. Note that each $t_{1/2}$ reduces the level of radioactivity by one-half.

We may now plot activity against time (Fig. 10.15) and we obtain exactly the same curve as in Fig. 10.14. The equation for this curve is expressed as:

$$A_t = A_0 e^{-\lambda t} \qquad \textbf{Equation 10.10}$$

where A_t is the activity after a time t, A_0 is the initial activity, e is the exponential constant, λ is the decay constant and t is the time after the initial measurement.

INSIGHT

In practice it is often easier to use Equation 10.10 in its logarithmic form. (For more information on logarithms, see Appendix.) Consider Equation 10.10:

$$A_t = A_0 e^{-\lambda t}$$

If we take logarithms to the base e of both sides of the equation, we get:

$$\log_e A_t = \log_e A_0 - \lambda t \qquad \textbf{Equation 10.11}$$

An illustration of the half-life of a particular radionuclide is shown in Fig. 10.15. The activity of the sample when $t = 0$ is A_0. When the activity is reduced to $A_0/2$, the radionuclide has undergone one half-life. This is indicated by the time $t_{1/2}$. If another half-life passes, the activity is reduced by a further factor of two and is now $A_0/4$, and so on for further half-lives.

If we now consider Equation 10.10, we can use this to establish a relationship between the decay constant and the half-life:

$$A_t = A_0 e^{-\lambda t_{1/2}}$$

Now, by definition, at the half-life, $A_0/2 = A_0 e^{-\lambda t_{1/2}}$. Thus the equation can be rewritten in the form:

$$\frac{A_0}{2} = A_0 e^{-\lambda t_{1/2}}$$
$$\frac{1}{2} = e^{-\lambda t_{1/2}}$$
$$2 = e^{\lambda t_{1/2}} \qquad \textbf{Equation 10.12}$$
$$\log_e 2 = \lambda t_{1/2}$$
$$0.693 = \lambda t_{1/2}$$
$$\lambda = \frac{0.693}{t_{1/2}}$$

The decay constant is thus measured in time^{-1} because it is inversely related to the half-life. The decay constant is simply a constant of proportionality (see Appendix).

SUMMARY

In this chapter you should have learnt:
- The mechanism for alpha decay and alpha-particle emission (see Section 10.4).
- Beta decay leading to negatron emission (see Section 10.5.1).
- Beta decay leading to positron emission (see Section 10.5.4).
- The fact that a neutrino or an antineutrino forms part of beta emission (see Section 10.5.4).
- The mechanism of gamma decay and gamma-ray emission (see Section 10.6).
- The meaning of metastable nuclei and isomeric transitions (see Section 10.6.1).

- The mechanism of the process of internal conversion (see Section 10.6.2).
- The mechanisms involved in the emission of X-rays and Auger electrons from the atoms of radionuclides (see Section 10.6.3).
- The mechanism of electron capture and the subsequent changes within the atom (see Section 10.7).
- Branching decay programmes (see Section 10.8).
- The processes involved in nuclear fission (see Section 10.9).
- Summary of radioactive nuclear transformations (see Section 10.10).

FURTHER READING

Ball, J.L., Moore, A.D., & Turner, S. 2008. *Ball and Moore's Essential Physics for Radiographers*. 4th edn. London: Blackwell Scientific. (Chapter 20.)

SECTION 2

X-rays and their applications

X-ray production

CHAPTER CONTENTS

11.1 AIM

X-ray production is a key topic in radiological physics as in underpins the operation of 'plain' or conventional X-ray imaging, as well as computed tomography (CT). X-rays are produced when highly energetic electrons lose energy, in the form of electromagnetic radiation. According to the law of conservation of energy, energy cannot just disappear, but can be transfigured from one form into another. Hence the lost electron energy can be converted into X-ray photons. In Chapter 10 we saw that unstable atomic nuclei can also lose energy, but in that instance the energy loss resulted in energetic gamma rays, or alpha- or beta-particle emissions, not X-rays, during the radioactive decay process. This chapter will describe the two mechanisms of X-ray production, namely Bremsstrahlung ('braking radiation') and characteristic radiation. The energy of Bremsstrahlung X-rays is determined by the electrical potential difference across an X-ray tube, which is often termed the peak kilovoltage or kVp. The energy of characteristic X-rays is determined by the elemental composition of the X-ray tube target material, which is normally tungsten but can be molybdenum or rhodium in mammography X-ray tubes. The detailed working of X-ray tubes will be covered in Chapter 12. At diagnostic X-ray energies (up to 150 keV), Bremsstrahlung is normally the most important X-ray production process, and may provide about 90% of the X-rays. However, characteristic X-ray production is especially important in mammography (see Chapter 18).

11.2 INTERACTIONS IN THE TARGET OF AN X-RAY TUBE

The 'target' of an X-ray tube is that portion of the positively charged anode which is actively bombarded by the high speed electron beam emerging from the negatively charged cathode filament (see Chapter 12). It usually consists of tungsten atoms, often with some rhenium atoms added to increase its hardness and durability. The term 'target' often causes confusion. Note that it is a part of the X-ray tube, not a target area in a patient's body and should not be mixed-up with the term 'target volume' which is used in radiotherapy. At any moment in time, all of the electrons passing through the vacuum of the X-ray tube insert will strike the target with the same velocity and hence the same kinetic energy. Kinetic energy is the energy of a mass moving at a particular velocity (see Chapter 3) and is equal to $\frac{1}{2}mv^2$, where m is the mass of the electron and v is its velocity. The electrons will all arrive at the target with the same velocity because the accelerating force applied to them is proportional to the electrical potential difference, V, across the X-ray tube. Because of this, the energies of the arriving electrons can also be expressed in kiloelectron volts, keV, where e is the charge on an electron and V is the electrical potential difference. So as V increases, the energy of the speeding electrons will also increase and this can produce more energetic X-rays. Interestingly, electrons striking the X-ray tube target with the same energy result in the production of X-rays with a range of energies, as illustrated by Fig. 11.1. This must be explained by the different interactions that can occur within the target.

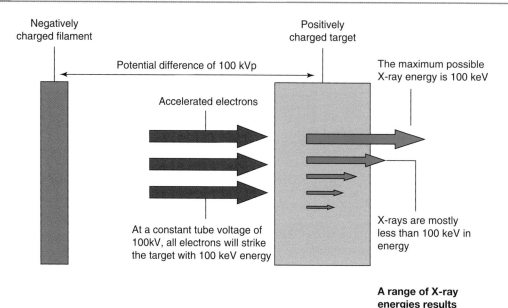

Negatively charged filament

Positively charged target

Potential difference of 100 kVp

The maximum possible X-ray energy is 100 keV

Accelerated electrons

At a constant tube voltage of 100kV, all electrons will strike the target with 100 keV energy

X-rays are mostly less than 100 keV in energy

A range of X-ray energies results

Fig. 11.1 Showing how electrons that strike the target with a constant kinetic energy result in X-rays with a broad range of energies.

INSIGHT

Although the dense material of a tungsten X-ray tube target may appear very solid, it is not in fact an impenetrable wall consisting of atoms packed together like golf balls. At the submicroscopic level, matter is mostly just empty space, through which electrons, other particles and X-rays can pass through very easily. The diameter of a tungsten nucleus is about 10^{-14} m across, whereas the diameter of a tungsten atom is about 10^{-10} m. This size difference of about 10,000 is rather like the size of a pea relative to the size of a football stadium. So electrons from the X-ray tube filament pass through the outer layer of the target—they don't 'bounce' off it.

As mentioned earlier, most of the volume of an atom is empty, although occupied by atomic electrons in various shells, labelled $K, L, M \ldots$ in increasing distance from the atomic nucleus. Tungsten has an atomic number of 74 and hence there will be 74 electrons contained in the electron shells. Because the size of the atomic nucleus is small compared with the size of the atom, it follows that the speeding electrons arriving from the cathode filament are more likely to interact with the shell electrons than with the nucleus. Any electron–electron interaction resulting in a loss of kinetic energy from the incoming filament electron is termed *inelastic*. The atomic shell electrons will be briefly 'excited' but then will drop back down to their original

states, with the emission of heat energy. In fact about 99% of the energy transfer that occurs in an X-ray tube target results in heat emission. This explains why the target and anode of an X-ray tube becomes so hot during use in the imaging department. More rarely, in about 1% of cases, an inelastic interaction between a filament electron and the target will result in X-ray emission, as described in Sections 11.3 and 11.4. Fig. 11.2 shows some of the various

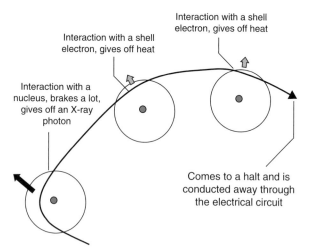

Interaction with a shell electron, gives off heat

Interaction with a shell electron, gives off heat

Interaction with a nucleus, brakes a lot, gives off an X-ray photon

Comes to a halt and is conducted away through the electrical circuit

Fig. 11.2 Some possible interactions between electrons from the filament and tungsten atoms in the target of an X-ray tube. An extra possible interaction (not shown here) involves ionisation of shell electrons, resulting in the release of characteristic X-rays.

interactions that can occur during a filament electron's passage through the X-ray tube target. An electron from the filament may experience many interactions before it is brought to rest within 0.25 to 0.5 mm of the target surface. 'Elastic' interactions, during which a filament electron may alter direction but will not lose energy, may also occur, but these are not of much practical consequence.

11.3 THE BREMSSTRAHLUNG PROCESS— THE CONTINUOUS X-RAY SPECTRUM

The term Bremsstrahlung means *braking radiation* in German and involves the braking or slowing down of filament electrons as they pass through the X-ray tube target. In so doing the electron will lose kinetic energy, which may be converted to photon energy in the form of an X-ray, as a 'radiative' emission. Note that the term 'braking' has nothing to do with breaking or shattering, although the words do sound the same. Imagine a situation where you suddenly brake hard when driving a car. All of that energy of momentum does not disappear; it is transferred to frictional heat in your car tyres and perhaps to any object that you accidentally hit. In a similar way, the speeding electrons will transfer some or all of their energy as they brake. The braking force exerted on the filament electrons is caused by electrostatic attraction between them and the tungsten nuclei in the X-ray tube target. Opposite charges attract and the single negative charge on an electron is powerfully drawn towards the 74 positively charged protons in a tungsten nucleus. The high atomic number of tungsten is one of the reasons why it is such a good material for an X-ray tube target because it will produce a lot of electron braking and hence many X-rays. According to Coulomb's law (see Chapter 5) the electrostatic force between two charges is directly proportional to the product of their magnitudes and inversely proportional to the square of the distance between them. Put simply, the electron will experience a much greater attractive force as it travels closer to a tungsten nucleus.

Imagine for a moment that the incoming filament electron is like an arrow and the tungsten atom is like an archery target. The atom is shown schematically in Fig. 11.3.

It can be seen in Fig. 11.3 that the bull's eye of the diagram, which is the atomic nucleus, is very small relative to the rest of the atom. It is not very likely statistically that the filament electron will head straight into the nucleus. If it did, it might brake completely to a halt because of electrostatic attraction and transfer all its kinetic energy to an X-ray photon. This photon would have the maximum possible energy in kiloelectron volts. If the X-ray tube voltage was 100 kVp, the maximum possible X-ray energy would

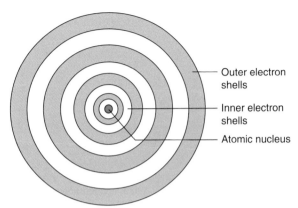

Fig. 11.3 A tungsten atom as viewed by an incoming filament electron. This electron is much more likely to pass through the outer parts of the atom than close to the nucleus.

be 100 keV. The electron, now brought to a standstill, would be conducted away through the tungsten metal as part of the flow of electricity through the X-ray tube circuit. Not many X-rays of the maximum possible energy will be produced. Looking again at Fig. 11.3, it can be seen that it is much more likely statistically that the filament electrons will pass by some distance from the nucleus, and this likelihood increases with distance because the outer area of the atom is greater than the inner area. The braking effect will decrease with greater distance from the nucleus, attributed to Coulomb's law as mentioned previously, and thus less energetic X-ray photons will result from braking events further out from the nucleus. The overall result of this is that X-rays resulting from the Bremsstrahlung process will be produced with a continuous range of energies and there will be many more low energy X-rays than high energy X-rays. This is not an ideal result, as will be seen in Chapter 14, but it is an inevitable effect of Bremsstrahlung. Figs. 11.4 and 11.5 show the braking effects on filament electrons that interact with tungsten nuclei.

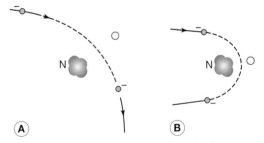

Fig. 11.4 The deflection of an electron from the filament when it interacts with the nucleus (N) of a target atom in the X-ray tube. (A) A small deflection; (B) a large deflection.

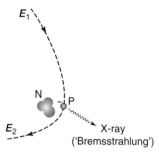

Fig. 11.5 The production of Bremsstrahlung X-rays. An electron at point P suddenly loses energy by the emission of an X-ray photon. The electron continues with a reduced energy E_2.

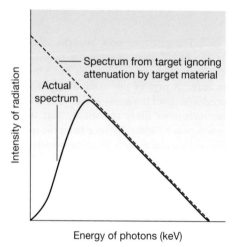

Fig. 11.6 The continuous X-ray spectrum, taking account of X-ray attenuation in the tungsten target.

INSIGHT

Filament electrons can also be braked to a small degree by interactions with electrons orbiting the tungsten nucleus in the various electron shells. The electrostatic force of this interaction will be relatively small because both electrons will have just a single negative charge, but there are 74 electrons in a tungsten atom and thus such interactions will be common. The overall effect may be the emission of large numbers of very low-energy (such as infrared) electromagnetic photons, contributing to X-ray tube target heating but not to X-ray production. Target heating can also result from temporary excitation of shell electrons which then drop back to their original lower energy level, with the emission of heat and light energy.

The quantity (often referred to as 'intensity' in radiological physics) of Bremsstrahlung X-ray emission is proportional to the target atomic number and also to the square of the voltage across the X-ray tube. The atomic number effect is attributed to Coulomb's law, as described previously in this section. Increasing tube voltage has the effect of accelerating the filament electrons to greater speeds across the X-ray tube. Thus the electrons will possess more kinetic energy. As their kinetic energy increases, it becomes more likely that this energy will be lost via X-ray emission than via heat emission. The likelihood of the filament electrons interacting with the orbital electrons surrounding the target's tungsten atoms will decrease. This effect is seen more dramatically in radiotherapy linear accelerators (LINACs), where bombarding electrons are accelerated to very high speeds and more than 40% of the energy transferred in the target results in X-rays being produced (compared with 1% in a diagnostic X-ray tube).

So the overall effect of Bremsstrahlung is a continuous X-ray spectrum, as shown by Fig. 11.6. Fewer X-rays of high energy are produced, and very few have the maximum possible energy. The figure shows the spectrum that is actually emitted from an X-ray target. Many of the low energy X-rays are absorbed in the dense metal of the X-ray tube target and anode, as well as in any added filtration, and hence do not emerge from the X-ray tube. The vertical axis of the graph refers to X-ray 'intensity' which is commonly used in radiological physics as a term relating to the 'number of X-ray photons'. Note that more generally in physics, 'intensity' refers to the total energy passing through a unit cross-sectional area per unit time, thus incorporating both the number and energy of photons.

11.4   THE CHARACTERISTIC RADIATION PROCESS—THE X-RAY LINE SPECTRUM

Some X-rays are emitted at fixed energies, giving a 'line spectrum' rather than the continuous spectrum described in the previous section. This process typically provides only about 10% of the X-ray photons produced in diagnostic imaging procedures, although it is more important in mammography (see Chapter 18). The fixed energies of the emitted rays are 'characteristic' of the element found in the X-ray tube target and are proportional to the atomic number of that element, as shown in Table 11.1. In this chapter, we are concerned only with those elements found in the

TABLE 11.1 The characteristic X-ray energies of some elements

Element	Atomic number Z	Main characteristic X-ray energies, keV
Carbon	6	0.3
Copper	29	8
Molybdenum	42	17, 19
Rhodium	45	20, 22
Tungsten	74	59, 67
Rhenium	75	60, 69
Lead	82	75, 85

Only molybdenum, rhodium, tungsten and rhenium may be found in diagnostic X-ray tube targets. The first two may be used in mammography whereas small amounts of rhenium may be added to tungsten targets for general radiography and computed tomography. Where two X-ray energies are listed, it is the lower energy one which has the highest intensity.

targets of X-ray tubes and involved in X-ray production. The main element used is tungsten.

To understand characteristic X-ray production, we need to consider the electron structure of atoms. Electrons are arranged in shells, with the K-shell electrons being those that are closest to the atomic nucleus. Tungsten, being a large atom, has electrons in K-, L-, M-, N-, O and P-shells, with the outer shell electrons being those that are involved in chemical bonding. The electron shells have fixed energy levels, these levels being characteristic of tungsten. Fig. 11.7 illustrates two important concepts that are easily confused—electron binding energy and electron potential energy.

Concept 1. Electron binding energy is the amount of energy that must be applied to eject an electron from its shell. Electrons are held in proximity to the atomic nucleus by the electrostatic attraction that exists between opposite charges and so the innermost (K-shell) electrons are the most tightly bound. Imagine them as being deep down a well—it would take a lot of energy to pull them out of the well and set them free. The binding energy of K-shell electrons increases with the atomic number of the element, because the greater number of protons in the nucleus will exert a greater attractive force on them. Thus binding energy increases with atomic number, and the binding energy of K-shell electrons in tungsten is greater than that in molybdenum. Binding energy increases with shell distance from the atomic nucleus, as shown by Table 11.2.

Concept 2. Electron potential energy is the amount of energy that an electron has by virtue of its location in an atom's electron shells. Electrons in outer shells are less

TABLE 11.2 Approximate binding energies of electrons held in the electron shells of a tungsten atom

Electron shell	Approximate electron binding energy, keV
P	0.02
O	0.1
N	0.6
M	3
L	11
K	69

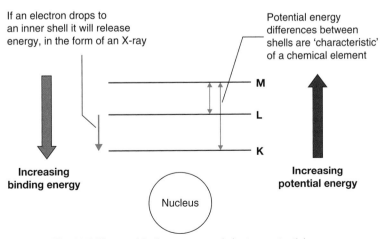

Fig. 11.7 Electron binding energy and electron potential energy.

tightly bound to the atomic nucleus and can be considered to be more 'energetic'. Imagine them as being higher up in a well, having been pulled up against the attractive force of the nucleus. If they are 'let go' and drop down to a lower position in the well, they will release potential energy. If a hole suddenly appears deeper down the well, one of these outer electrons will drop down into it, with the release of energy. This process within electron shells results in the production of characteristic X-rays, whose energy is characteristic of the potential energy difference between two electron shells, and hence of the element. The concept of electrons occupying fixed energy levels and being able to drop between these levels with a release of an X-ray photon can be considered to be a part of quantum theory, in which energy can be regarded as little packets of energy called 'quanta'.

In the process of characteristic X-ray production, an innermost (K-shell) electron from a tungsten atom in the X-ray tube target is ejected by an inelastic interaction with a fast-moving filament electron. This leaves a vacancy in the K-shell which is unstable and is immediately filled by an electron 'dropping down' from the L-shell or M-shell, with the release of electron potential energy in the form of an X-ray. Because the potential energy difference between the M- and K-shells is greater than the potential energy difference between the L- and K-shells, an electron dropping from the M-shell to the K-shell will produce a higher energy X-ray than will an electron dropping from the L- to the K-shell. These transitions will produce Kβ and Kα characteristic X-rays, as shown by Fig. 11.8.

In the case of tungsten, these characteristic emissions will produce spectral lines at about 67 keV and 59 keV respectively, as shown by Fig. 11.9. The lower energy line will be of greater intensity because electron transitions between the L- and K-shells, producing X-rays of about 59 keV, are

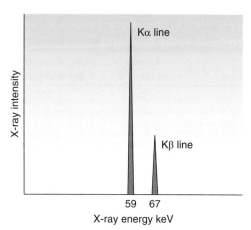

Fig. 11.9 The characteristic X-ray spectrum for tungsten.

the most likely. This is because the L- and K-shells are in close proximity. Note that characteristic X-rays can only be produced if the energy of the speeding filament electron is greater than the binding energy of the K-shell electron. Thus characteristic X-rays from tungsten can only be produced if the filament electron has 69 keV energy or above (see Table 11.2). This means that characteristic X-rays from a tungsten target can only result when the voltage across the X-ray tube is 69 kVp or higher.

Only characteristic X-rays resulting from the ejection of K-shell electrons are of practical consequence in medical imaging. These 'K lines' of about 59 to 67 keV energy for tungsten are energetic enough to penetrate through a patient's body and contribute to the radiographic image. But it should be mentioned that the speeding electrons from the filament can also eject electrons from any of the other tungsten shells. Electron shell transitions will also occur in these cases, but the resulting characteristic X-rays are too low in energy to escape from the X-ray tube. The energies of these other characteristic X-ray emissions for tungsten are shown in Table 11.3.

INSIGHT

The characteristic K lines for tungsten and for other elements, when examined closely, can be split into several peaks that are quite close together in terms of their X-ray energy. This is because the electrons occupying the L-, M- and other shells of an atom are found occupying subsidiary potential energy levels. For example, the L-shell comprises electrons found in s and p orbitals, at slightly different energies. Any of these electrons can 'drop down' to fill a vacancy in the K-shell, giving very slightly different X-ray energies. For this reason it can be hard to state a precise single energy for a characteristic X-ray emission. The practical consequence of this is small, however.

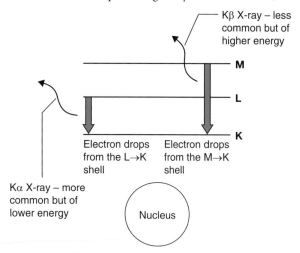

Fig. 11.8 Production of Kα and Kβ characteristic X-rays.

TABLE 11.3   Characteristic X-ray emissions for tungsten

Electron shell	Electron transition	X-ray energy, keV
K-shell	L → K Kα line	59
	M → K Kβ line	67
L-shell	M → L Lα line	9
	N → L Lβ line	11
M-shell	N → M Mα line	2
	O → M Mβ line	3
N-shell	O → N Nα line	0.5
	P → N Nβ line	0.6

Only the K-lines are of practical importance in medical imaging

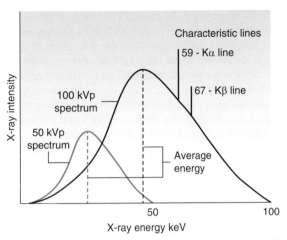

Fig. 11.10 The complete X-ray spectrum for tungsten, at kVp values of 50 and 100.

11.5   THE COMPLETE X-RAY SPECTRUM

So far in this chapter we have considered the production of X-ray quanta by two major mechanisms:

1. Bremsstrahlung. Energetic electrons from the filament interact with the nuclei of target atoms and are slowed down, thus giving off energy in the form of X-ray quanta—Bremsstrahlung radiation. As we mentioned earlier, the energy of the quantum may be very small if the interaction with the nucleus is small, or it may be up to the energy of the incoming electron if this electron is brought to rest by the nucleus. All energies between the two extremes are possible and so it can be seen that the Bremsstrahlung radiation will form a continuous X-ray spectrum.

2. Characteristic radiation. Vacancies created in inner electron shells (especially the K-shell for practical purposes) are filled by the electrons from shells further away from the nucleus making a quantum drop to fill the vacancy and giving off a photon of radiation in the process. This is the characteristic radiation from the atom. As the energy differences between specific shells is constant for an atom, this will take the form of a series of line spectra.

If the overall X-ray intensity is plotted against the energy of the radiation, a summation of the two effects known as the *X-ray spectrum* is produced. Such a spectrum produced at the tungsten target of an X-ray tube is shown in Fig. 11.10. Spectra produced at two different kVp values are shown.

Certain important features of this spectrum are worthy of further discussion:

- The energy of the continuous or Bremsstrahlung radiation is expressed in keV and lies somewhere between zero and a maximum value. This maximum photon energy is achieved if an electron which has the maximum kinetic energy gives up all its energy to form a single photon. The value of this photon for a specific beam may be deduced as follows. Suppose the potential difference across the X-ray tube is 100 kVp. An electron accelerated across the tube when the peak voltage is applied would have achieved a kinetic energy of 100 keV at its point of contact with the anode. If it now gives up all this energy as a single photon, the energy of the photon will be 100 keV and this will be the maximum photon energy for a tube operating at this kVp. Similarly, for an X-ray tube operating at 50 kVp, the maximum photon energy will be 50 keV. Thus it can be seen that the maximum photon energy is dependent on the potential difference across the tube (kVp) but is independent of the material of the target.

- The average energy of the X-ray beam is about one-third to one-half of its maximum; this is related to the 'quality' of the X-ray beam.

- The total intensity of the beam—the quantity of the radiation—is given by the area under the curve.

- The energies of the *K, L, M*, and so on lines are always in the same position for a given target element, although the energy of lines from L onwards is so small that it is likely to be totally absorbed in the X-ray tube. These discrete energies form a line spectrum.

- The line spectra will not be produced unless the energy of the electron beam from the filament exceeds the binding energy of the appropriate electron shell of the atom. To produce the K characteristic lines at a tungsten target, electrons must have an energy of 69 keV or higher, and to produce L lines, electrons must have an energy 11 keV or higher. In practice, this means that K lines are not produced when the potential across the tube is less than 70 kVp.

In the spectrum shown in Fig. 11.10 we have plotted the intensity of the radiation plotted against the photon energy. Note that 'intensity' is often considered in terms of numbers of X-rays in medical imaging. It is sometimes useful to calculate the wavelength of the radiation rather than know its photon energy. As you may remember from Section 8.6, the photon energy and its associated wavelength are related by Planck's equation (see Equation 8.2). From this we can see that the maximum photon energy corresponds to the minimum wavelength. Because the numerical value of the maximum photon energy expressed in keV is the same as the kVp, we can calculate the minimum wavelength from the equation:

$$\lambda_{min} = \frac{1.24}{kVp} \qquad \textbf{Equation 11.1}$$

INSIGHT

Speeding electrons from the X-ray tube filament will be brought to a halt in the tungsten target in quite a short distance, less than a millimetre. They will have more kinetic energy initially and thus the most energetic X-rays will be emitted in the very shallow layers of the target. Deeper into the target material, the kinetic energy of the filament electrons will have dropped to the point where only lower energy X-rays, which are more likely to be absorbed in the target itself, are emitted. Thus the 'useful thickness' of the target material is quite small. This can become an issue if a target becomes 'pitted' and worn as a result of heat damage from long-term use.

Fig. 11.10 also shows the effect of increasing the kVp on an X-ray spectrum. The following things occur as we increase the kVp:

- The total number of X-rays produced ('intensity') increases greatly. In fact this increase is proportional to the kVp squared, as was mentioned in Section 11.2.
- The maximum possible X-ray energy (or peak energy) increases.
- The average X-ray energy increases (as shown by the shift to the right of the highest point or 'hill' on the continuous X-ray spectrum curve).
- Characteristic lines may now appear (these will have been absent at a kVp <69).
- Note that the energy of characteristic lines is not affected by the kVp.

Table 11.4 shows the effect of various factors on a complete X-ray spectrum.

Increasing either the current across the X-ray tube (mA) or the exposure time(s) or the two in combination (mAs) will provide a greater number of electrons striking the X-ray tube target. This in turn will produce more X-rays. The relationship is direct and so a doubling of electrons will double the number of X-rays produced.

Increasing the atomic number of the X-ray tube target material (e.g., using tungsten instead of molybdenum) will increase the efficiency of Bremsstrahlung, because of greater braking of radiations. This will increase the number of X-rays produced and will also shift the average energy of the Bremsstrahlung a bit higher. In addition, any emitted characteristic rays will be of higher energy.

TABLE 11.4	**Effects of various factors on the complete X-ray spectrum**		
Factor	Effect on the number of X-rays (intensity)	Effect on the energy of the X-rays	Effect on the characteristic X-ray K lines
Increasing kVp	Large increase, proportional to kV²	Increase in peak and average energy	K lines will not be present <69 kVp. whereas >69kVp, K-line intensity will be affected by kVp
Increasing mA	Increase	No effect	Increase in intensity but no change in energy
Increasing exposure time(s)	Increase	No effect	Increase in intensity but no change in energy
Increasing the atomic number of the X-ray tube target	Increase	No effect on the peak energy but an increase in the average energy	The energy of the K lines will increase
Increasing X-ray beam filtration	An overall decrease, but especially for low-energy X-rays	Average energy will increase	No effect on energy but intensity may decrease

Increasing the filtration of the X-ray beam, for example, using an aluminium sheet attached to the X-ray tube assembly, will remove lower energy 'soft' X-rays preferentially. This has the effect of 'hardening' the beam, which means increasing its average energy and penetrating power. This in turn can help to reduce a patient's absorbed radiation dose.

SUMMARY

In this chapter, you should have learnt the following:

- X-ray production occurs when high-speed electrons from the filament of an X-ray tube interact with atoms in the X-ray tube target.
- These filament electrons experience many interactions with the X-ray tube target atoms, about 99% of which only result in heat emission at diagnostic X-ray tube voltages.
- X-ray production mainly occurs via Bremsstrahlung, the 'braking' of these electrons, which accounts for most X-rays produced. This results in a continuous range of X-ray energies.

- A subsidiary process is called characteristic X-ray production. These X-rays are produced at fixed energies which are characteristic of the atomic number of the element contained in the X-ray tube target.
- The kVp, mA, exposure time, X-ray tube target element and filtration all affect the properties of an X-ray beam.

FURTHER READING

Allisy-Roberts, P.J., & Williams, J. 2007. *Farr's Physics for Medical Imaging*. 2nd edn. Edinburgh: Saunders.

Ball, J.L., Moore, A.D., & Turner, S. 2008. *Ball and Moore's Essential Physics for Radiographers*. 4th edn. London: Blackwell Scientific. (Chapter 16.)

Bushong, S. 2016. *Radiologic Science for Technologists: Physics, Biology, and Protection*. 11th edn. New York: Mosby. (Chapter 7.)

Dendy, P., & Heaton, B. 2011. *Physics for Diagnostic Radiology*. 3rd edn. Boca Raton, Florida: CRC Press. (Chapter 2.)

The diagnostic X-ray tube

CHAPTER CONTENTS

12.1 AIM

The aim of this chapter is to discuss the components and operations of diagnostic X-ray tubes. All X-ray tubes are descended from the cathode ray tube, which was used by Wilhelm Roentgen in 1895 to accidentally detect the mysterious invisible rays that were named *X-rays* because of their unknown nature. The cathode tube consisted of a partially evacuated glass tube with a negatively charged cathode and a positively charged anode, with a large electrical potential difference between them. The applied voltage caused electrons to be drawn from the cathode to the anode, acquiring kinetic energy as they travelled and producing X-rays plus heat when they struck the anode. William Coolidge improved on the design when he introduced his Coolidge tube in 1913, which contained a more complete vacuum as well as anode improvements. However, the glass tubes were still used without any protective lead casing in the early years of medical imaging, showing a lack of awareness of the damaging effects of ionising radiation. X-ray tubes have advanced a lot since the early 1900s but are still based on this fundamental cathode and anode design.

12.2 INTRODUCTION

The rotating anode X-ray tube is the most common type of X-ray tube found in diagnostic imaging departments. The reason for this is that it can produce higher intensities of X-rays than the stationary anode tube. This is the result of two factors:

1. The heat deposited in the anode during an X-ray exposure is spread over a larger area and so there is a smaller temperature rise at the anode surface.
2. The cooling characteristics of the rotating anode are superior to those of the stationary anode and this effective

dissipation of heat means that larger loads can be applied without causing thermal damage to the target.

The stationary anode tube has a very low rating (meaning that its heat capacity is low) and is found only in dental and some portable X-ray units. These units are connected to a single phase 240-volt mains supply. This limits the amount of electrical power that can be applied to it, preventing overloading of the tube.

12.3   CONSTRUCTION OF X-RAY TUBES

The X-ray tube assembly consists of two main components: the insert and the tube shield (housing).

These components and the light-beam diaphragm (the role of which will be discussed later in this chapter) are shown in Fig. 12.1. The components of this tube are dis-

cussed individually in Section 12.5. Although the inserts for the rotating anode tube and the stationary anode tube differ substantially, the shields for both types of tube are very similar in design and function.

12.4   CONSTRUCTION OF THE TUBE SHIELD (HOUSING)

It is necessary to protect the patient and the operator from the electrical and radiation hazards posed by the X-ray tube insert while in operation. The insert is incorporated within a suitable container—the shield—which must satisfy the following criteria:
- There must be no danger of electrical shock if the shield is touched during operation of the X-ray tube.

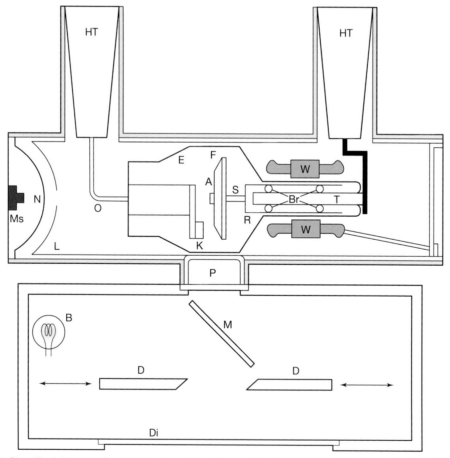

Fig. 12.1 Simplified diagram of a rotating anode X-ray tube and diaphragm assembly. *A*, Anode disc; *B*, light bulb; *Br*, bearings; *D*, moveable diaphragms (only one pair shown); *Di*, plastic diaphragm front; *E*, glass envelope; *F*, focal track; *HT*, high-tension socket; *K*, cathode assembly; *L*, lead lining; *M*, mirror; *Ms*, microswitch; *N*, bellows; *O*, oil; *P*, tube port and aluminium filter; *R*, rotor assembly; *S*, anode stem; *T*, rotor support; *W*, stator windings.

- No significant amounts of radiation should escape from the shield other than the radiation necessary for taking the radiograph.
- The shield must give secure support to the X-ray tube insert, the high-tension (high-voltage) cables and the other connecting cables within the shield.
- Adequate electrical insulation must be provided between the insert and the tube shield to avoid breakdown and 'sparking'.
- There must be adequate cooling of the insert and facilities to permit operation without overheating which would cause an automatic 'cut-out'.
- There must be facilities at the tube port to allow adequate filtration of the emergent beam so that low-energy radiations may be removed from the beam.

As can be seen from this list, the shield must satisfy many requirements. A schematic diagram of the shield for a rotating anode X-ray tube is shown in Fig. 12.1. Note that the insert is held in position by a support at the anode end.

The metal casing surrounding the insert is made of either aluminium or steel and is lined with about 3 mm of lead to provide sufficient radiation protection. This housing is filled with pure oil that acts as an electrical insulator and as a coolant. A neoprene rubber diaphragm at one end of the shield allows for expansion of the oil when the oil is heated. The assembly is usually fitted with a microswitch, which will prevent further exposures if the oil is very hot. Within the casing there is a radiolucent window—the tube port—which will allow the useful or primary beam of radiation to leave the tube via the light-beam diaphragm.

12.4.1   Electrical safety

Electrical safety is designed around four basic principles:
1. Insulation of live components.
2. Earthing of component housings.
3. Restricted access to live components.
4. Isolation of the circuits from the mains supply when not in use.

All these features are used in the design of the X-ray tube. Insulation exists between the live components and the housing in the form of the oil in the housing. The resistance of an electrical insulator (and so its insulating properties) diminishes as the temperature of the insulator increases and so the role of the oil in heat dissipation is also important from the point of view of electrical safety.

The tube shield is connected to earth via the outer braiding of the high-tension cables (Fig. 12.2) and so the casing will always remain at earth potential. If an electrically 'live' wire within the casing becomes disconnected and touches the shield, then the current will readily flow to

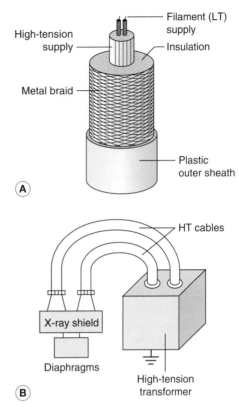

Fig. 12.2 (A) Structure of a high-tension (*HT*) cable. Note the thickness of the insulation surrounding the central conductors. (B) The X-ray tube shield is made electrically safe by connecting the copper braiding of the HT cables to both the shield and the casing of the high-tension transformer tank. The latter is securely earthed. *LT*, Low-tension.

earth and the casing will present minimal electrical hazard to someone touching it at the time.

The electrically 'live' components in the X-ray tube are secured inside the tube shield and the ends and the high-tension cable connectors are securely fixed. This means that, under normal circumstances, the operator has no easy access to the live components. In addition, the circuits may be isolated from the mains by switches, fuses or circuit breakers.

12.4.2   Radiation safety

Radiation safety is important for the operators of X-ray equipment and for patients and others who may be in the vicinity at the time of making an X-ray exposure. The lead lining of the tube housing (Fig. 12.1) limits the radiation leakage from the tube and so provides protection to both the operator and the patient. Remember that X-rays are emitted in all directions from the focus on the anode, but only those which pass through the tube port are allowed to leave the housing. The anode itself has a high X-ray absorption and so the lead lining at the anode end of the shield is often absent or thinner than at the cathode end.

The radiation leakage rate from the tube is normally measured at a distance of 1 metre from the housing and should not exceed an air kerma of 1.00 milliGray per hour, measured at a distance of 1 metre from the focus (for definitions of the kerma and the Gray, see Chapter 21). Any break in the lead lining will result in radiation leakage from the tube, so the leakage levels should be checked at regular intervals as part of the quality checks on the X-ray unit.

Radiation safety means exposing the patient only to the minimum dose necessary to produce a radiograph of acceptable quality. As we saw in Chapter 11, the spectrum of X-rays produced at the target is a continuous spectrum containing a mix of low-, medium- and high-energy photons. Some of the photons have very low energy and will not be able to pass through the patient to reach the image receptor. These photons would contribute to the patient dose but not to the image production. Some of these are removed by the glass envelope of the insert and the oil as the beam passes to the tube port. This is known as the *inherent filtration* of the tube. Further filtration takes place through the aluminium filters placed at the tube port (Fig. 12.1). These are known as *added filtration*. Thus, the total filtration of the beam is determined by the inherent filtration plus the added filtration. Details of this information are frequently marked on the end of the shield.

Scattered radiation contributes to the patient dose and the operator dose and causes degradation in the radiographic image quality. The amount of scatter produced at a given set of exposure factors is dependent on the volume of tissue irradiated. The volume can be reduced by reducing the area irradiated using a light-beam diaphragm (Fig. 12.1). This also means that parts of the body not required on the radiograph can be protected from radiation. In this way, adequate collimation using the lead shutters in the light-beam diaphragm will reduce the patient dose and the operator dose and produce an improvement in the image quality.

12.5 CONSTRUCTION OF THE ROTATING ANODE TUBE INSERT

12.5.1 Insert envelope

X-ray production is at its most efficient when a vacuum exists between the cathode and the anode of the X-ray tube, so these structures are enclosed within an evacuated metal or heatproof glass envelope, which must be sufficiently strong to preserve this vacuum. Where a glass enve-

lope is used, it is joined to the anode spindle at one end and to the nickel cathode support at the other end by reentrant seals—so called because the glass is shaped to point inwards at the area of contact. Slightly different glass seals are used at each end so that the thermal expansion of the glass is similar to that of the metal used in the construction of the anode spindle and cathode. This reduces the stress on the glass when the insert is hot and so limits the chance of cracking. The glass must be a good electrical insulator or a substantial current will flow through it when the high potential difference is applied between the anode and the cathode. However, electrical charges are built up on the inside of the glass during operation and so the glass must have sufficient electrical conductivity to allow these to leak away, usually between exposures, avoiding the buildup of high amounts of static charge. The glass is gently rounded so that there are no sharp corners, which would allow the buildup of high amounts of static charge.

During operation of the X-ray tube, a thin film of tungsten will be deposited on the inside of the envelope as a result of the release of tungsten vapour from the filament and the target. This film acts as a filter to emergent radiation and, where a glass envelope is used, may eventually cause electrical breakdown within the tube because it can act as an electrical conductor around the inside wall of the glass envelope. If this happens, the tube is classed as gassy and is of no further use. The rate of tungsten vaporisation can be reduced by not keeping the tube in the preexposure 'prep' (preparation) mode any longer than is required when using the exposure switch and by keeping exposures well within the heat rating of the tube.

Some modern X-ray tubes use a metal insert rather than a glass one. As shown in Fig. 12.3, metal envelopes do not completely surround the insert. The cathode end of the envelope is formed from a ceramic material to provide the necessary electrical insulation between the anode and the cathode. The metal component of the envelope is earthed and, as a result, there is no buildup of

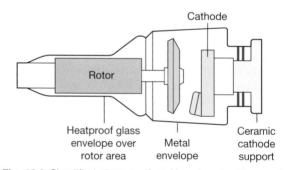

Fig. 12.3 Simplified diagram of an X-ray insert with a metal envelope.

static charges on the metal envelope. This improves the focusing of the electron beam within the insert and reduces the effect of the buildup of vaporised tungsten on the inner walls of the envelope.

12.5.2   The anode assembly

The simplest anode configuration is shown in Fig. 12.4 where the anode consists of a disc with an accurately bevelled edge on which is deposited a target track. A number of different materials are used in the design of the anode disc, as shown in Table 12.1. A small amount of rhenium, which has an atomic number and melting point similar to that of tungsten, is alloyed with the tungsten of the target track. This improves the thermal expansion of the target track, making it more resistant to pitting. Mammography X-ray tubes (see Chapter 18) may use molybdenum ($Z = 42$) as a target material because of its useful low-energy characteristic radiation K lines.

Tungsten is used as the main component in the target track for the following reasons:

- Tungsten has a high atomic number ($Z = 74$) and so is an efficient producer of X-rays (see Chapter 11).
- Tungsten has a high melting point (3387° C), so it can withstand the heat generated during the X-ray exposure without melting.
- Tungsten has a low vapour pressure, so it does not readily vaporise at its normal working temperature.
- Tungsten can be readily machined to give the smooth surface required for X-ray production.

The bevelled anode target edge permits the use of the line focus principle. This results in an effective focus that is smaller than the real focus. The real focus can be longer than the effective focus. Thus the filament may be relatively long without giving rise to excessive geometric unsharpness. Thermionic emission from the filament is proportional to its surface area and so a long filament will provide the high values of mA required by many exposures. The

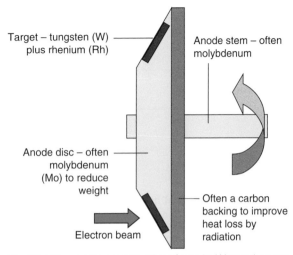

Fig. 12.4 The detailed construction of a typical X-ray tube rotating anode.

area over which the heat is deposited is the larger area of the real focus as shown in Fig. 12.5. This is smaller than the apparent focus. The advantage of the line focus principle is that the temperature rise experienced by a large area for a given amount of heat is less than that experienced by a small area because more atoms are able to take part in the heat dissipation processes. The line focus principle enables the anode to be designed so that the area of the real focus is about three times the area of the apparent focus. This enables a reasonable compromise between the need to minimise the temperature rise at the target (thus requiring a large focal area) and the need for minimising the geometric unsharpness (thus requiring a small focal area). The anode face is usually set at an angle between 7 degrees and 15 degrees to the central axis of the X-ray beam. This is called *the target angle.*

TABLE 12.1	Materials used in the design of X-ray tube anodes	
Material	**Use**	**Reason for use**
Molybdenum $Z = 42$	Anode disc and stem (also the target in mammography X-ray tubes)	Half the density and twice the specific heat capacity of tungsten. Melting point 2600° C
Tungsten $Z = 74$	Focal track (90%)	High atomic number. High melting point about 3400° C. Low vapour pressure. Strong, ductile
Rhenium $Z = 75$	Focal track (10%)	More elastic than tungsten, therefore less pitting of the focal track. High melting point 3180° C
Graphite $Z = 6$	Anode disc backing	Low density, light, strong. Acts as 'heat sink'. Radiates heat by black-body radiation. Melting point about 4000° C
Copper $Z = 29$	Stationary anode block	Electrically conductive, good heat transmitter, high heat capacity, melting point 1080° C

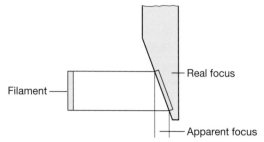

Fig. 12.5 The line focus principle. Because of the angulation of the anode, apparent focus is much smaller than the real focus.

The disc has a central hole in it through which it is connected to a molybdenum anode stem and hence to the rotor of the induction motor (see Fig. 12.1). The rotor, stem and anode disc are accurately balanced so that no appreciable wobble occurs when the whole assembly rotates. The rotor is made to spin by the rotating magnetic fields produced by the stator coils situated externally to the insert, using the principles of electromagnetic induction. The rotor moves smoothly on steel ball bearings coated in a soft metal, such as tin or silver, which acts as a lubricant but does not destroy the vacuum inside the envelope; a lubricant such as oil would evaporate and compromise the vacuum. The rotating magnetic field produced by the stator coils causes the rotor (and thus the anode disc) to rotate at the same frequency as the applied voltage.

The rotation of the anode during the exposure has the effect of lengthening the area bombarded by the electron beam (think of using a whole lap of a circular racetrack rather than just a part of it), reducing the amount of heat generated per unit area even further. The positive terminal from the high-tension supply is connected to the rotor support, and through this there is a continuous electrical connection to the anode disc.

The conduction of heat from the anode disc to the ball bearings is inhibited by the fact that the anode stem has a small cross-sectional area and is made of molybdenum (a relatively poor thermal conductor). However, some heat will inevitably reach the ball bearings and could cause sufficient expansion to produce a risk of seizure. This risk is reduced by applying a black coating to the outer surface of the rotor so that it loses heat efficiently by black-body radiation (see Chapter 3).

Many modern X-ray tubes also have carbon graphite backing on the anode disc, as shown by Fig. 12.4. This has a greater thermal capacity than molybdenum and draws heat from the anode and then dissipates it by black-body radiation. This results in the possibility of greater loads being applied to the anode and in reduced heat dissipation to the ball bearings.

12.5.3   The anode heel effect

Consider Fig. 12.6. X-rays are produced slightly below the surface of the target material. X-rays passing along path 1 will therefore pass through a smaller section of the target than those passing along path 2. There is absorption of the

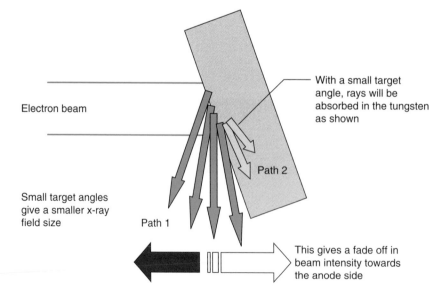

Fig. 12.6 The anode heel effect. An X-ray photon following path 2 is more attenuated than one following path 1, owing to its longer path through the tungsten target.

X-rays as they pass through the target and so the rays that pass through the greatest thickness of the target are the more heavily absorbed; there will be a lower intensity of X-rays along path 2 than along path 1. This means that the X-ray intensity at the anode end of the beam will be less than at the central axis, whereas the intensity at the cathode end will be greater than at the central axis. This is known as the *anode heel effect*. The effect increases as the target angle is reduced and increases with the age of the X-ray tube. This latter increase is the result of the target becoming pitted with use.

12.5.4   The cathode assembly

The terms 'cathode' and 'filament' are often interchanged when discussing the X-ray tube. However, the correct usage of the term cathode implies the whole cathode assembly, including the filament, focusing cup, supporting wires and cathode support. The filament is therefore part of the cathode, but the cathode is not part of the filament.

The focusing cup, which supports the filaments, is offset from the central axis of the tube so that the electrons emitted from the filaments are aligned with the bevelled edge of the anode disc. It is made of either nickel or stainless steel, each of which has a high melting point and is a relatively poor thermionic emitter—each has a high thermionic work function. In addition, the thermal expansion of these materials is close to that of certain types of glass, thus reducing the stress on the seals during operation of the tube. When the filaments produce electrons by thermionic emission, these would repel each other by electrostatic repulsion—'like' charges repel—and so would strike a large area of focal spot. The area of the focal spot is reduced by the negative bias on the focusing cup which 'squeezes' the electrons together.

The filaments are made of a thin tungsten wire for the following reasons:

- Tungsten has a low thermionic work function and so will readily emit electrons by thermionic emission.
- Tungsten has a low vapour pressure and so does not easily evaporate. This helps prolong the life of the filament, as evaporation would cause the wire to become thin. It also prolongs the life of the tube as it prevents the formation of a tungsten film on the inner wall of the glass envelope.
- Tungsten is a strong metal that can be drawn into a thin wire that will not easily distort. This helps to maintain the shape of the filament helix over a period of time.

A rotating anode X-ray tube usually has two filaments. They may be positioned side by side, as shown in Fig. 12.7. This is known as a *dual-focus tube*. Alternatively they may be positioned end to end, which means that the electron beams fall on different parts of the bevelled surface of the anode disc, which can be set at differing angles. This in-line

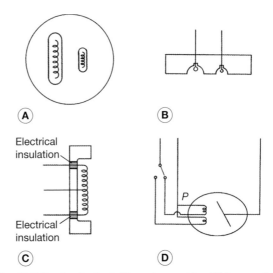

Fig. 12.7 Details of cathode filament assemblies. (A) Face-on view of dual filaments; (B) dual filaments viewed from above; (C) in-line filaments viewed from the side; (D) electrical connections.

configuration with different anode angles is referred to as a *biangular tube*. Smaller anode target angles are often associated with smaller effective focal spot sizes, as shown by Fig. 12.8. In both instances, the differing sizes of filament result in differing sizes of electron foci on the anode. The larger is known as the *broad* focus and would be used in situations where a high radiation output was required from the tube, whereas the smaller (the *fine* focus) would be used in situations where it is desirable to keep geometric unsharpness to a minimum. One side of each filament is connected to the focusing cup whereas the other is insulated from it (Fig. 12.7C). This connection between both filaments also forms the common connection between the filament circuit and the high-tension circuit. This is represented by point *P* in Fig. 12.7D. From this diagram, it can be seen that three conductors are required in the high-tension cable coming to the cathode end of the X-ray tube. The secondary side of the filament transformer is also connected to one side of the high-tension circuit, and this transformer could be a source of electrical hazard to the operator of the X-ray unit. For this reason and for reasons of ensuring good electrical insulation and heat dissipation, the filament transformer is contained in the same oil-filled tank as the high-tension transformer. All high-tension cables for X-ray units contain at least three conducting wires, even though only one is required at the anode end of the tube. This means that manufacturers only need to make (and X-ray departments only need to stock) one type of cable. Only one of the three wires at the anode end is used to make an electrical connection to the tube.

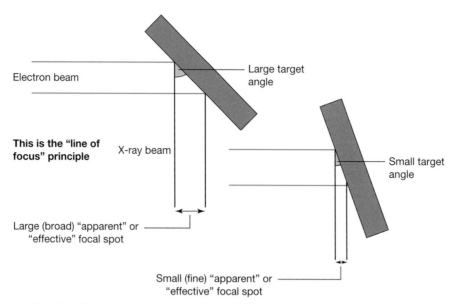

Fig. 12.8 Showing how the target angle can affect the size of the apparent focal spot.

12.6   CONSTRUCTION OF THE STATIONARY ANODE TUBE INSERT

12.6.1   The anode

The anode of the stationary anode tube, like the rotating anode, is constructed of two materials, copper and tungsten, and so is known as a *compound anode*. The main part of the anode assembly is made of copper because of its good thermal conductivity. The face of the anode is inclined at an angle of about 15 degrees to the central axis of the insert and has an inset of a thin (about 2–3 mm) tungsten plate known as the *target* on which the electrons are focused. This type of anode is suitable for relatively small X-ray exposures only because of its limited heat capacity and is shown by Fig. 12.9.

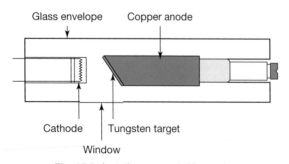

Fig. 12.9 A stationary anode X-ray tube.

12.6.2   Cathode and filament

The basic construction of the cathode is the same as that of the cathode of a rotating anode tube. The main differences in construction are that the focusing cup is aligned along the central axis of the insert and there is only a single filament present.

12.7   PRINCIPLES OF OPERATION OF THE X-RAY TUBE

As we have seen in Chapter 11, X-rays are produced by electrons which are accelerated from the cathode to the anode of the X-ray tube. The number of electrons crossing the tube is controlled at the mA selector, whereas the kinetic energy of the electrons (and thus the photon energy of the X-ray beam) is indicated by the kV selector.

12.7.1   Thermionic emission

The electrons are emitted by the heated filament by a process termed *thermionic emission*. In atoms, the outer shell electrons are more loosely bound than the inner electrons because they are further away from the nucleus (remember $F \propto 1/d^2$). The application of heat to a body increases the kinetic energy of its atoms and so increases the violence of their collisions. Because of these collisions, the outer electrons may be dislodged from the atom. Electrons so released near the centre of a body travel only a relatively short distance, but if they are released near the surface of the material, they may have sufficient kinetic energy to leave the body.

The higher the temperature of a body, the greater the kinetic energy of the atoms, and the greater number of electrons with sufficient energy to break free from the influence of the surface atoms of the body. The electrons, which are released by thermionic emission, are released from the surface atomic layers of the body. It follows that any alteration to these outer layers will alter the ability of a body to perform as a thermionic emitter. This has two practical consequences in radiography:

1. All the surfaces involved in thermionic emission (e.g., the tube filament) must be manufactured to a high degree of purity and must be kept scrupulously clean during assembly.
2. The thermionic emission characteristics of a body may be altered by the deliberate addition of 'impurities' either to the whole body or just to the body surface.

The efficiency of thermionic emitters may be evaluated by comparing their work function, which is normally expressed in electron volts (eV). The work function is the amount of work that must be performed by an electron in escaping from the body. Alternatively, it can be considered as the amount of work that must be performed on an electron to enable it to escape from the body. Substances which are good thermionic emitters have a lower work function than those that are poor thermionic emitters because, in the former, less work is required to allow the electrons to escape.

From this discussion, it should be apparent that the amount of thermionic emission from a body is controlled by:

• the temperature of the body
• the material of the body
• the surface area of the body.

The relationship between the temperature of a tungsten filament and the number of electrons liberated in unit time is shown in Fig. 12.10.

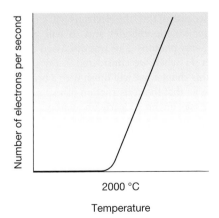

Fig. 12.10 Graph of thermionic emission against temperature for a tungsten filament. Note that a small change in temperature produces a large change in emission.

12.7.2 The space charge effect

If we assume that a body is electrically neutral before the application of heat, then each electron which leaves the body by thermionic emission will cause the body to have a net positive charge. After a very short time, a state of equilibrium is set up where electrons leave the body and enter a 'cloud' of electrons near its surface and are then attracted back to the body, that is, electrons are attracted back to the body as fast as they are emitted. The number of electrons in this cloud remains fairly constant because electrons are entering and leaving the cloud at equal rates. This cloud of electrons is known as the *space charge*. If the temperature of the body is increased, then the number of electrons in the space charge will also increase because of the increased electron emission from the body. If the body is left to cool, it will reduce the space charge to zero by attracting electrons from it back to the body.

INSIGHT

If we take a normal tungsten filament light bulb and switch it on, then the filament of this bulb is producing significant numbers of electrons by thermionic emission. These electrons form a space charge around the filament and return to it in the process described above. If we bring a large positive charge close to this light bulb, we can cause these electrons to 'flash over' to this positively charged body. If we switch off the power supply to the bulb, the filament cools down almost immediately, thermionic emission ceases and no further flash over occurs until the bulb is switched on again. If a positively charged body is placed close to the space charge, then some of the electrons within the space charge will be attracted towards that body and so an electrical current flows between the heated body and the positive body via the space charge.

12.7.3 Tube current and filament current

Fig. 12.11 shows a circuit diagram of the X-ray tube and high-tension circuit which has been greatly simplified to illustrate the difference between the tube current (mA) and the filament current (I_f). The relationship between the temperature of the tungsten filament and the number of electrons released by thermionic emission has already been discussed in Section 12.7.1. This section will look at the application of this information to the X-ray tube. In Fig. 12.11, B_1 represents the power supply across the X-ray tube and B_2 represents the power supply across the filament. Suppose B_2 causes a current I_f to flow through the filament circuit. The passage of this current through the filament causes the filament to heat and the subsequent temperature rise will cause electrons to be emitted by thermionic emission. These electrons are drawn towards the positive anode and constitute the tube current (mA).

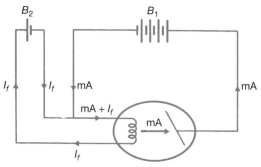

Fig. 12.11 Simplified diagram to show the difference between tube current (mA) and filament heating current (I_f).

When all the electrons in the space charge are 'in use', it is said to be operating under saturation conditions. This is the normal operating condition of the X-ray tube. The only method of increasing the tube current is to increase the number of electrons in the space charge by increasing the temperature of the filament, causing more electrons to be released. Thus, the selection of a given mA by the radiographer determines the filament heating current required to produce that mA. A typical set of filament currents for an X-ray tube is shown in Table 12.2.

12.7.4   Electron focusing

During X-ray exposure, the anode of the X-ray tube is positively charged, and the cathode is negatively charged. As a result of this, the electron space charge emitted from the filament is repelled from the negative cathode and attracted to the positive anode. The situation, which would arise if both the cathode and the anode were flat plates, is shown in Fig. 12.12A. The electric force field (see Chapter 5) consists of parallel lines starting at the anode and finishing at the cathode. Electrons are emitted from the filament, F, and are attracted to the positive anode. However, the electrons repel each other, so the beam of electrons will increase in size as it travels across the X-ray tube. The area, W, on the anode represents an unacceptably large focal area as this would produce a large geometric unsharpness on the resultant radiograph. This problem is overcome by the use of a focusing cup (see Section 12.5.4), as shown in

TABLE 12.2 Filament heating currents for different tube currents for a typical X-ray tube	
Filament heating current (A)	Tube current (mA)
5	200
7.5	400
9	800

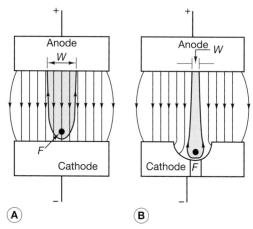

Fig. 12.12 Simplified explanation of the focusing of electrons in the X-ray tube. (A) The result of no focusing cup on the cathode; (B) the electrostatic charge around the concave focusing cup directs the electrons from the thermionic emitter. F, Towards the central axis so they strike a smaller area; W, on the anode.

Fig. 12.12B. The thermionic electrons from F now experience two forces—one towards the anode and the other towards the central axis of the beam. The force towards the central axis of the beam is greater than the force of electrostatic repulsion between the electrons and so the beam of electrons is focused onto a small area of the anode—W in Fig. 12.12B. The interactions between the electron beam and the anode are discussed in more detail in Chapter 11.

12.7.5   Tube voltage

The kVp selected by the radiographer controls the peak potential difference across the X-ray tube. The higher the kVp, the higher the peak potential difference and so the greater the force of attraction between the anode and the cathode. Because of this, the electrons will strike the anode with greater kinetic energies and so will produce more energetic X-ray photons. This was discussed in more detail in Chapter 11 when we considered X-ray production in detail. In this chapter, we will finish with a brief synopsis of the process so that the construction of various parts of the X-ray tube may be more clearly understood.

12.7.6   X-ray production

In the X-ray tube, electrons are produced at the cathode by thermionic emission. These electrons are then accelerated towards the anode and are made to give up their energy when they collide with the atoms of the target material. The main mechanism of X-ray production is when the electron is made to lose kinetic energy because of the pull of the positive nucleus of the target atoms. This is known as *Bremsstrahlung radiation*. The intensity (I) of the Bremsstrahlung radiation varies with both the energy (E) of the electrons striking the target and with the atomic number (Z) of the target material, as shown in the following equations:

$$I \propto Z \times E^2 \qquad \textbf{Equation 12.1}$$

or

$$I \propto Z \times kVp^2 \qquad \textbf{Equation 12.2}$$

The process of X-ray production is very inefficient and up to 99% of the energy of the electrons may be converted into heat, which must rapidly be transferred from the focal area to avoid damage to the target of the tube.

12.8   X-RAY TUBE RATING

12.8.1   Definition of rating

The general term *rating* is used to describe the practical limits that are inherent in any device. An example of this is that a fuse rated at 5 amperes will tolerate currents up to 5 amperes. If a current above 5 amperes passes through the fuse, then the fuse will melt, causing a break in the circuit. Similarly, the rating of an X-ray unit (the X-ray tube and the associated equipment) depends both on how it is constructed and how it is being used. The rating may be defined as follows:

DEFINITION

The rating of an X-ray unit is the combination of exposure settings that the unit can withstand without incurring unacceptable damage.

All radiographic exposures cause slight wear and tear on the X-ray tube; the anode becomes more slightly pitted and the filament becomes slightly thinner as a result of any exposure. However, in this context, unacceptable damage means damage that would seriously impair the performance of the unit for further exposures or might indeed make it inoperative. In this context, a single short exposure where the mA was above the rating of the tube might damage the anode by melting the focal track. Alternatively, a long exposure at low mA may again damage the anode if the total amount of heat generated in the anode caused a sufficient temperature rise to melt the tungsten. It is also true that multiple exposures, each of which is individually within the tube rating, might damage the tube because of the total heat accumulated in the anode by the exposure series. Because the anode takes a finite time to cool after an exposure, the closer the exposures follow each other, the more likely the anode is to suffer thermal damage. For this reason, the ratings for single and multiple exposures will be considered separately in this chapter.

12.8.2   Single exposures

The rating for a single exposure is affected by a number of different factors; some of these are under the control of the operator whereas others are not. In any particular unit, the nonselectable factors are fixed, so a rating must be used which is applicable to that set of circumstances. The rating can be plotted as a graph showing the effect on the rating of varying the quantities in the selectable group. A simplified form of such a graph is shown in Fig. 12.13. Here the rating curve corresponds to a 1.2-mm focus selection and a kVp selection of 80 kVp. The curve indicates the upper limit for all combinations of mA and time for this value of kVp. The points below the line are safe, whereas points above the line are unsafe because they would result in unacceptable damage to the X-ray tube. If we consider an exposure of 80 kVp, 100 mA and 0.2 seconds, then we can see that this exposure may be safely made, as the point P is below the 80-kVp line. Note that because of the wide range of exposure times possible, it is usual to use a logarithmic scale on the x-axis.

It can also be seen from the graph that higher values of mA will be tolerated for short exposure times (150 mA at a time of 0.1 second is within the rating) whereas, at long exposure times, only lower values of mA are within the rating—for an exposure time of 2 seconds, the maximum mA permissible within the rating is 50 mA. In each case, the limiting factor is the anode temperature. For longer exposure times, there can be significant cooling of the anode during the exposure. This is shown by the flattening off of the curve at longer exposure times.

In clinical practice, a range of kVp values is applied to the X-ray tube. Rating calculations take this and the focus size into account, producing separate rating graphs for broad and fine focus. Examples of such graphs are shown

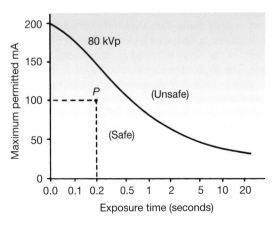

Fig. 12.13 Graph of rating at a single kVp.

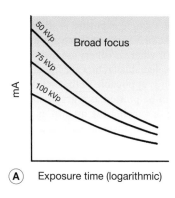

(A)   Exposure time (logarithmic)

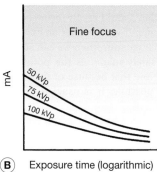

(B)   Exposure time (logarithmic)

Fig. 12.14 Graphs showing the effect of tube focus on rating.

in Fig. 12.14. Fig. 12.14A in the chart is for the broad focus and Fig. 12.14B is for the fine focus. As can be seen from these graphs, the rating of the tube is lower for the fine focus than for the broad focus. This is because, for a fine focus, the electron beam is concentrated onto a smaller area, thus producing a higher temperature rise for the same value of mA.

The figure also shows that larger values of mA are permitted as the kVp is reduced; the difference between the curves is most marked for the shorter exposure times. As was discussed in Chapter 11, electrons are produced at the filament of the X-ray tube and are accelerated towards the anode. The higher the kVp across the tube, the more kinetic energy each electron possesses when it interacts with the anode target. Thus, the same number of electrons per second (mA) will deliver more energy per second to the target and so will increase the possibility of thermal damage. The graph shows this inverse relationship between the kVp and the mA.

For longer exposure times, the thermal capacity (see Chapter 3) of the anode disc is the dominating factor. This is independent of the type of rectification and so the curves all tend to come closer together as the exposure time increases. Also, note that for longer exposure

times the cooling of the tube shield and the heat dissipation within the high-tension transformer are significant factors in determining the rating of the tube and X-ray unit.

12.8.3   Rating of stationary anode and rotating anode X-ray tubes

In the stationary anode X-ray tube, the process of conduction loses heat from the target through the copper anode and thence to the oil surrounding the insert in tube shield. The process is limited by the melting point of copper (1083° C) and the rate at which conduction occurs. As a result, the rating of stationary anode X-ray tubes is much lower than that of rotating anode X-ray tubes. Such X-ray tubes have a very limited application. In the rotating anode X-ray tube, heat loss by conduction is discouraged by the design of the anode stem and the main method of heat loss from the anode is by radiation. Efficient heat loss by radiation is achieved by designing the anode disc so that it can tolerate high temperature rises (remember that the rate of heat loss by radiation is proportional to the fourth power of the kelvin temperature). During large exposures, the anode disc often becomes incandescent and at such temperatures can lose heat effectively by radiation, hence the higher rating of the rotating anode tube.

12.8.4   Effects of anode diameter and speed of rotation on tube rating

When we consider the rating of the rotating anode tube, we must consider not only the material used in its construction and its mass but also the effects of the anode diameter and the rate of anode rotation. In the rotating anode tube, the electrons land on the focal track around the bevelled circumference of the disc. This means that the heat is deposited around the whole disc instead of in the same area, as in the case of the stationary anode tube. Because this heat energy is now deposited over a larger area, there is a smaller temperature rise per unit area and rating is improved.

If we increase the anode diameter, we may increase its mass, but this change also increases its circumference. This means that the heat energy is now deposited over a larger area and, as more atoms are involved in cooling, this leads to more efficient cooling, improving the rating. Doubling the diameter of the disc will increase its rating by 40% to 50%, but this has practical limitations because of the extra mechanical stress this imposes on the bearings. As mentioned in Section 12.9, this can be addressed in modern X-ray tube designs by anchoring the anode spindle at both ends. Doubling the speed of rotation will again increase the rating by about 40% to 50%.

12.8.5   Multiple exposures

When single exposures are made, there is a comparatively long interval between exposures. If a series of exposures is made, there may be insufficient time for the anode disc to cool between exposures. Although every single exposure in this series may be within the rating of the tube, the heating effect of subsequent exposures could raise the temperature of the anode above the permitted level, resulting in thermal damage to the focal track. In such cases, it is necessary to consider additional factors to be able to predict the safety of any combination of exposures.

12.8.6   Anode heating

The anode disc has a given mass and thermal capacity and so there is a given quantity of heat which will raise the whole anode disc to its maximum desirable operating temperature. This is known as the *heat storage capacity* of the anode and is expressed in kilojoules (in the example shown in Fig. 12.15, this is 80,000 kilojoules).

For long exposures such as during fluoroscopy, the cooling, which occurs during the exposure, becomes important in calculating tube ratings. The anode initially heats up fairly quickly but then tends towards a thermal equilibrium, which occurs when the rate of heat generated in the anode by the electron beam is exactly balanced by the rate of heat loss from the anode. Examples of anode heating curves for a particular tube are shown in Fig. 12.15, where the number of kilojoules stored by the anode at any moment is plotted against time. The maximum heat storage capacity of this anode is 80,000 kilojoules. Three different exposure rates are shown:

1. The rate of 1000 kilojoules per second fairly rapidly exceeds the heat storage capacity of the anode, and further exposure beyond this time would result in thermal damage.

2. The rate of 500 kilojoules per second establishes thermal equilibrium at the maximum heat storage capacity of the anode.

3. The exposure at 100 kilojoules per second—this would be the rate of heat production for a fluoroscopic kV of 100 kVp and a fluoroscopic current of 1 mA—produces thermal equilibrium with the anode at a fairly low temperature.

Note that in many cases it is convenient to show the heating and cooling curves on the same graphs.

12.8.7   Anode cooling

The heat stored in the anode is lost at a finite rate and a cooling curve showing the rate at which this heat is lost plotted against time (assuming that the anode has received its maximum permitted number of kilojoules at $t = 0$) is shown in Fig. 12.5. Suppose an exposure of 40,000 kilojoules is made: the point P shows this in the figure. The anode loses heat, as given by the curve below P, such that 5 minutes later, at point Q, only 20,000 kilojoules remain stored in the anode.

12.9   MODERN TRENDS IN X-RAY TUBE DESIGN

There are a number of improvements in X-ray tube design that have occurred over the past few decades. Many of these have been intended to improve X-ray tube performance for the large exposure requirements of computed tomography (CT).

Some tubes have achieved a more frictionless anode rotation by replacing the traditional silver-coated or lead-coated steel ball bearings with a liquid metal alloy layer, composed of gallium, indium and tin, between the anode rotor and the rotor support. Philips introduced this innovation in 1989. The liquid metal alloy is contained in spiral grooves and gives several advantages, such as noiseless rotation, longer tube life and improved heat conduction, thereby improving the tube rating.

Anode grounding was introduced by Varian in 1998, principally for radiotherapy X-ray tubes and permits the anode to operate at an earth (i.e., zero) electrical potential whereas the cathode retains a high negative potential. This maintains a high potential difference between the two electrodes and also permits water or air cooling of the anode. This principle has also been used in some diagnostic X-ray tubes, such as the Toshiba Aquilion.

The single end anode spindle attachment of traditional rotating anode X-ray tubes is a limitation because it reduces the maximum possible size and weight of the anode disc. Too great a load would put strain on the rotor assembly, especially

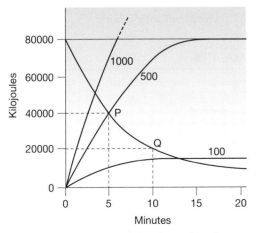

Fig. 12.15 Graph showing anode heating and cooling curves.

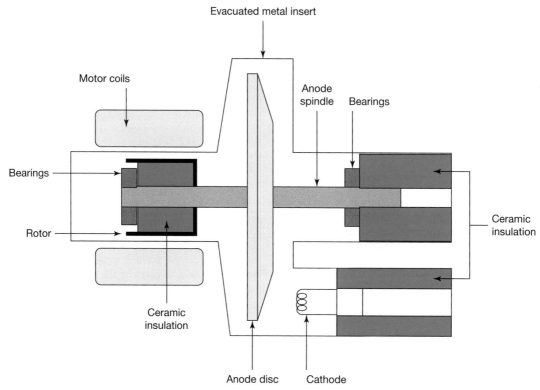

Fig. 12.16 A schematic diagram of the Philips Super Rotalix X-ray tube for computed tomography, based on an anode spindle that is anchored at both ends. Also note the metal insert and use of ceramic electrical insulation.

at high speed rotation. To alleviate this, manufacturers have brought in anode spindles that are attached to the X-ray tube assembly at both ends, permitting larger anodes and improved exposure capacity. An example of such a design is shown in Fig. 12.16.

Many modern X-ray tubes have replaced glass tube inserts (envelopes) with metal designs, made of chromium and iron. In conjunction with ceramic insulators at both the anode and cathode ends of the tube, this removes the problem of electrical 'arcing' and insulation breakdown which could occur when tungsten vapour gradually deposits on the inside of glass inserts. The metal insert also attracts 'off focus' electrons which might otherwise produce unwanted X-rays from outside of the anode target. The ceramic insulators are composed of metal oxides such as aluminium oxide.

Siemens introduced a rotating envelope X-ray tube, named the Straton, in 2003 for CT applications. In this design the entire metal envelope (or insert) rotates during

the X-ray exposure and is anchored at both ends to improve stability. This design is made possible by electromagnetic deflection of the electron beam, which is angled to strike the anode target. This arrangement is illustrated by Fig. 12.17. The backing of the anode is in direct contact with oil, thereby improving cooling.

SUMMARY

In this chapter, you should have learnt the following:
- The differences between stationary and rotating anode designs.
- The design features of the components of a standard rotating anode X-ray tube.
- Principles of electrical and radiation safety.
- Factors affecting the cooling and 'rating' of X-ray tubes.
- Developments in X-ray tube design.

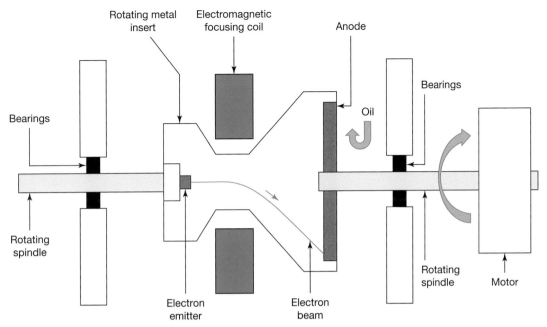

Fig. 12.17 A schematic diagram of the Siemens Straton X-ray tube for computed tomography. Note the whole inset rotation as well as the deflected electron beam. Ceramic insulation is not shown.

FURTHER READING

Ball, J.L., Moore, A.D., & Turner, S. 2008. *Ball and Moore's Essential Physics for Radiographers*. 4th edn. London: Blackwell Scientific. (Chapter 4.)

Bushong, S.C. 2016. *Radiological Science for Technologists: Physics, Biology and Protection*. 11th edn. New York: Mosby. (Chapter 6.)

Dendy, P., & Heaton, B. 2011. *Physics for Diagnostic Radiology*. 3rd edn. Boca Raton, Florida: CRC Press. (Chapter 2.)

Dowsett, D.J., Kenny, P.A., & Johnston, R.E. 1998. *The Physics of Diagnostic Imaging*. London: Chapman & Hall Medical. (Chapter 3.)

Webb, S., (Ed.). 2000. *The Physics of Medical Imaging*. 2nd edn. Bristol: Institute of Physics. (Chapter 2.)

X-ray attenuation

CHAPTER CONTENTS

13.1 AIM

Chapter 11 and 12 covered the production of X-rays. In this chapter we will review the processes that occur when X-rays (and also gamma rays) interact with matter, such as body tissues and metal filters. This causes ionisation of atoms and molecules, which has the harmful effect of causing radiation dose in body tissues, as covered in Chapter 21. It should be noted that this ionisation does not cause heating of body tissues; the radiation erythema ('skin-reddening') that can occur when high doses of radiation are absorbed is caused by cell death, not warming. A helpful effect of attenuation is the production of X-ray images, which is made possible by the differential interactions of X-rays with the human body.

13.2 WHAT IS ATTENUATION?

Attenuation means a reduction, in this case the reduction in intensity, that occurs to an X-ray beam as it passes through matter. In diagnostic imaging, this occurs via two important processes—absorption and scatter.

During absorption, an X-ray photon transfers all of its energy to an atom, for example via the ionisation of that atom and is effectively 'stopped'. In other words, it disappears. Substances that are dense and of a high effective atomic number, such as bone, will absorb a lot of X-rays and produce a white 'shadow' image on an imaging plate, whereas low-density substances will permit many X-rays

to pass through and will appear black. Absorption occurs most at relatively low X-ray energies, particularly when X-ray tube kVp values are less than about 70.

During scatter, which is more technically called *Compton scatter*, an X-ray photon transfers energy to an atom, for example via ionisation, but retains some energy and continues in a different direction, which is termed the *scattering angle*. Scatter is not a useful process in terms of X-ray image production, as it causes an overall 'fogging' or loss of contrast in the image, as explained in Chapter 16.

Some X-rays will pass straight through matter in a straight line without being absorbed or scattered and are termed *transmitted* rays. These are useful for forming a diagnostic image.

It is important to know that X-ray attenuation occurs to any appreciable extent only in solids and liquids. It is negligible in air or other gases and does not occur at all in a vacuum. However attenuation via ionisation in air is employed in radiation dosimetry (see Chapter 21) and has also been used in gas-filled X-ray or gamma ray detectors. So in practice we cannot describe an X-ray beam as being attenuated as it passes across an X-ray room, during its travel from the X-ray tube to the patient's skin surface. Loss of X-ray intensity does occur in the air of the room, but this is because of the inverse square law (see Chapter 14), a process by which the divergence of X-rays travelling away from a point source leads to a reduction in their number per unit cross-sectional area as distance increases. X-rays do not disappear via the inverse square law—they only diverge further away from

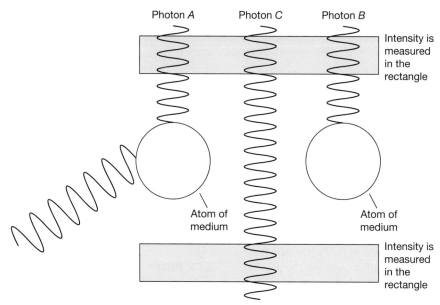

Fig. 13.1 Mechanisms of interaction of X-ray photons with matter. Photon *A* is scattered, photon *B* is absorbed and photon *C* is transmitted. Note that the number of photons passing through the lower rectangle is less than the number passing through the upper rectangle and so attenuation has taken place.

each other as they travel. In the same way, the light received by your eye from a distant star is dim only because your eye is small and far away from the star.

The processes of X-ray absorption, scattering and transmission, all important in diagnostic imaging, are shown in Fig. 13.1.

In addition to absorption and scatter, there are two further X-ray attenuation processes that can take place. Neither of these are of practical relevance to diagnostic imaging but will be mentioned for the sake of completeness. *Coherent scattering*, sometimes called *Rayleigh scattering*, occurs at very low X-ray energies and involves scattering (change in X-ray direction) without loss of energy. X-rays of such a low energy will not pass through body tissues. The second process is termed *pair production* and results in the formation of a positively charged and negatively charged electron pair (termed a *positron* and *negatron*) when energy is transferred from an X-ray of 1.02 MeV energy or above. This is very interesting from a physics perspective but will occur only when using radiotherapy linear accelerators (LINACs) because diagnostic imaging does not produce X-rays of megaelectron volt energy. However a reverse process, during which a positively charged electron emitted from an artificially manufactured radioactive isotope meets a negatively charged electron and produces a pair of 511 keV gamma rays, is employed in positron emission tomography (PET) scanning (see Chapter 23).

The two important processes of X-ray absorption (termed *photoelectric absorption*) and Compton scatter both involve interactions between X-rays and the orbiting electrons in atomic shells. It is easy to get a bit confused between X-ray production and X-ray attenuation processes. So to clarify:
- X-ray production involves fast-moving electrons from an X-ray tube filament, which interact with electrons in the shells of X-ray tube target atoms such as tungsten.
- X-ray attenuation involves X-rays from the X-ray tube target, which interact with electrons in the shells of atoms in body tissues and other materials.

We will now consider X-ray attenuation coefficients, which are formal ways of measuring the amount of X-ray attenuation that occurs in different materials. These coefficients make some assumptions, such as X-ray photons being all of the same energy, and the material being homogeneous, as in a sheet of metal for example, but are useful in radiation physics.

13.2.1   The linear attenuation coefficient (μ)

A parallel beam of monoenergetic radiation (radiation where all the photons have the same energy) will undergo exponential attenuation as it passes through a uniform medium. The intensity of the beam (I_x) is given by the equation:

$$I_x = I_0 e^{-\mu x}$$

Equation 13.1

where I_0 is the initial beam intensity, e is the exponential function, x is the thickness of attenuator and μ is the total linear attenuation coefficient. As the probability of an interaction increases, (e.g., as the density of a material increases), the linear attenuation coefficient μ will also increase. The exponential relationship means that equal extra thicknesses of attenuating material will produce equal fractional reductions in X-ray intensity, assuming a monoenergetic beam and a homogeneous attenuator. For example, the X-ray intensity could be one-half after 1 cm, one-quarter after 2 cm, one-eighth after 3 cm and so on. Linear attenuation coefficients decrease as beam energy increases, as a result of the greater penetrative capability of the beam. The linear coefficient may be defined as follows:

> **DEFINITION**
>
> The linear attenuation coefficient, μ, is the fraction of X-rays removed from a beam per unit thickness of the attenuating medium. Units are cm^{-1} (for example, a value of 0.25 cm^{-1} would give a fractional reduction of 25% in beam intensity per centimetre).

The linear attenuation coefficient is very important for the determination of radiation dose distributions, both in radiation dosimetry and in radiotherapy planning. It is also used in computed tomography (CT) (see Chapter 20) to calculate Hounsfield units that depict the relative X-ray attenuation values of body tissues as a scale of signal intensities.

13.2.2 The mass attenuation coefficient (μ/ρ)

If we divide the linear attenuation coefficient μ by the density ρ of a material, then we have a property which is affected by the atomic number of that material but is independent of its density. This ratio μ/ρ is known as the *total mass attenuation coefficient* and is defined as follows:

> **DEFINITION**
>
> The total mass attenuation coefficient, μ/ρ, is the fraction of the X-rays removed from a beam of unit cross-sectional area by unit mass of the medium.

This means that the same mass of a substance will have the same X-ray mass attenuation coefficient, regardless of whether it is a solid, liquid or gas. The mass attenuation coefficient is less relevant than the linear attenuation coefficient in medical imaging, because X-ray images are based on the relative amounts of attenuation that occur in different densities of tissue.

13.3 PHOTOELECTRIC ABSORPTION

Photoelectric absorption is a very important process in medical imaging as it is proportional to the atomic number cubed of the atoms in the absorbing medium. Because soft tissue has an average (or 'effective') atomic number of about 7 and bone an average atomic number of 14; this means that there will be a very large signal difference (contrast) between soft tissue and bone on an X-ray image. This is particularly true using low kVp values, at which photoelectric absorption is a major attenuation factor. So the relative magnitudes of photoelectric absorption in soft tissue and bone attributed to the contribution of atomic number will be $(7 \times 7 \times 7) = 343$ and $(14 \times 14 \times 14) = 2744$, respectively, a difference of eight times.

In photoelectric absorption, the X-ray photon is involved in an inelastic collision with an orbiting electron of an atom in the absorbing material. (The term 'inelastic' means that energy is lost from the X-ray photon, as opposed to an elastic collision in which its energy is retained.) During photoelectric absorption, the X-ray photon gives up all its energy to the electron (and thus disappears) and the electron is ejected from the atom, resulting in ionisation. As ejection of the electron from the atom is a necessary part of the process, photoelectric absorption can take place only if the photon energy is equal to, or greater than, the binding energy of the electron. The concept of electron binding energies was discussed in Chapter 11.

The process of photoelectric absorption is shown schematically in Fig. 13.2, where it is assumed that the X-ray photon of energy $h\nu$ ejects an electron from the K-shell of

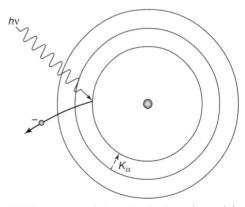

Fig. 13.2 The process of photoelectric absorption and the subsequent emission of a quantum of characteristic radiation. The incoming photon ($h\nu$) is absorbed by the K-shell electron which is then displaced from that shell. The vacancy is filled from the L-shell with the emission of $K\alpha$ characteristic radiation.

the atom. Some of the energy of the photon is used in overcoming the binding energy of the electron and the rest is given to the electron as kinetic energy. If we assume that the electron has a binding energy of B, then the kinetic energy after ejection (it is then referred to as a *photoelectron*) is $(hv - B)$. The vacancy thus created in the K-shell will be filled by electrons in orbitals further from the nucleus performing a series of quantum jumps downwards, producing characteristic radiation (a similar process to that which occurs in characteristic X-ray production—see Chapter 11) and the possible emission of Auger electrons. From orbitals further out from the nucleus. The ejected photoelectron is quickly brought to rest by the surrounding atoms and delivers its energy to them in the process. A similar thing happens with the Auger electrons.

INSIGHT

In diagnostic imaging, photoelectric absorption is an important X-ray attenuation process. When K-shell electrons are ejected from body tissue atoms, there is some associated minor characteristic X-ray production as outer shell electrons 'drop down' to fill the K-shell vacancy, but these rays are of very low energy and not of practical importance, when considering body tissue atoms such as hydrogen, carbon and oxygen, or even calcium and phosphorus. This is because the energy of characteristic X-rays is proportional to the atomic number of an atom (see Table 11.1). Characteristic X-ray production is of some practical consequence when the absorbing materials are high atomic number elements such as lead. The take-home message is: do not confuse the minor characteristic X-ray production that occurs during photoelectric absorption with the more important characteristic X-ray production that occurs in an X-ray tube target. Also remember that characteristic X-ray production in an X-ray tube target mainly occurs when K-shell electrons in tungsten atoms are ejected by high-speed electrons from the filament.

The energy of the characteristic radiation is equal to the difference in energy of the electron before and after the quantum jump. In the case of X-ray photons interacting with atoms of body tissue, this energy difference is very small (normally between 1.2×10^{-2} eV and 1.8×10^{-2} eV) and so is in the infrared part of the electromagnetic spectrum.

The probability of a photoelectric interaction occurring at a particular shell depends on the binding energy of the electrons in the shell and the energy of the incoming photon. The probability is zero when the energy of the photon is less than the binding energy of the electron; it is greatest when the photon energy is equal to the binding energy and thereafter decreases rapidly with increasing photon energy. A graph of the mass absorption coefficient for photoelectric absorption in lead is shown in Fig. 13.3 to illustrate these points.

The outer electron shells of the atom are affected by the lower photon energies, only to have a reducing absorption as the photon energy increases. When the photon energy reaches the binding energy of the shell, electrons in that shell can take part in photoelectric absorption, thus producing a sudden increase in the amount of absorption. Such an increase is shown for the K-shell electrons of the lead atom in Fig. 13.3. This sudden increase is known as an *absorption edge* and Fig. 23.4 shows the K absorption edge for the lead atom. Between the absorption edges, the linear attenuation coefficient attributed to the photoelectric effect (τ) is approximately proportional to $1/E^3$.

INSIGHT

K-shell X-ray absorption edges are not of much consequence in soft tissues because the K edge energy is very low in soft tissue atoms such as hydrogen, carbon and oxygen, or even in bone atoms such as calcium and phosphorus. However, the K absorption edges of contrast agent atoms such as iodine and barium are of sufficient energy to be important, being of 33 keV and 37 keV respectively. It was mentioned in Chapter 11 that X-rays emitted from an X-ray tube via Bremsstrahlung, forming the continuous X-ray spectrum, are most commonly produced at about one-third to one-half of the peak X-ray energy. This means that a kVp of about 80 will be very good at producing lots of X-rays in the 30 to 40 keV energy range and will therefore create a lot of X-ray absorption in iodine or barium, thereby increasing 'contrast enhancement'. A kVp of 80 is often recommended in CT for enhancing the visualisation of contrast media.

13.3.1   Factors affecting photoelectric absorption

The linear attenuation coefficient for the photoelectric effect (τ) is related to the atomic number (Z) of the absorber, the density of the absorber (ρ) and the photon energy of the X-rays (E). This relationship is shown by the equation:

$$\tau = \left(Z^3 / E^3 \right) \times \rho \qquad \textbf{Equation 13.2}$$

This equation applies to energies up to about 200 keV, covering the energies that are used in diagnostic X-ray imaging. It can be seen from Equation 13.2 that photoelectric absorption increases very greatly with the atomic number

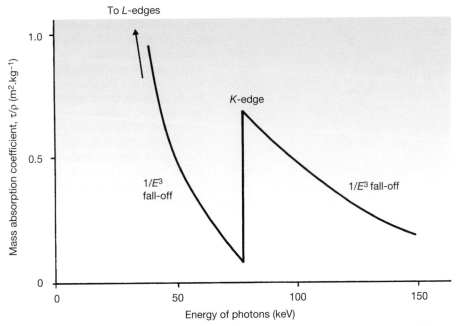

Fig. 13.3 The mass absorption coefficient for the photoelectric absorption effect in lead and its variation with photon energy.

of the absorber and also falls off very much as X-ray beam energy increases. In addition, it is proportional to the density of the absorber. Bone is approximately twice as dense as soft tissue and its atomic number is also approximately twice that of soft tissue (giving an eight times increase in X-ray absorption owing to the effects of atomic number). For these reasons, the linear attenuation coefficient for photoelectric absorption in bone is approximately 8 × 2 which equals 16 times that of soft tissue. Table 13.1 illustrates the effective atomic numbers and densities of some different body tissues.

The atomic number and density of most soft tissues is similar to that of water. It can be seen that there will be large photoelectric absorption differences between bone and soft tissue. Fat will absorb fewer X-rays than other soft tissues.

13.4   COMPTON SCATTER

If the energy of an X-ray photon is very much higher than the binding energy of an electron circling an atom in the attenuating material, then the electron may be regarded as a 'free' electron. The interaction between an X-ray photon and a free electron is known as *Compton scattering* and results in the partial absorption of the energy of an X-ray photon which undergoes such scatter. During the process the electron will gain energy and may be ejected from the atom, resulting in ionisation. Because the interaction is between a photon and a free electron, the electron density of the material is the most important factor in determining the probability of Compton scatter occurring. Compton scatter is the main X-ray attenuation process in body tissues at higher beam energies, (e.g., at kVp values >70).

The Compton scattering process is shown diagrammatically in Fig. 13.4. The incident X-ray photon has an energy $E_1 (= h\nu_1)$ and collides with the electron, which receives some of the photon energy. The energy remaining, $E_2 (= h\nu_2)$, is the energy of the scattered photon. Because E_2 is less than E_1, then the wavelength of the scattered photon must be greater than the wavelength of the incident photon, as shown

	Effective atomic	Density
Tissue	number, Z	(grams/cm³)
Air	7.6	0.0013
Fat	5.9	0.91
Water	7.4	1.00
Bone	13.8	1.85

TABLE 13.1   Effective atomic numbers and densities of body tissues

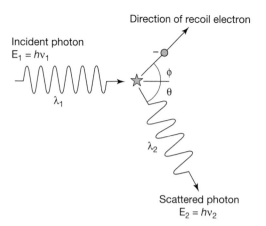

Fig. 13.4 The process of Compton scattering. The scattered photon has less energy than the incident photon and may be scattered through any angle. The recoil electron is always scattered in a 'forward' direction.

in Fig. 13.4 (see Section 9.3.1 for the relationship between photon energy and wavelength). Compton scattering interactions are termed *inelastic* in that the X-ray photon loses some energy during the process, although the total energy of the entities involved in the interaction (the X-ray photon and the electron) remains the same.

After a Compton scattering interaction, the X-ray photon may travel in any direction, but the ejected electron can only travel in a forward direction relative to the incident photon. Thus, in Fig. 13.4, the scattering angle θ of the X-ray may be any value, while Φ is always in a forward direction, in order to conserve momentum. The division of the energy of the original photon between the electron and the scattered photon depends on the original photon energy (E_1) and the angle θ through which it has been scattered. It may be shown that to preserve both energy and momentum, the following equation must be obeyed:

$$\lambda_2 - \lambda_1 = \frac{\left(h\left(1-\cos\theta\right)\right)}{mc} \qquad \textbf{Equation 13.3}$$

where the quantity $\lambda_2 - \lambda_1$ is called the Compton wavelength shift, h is Planck's constant, θ is the X-ray scattering angle, m is the mass of the electron and c is the velocity of electromagnetic radiation.

Two important conclusions may be drawn from Eq. 13.3:
1. $\lambda_2 - \lambda_1$, which is the change in X-ray wavelength (and hence relates to the change in X-ray energy), depends only on h, m, c and θ and so is not dependent on the wavelength of the incident photon or the composition of the attenuating material.
2. For a given value of scattering angle, θ, the value of $\lambda_2 - \lambda_1$ is constant (see Table 13.2). Low-energy photons have longer wavelengths, so that the wavelength change represents a smaller *fractional* change in λ and hence only a slight reduction in the energy of the scattered photons. By applying the same argument, high-energy photons scattered through the same angle will experience a much larger fractional change in their wavelength and energy.

Equation 13.3 shows what happens to the photon wavelengths when scattered through an angle of θ. It does not give any information on the relative probability of a photon actually being scattered through that angle. Low-energy X-ray photons tend to be scattered fairly equally in all directions, whereas scatter becomes more forward in direction as X-ray energy increases. This is particularly the case at the high energies used in radiotherapy. The increasingly forward direction of scatter (i.e., with a small scattering angle) is one factor which contributes to the increased 'fogging' from scatter which may affect imaging plates at high kV. The magnitudes and directions of X-ray scatter at different X-ray beam energies are shown in Fig. 13.5.

13.4.1   Compton attenuation, absorption and scatter coefficients

The linear attenuation coefficient for Compton scattering (σ) is given by the equation:

$$\sigma = \left(\text{Electron density} \,/\, E\right) \times \rho \qquad \textbf{Equation 13.4}$$

TABLE 13.2 Relationships between Compton scatter angle and scattered X-ray photon energy			
	Scattered X-ray energy at different scattering angle, θ		
Primary X-ray energy	30 degrees (forward scatter)	60 degrees	90 degrees (side scatter)
50 keV	49.6 keV	48 keV	46 keV
100 keV	98 keV	91 keV	84 keV
150 keV	146 keV	131 keV	116 keV

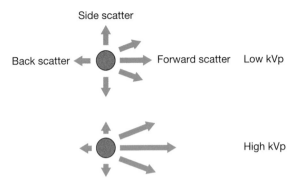

Fig. 13.5 Effects of X-ray beam energy on the magnitude and direction of X-ray scatter. Note that scatter is more forward in direction at high kVp.

TABLE 13.3 **The electron densities of some tissues**

Tissue	Electron density (electrons/cm³)
Air	0.004×10^{23}
Fat	3.27×10^{23}
Water	3.34×10^{23}
Bone	5.55×10^{23}

Where E is the photon energy of the X-rays, ρ is the density of the absorber. Electron density refers to the number of electrons per cm³ of absorber.

INSIGHT

The electron density of a material is based on including all of the electrons in the electron shells of the atoms within that material. Within the Compton scatter process, an X-ray can be scattered by any electron, regardless of which shell it occupies, or its binding energy. This means that Compton scatter is unaffected by the atomic numbers (Z) of the atoms in the attenuating material. In fact, electron density (numbers of electrons per cm³) is fairly constant for elements other than hydrogen. This is because the number of electrons in an atom increases roughly in line with the volume of that atom as atomic number increases. In practice, the electron density of materials is affected more strongly by how close the atoms are packed together within it, rather than by the size of the atoms. So densely packed tissues like bone have a higher electron density than do soft tissues.

The electron densities of some tissues are shown by Table 13.3. Note that the electron density of water is similar to that of most soft tissues.

Table 13.3 shows that unsurprisingly the electron density of air, being a gas, is much less than that of liquids or solids. There is a notable electron density difference between bone and air, meaning that there will still be some X-ray attenuation difference (i.e., image contrast) between bone and air even at high kVp, where Compton scatter is the main X-ray attenuation process. However this image contrast will be reduced at low kVp when compared to high kVp because photoelectric absorption will not be such a big contributor to X-ray attenuation.

As shown in Equation 13.4, the probability of Compton scattering occurring is inversely proportional to the energy of the photon; the amount of Compton scattering decreases as the photon energy increases. This is not a surprise because both photoelectric and Compton scatter attenuation decreases with X-ray beam energy. High-energy beams are more penetrating.

In diagnostic radiography, many consider that the Compton process only produces scatter which degrades the radiograph and so makes no contribution to contrast. However, remember that linear X-ray attenuation is also affected by the density of the tissue and so the Compton process is responsible for the differences in attenuation (and hence contrast) which we get between soft tissue and air or between contrast agents and air in high kV radiography. Electron density differences (which do relate to tissue density differences) are a contributor to Compton attenuation, as mentioned previously in this section.

13.5 RELATIVE IMPORTANCE OF THE DIFFERENT X-RAY ATTENUATION PROCESSES IN DIAGNOSTIC IMAGING

At diagnostic X-ray energies of up to 150 keV, both photoelectric absorption and Compton scatter will contribute to the total X-ray linear attenuation coefficients of body tissues. However the contribution of photoelectric absorption falls off as beam energy increases, and is most important at low kVp. However, photoelectric absorption is still an important contributor even at high kVp in high atomic number contrast media elements such as iodine and barium. This is because photoelectric absorption is proportional to Z^3, as shown previously by Equation 13.2.

Table 13.4 shows the relative contributions of photoelectric and Compton attenuation at different X-ray energies and in different tissues. It is important to note that the average X-ray energy of a beam in keV is about one-third to one-half of that of the peak X-ray energy (which is set by the kVp).

In Table 13.4, it can be seen that photoelectric absorption falls off more rapidly in water (which is equivalent to soft tissues) than in bone as X-ray energy increases. The

TABLE 13.4   Relative contributions of photoelectric absorption and Compton scatter at different X-ray energies and in different tissues

X-ray energy	In water	In bone	In iodine contrast media
20 keV (at 40–50 kVp)	Photoelectric 65%	Photoelectric 89%	Photoelectric 94%
	Compton 35%	Compton 11%	Compton 6%
60 keV (at 120–150 kVp)	Photoelectric 7%	Photoelectric 31%	Photoelectric 95%
	Compton 93%	Compton 69%	Compton 5%

maintenance of photoelectric absorption in iodine contrast media at higher kVp is explained by its K-shell absorption edge (see Section 13.3). Coherent scatter (Rayleigh scatter) is insignificant at diagnostic X-ray energies and pair production is not a factor because it occurs only at X-ray energies greater than 1.02 MeV, whereas 0.15 MeV (i.e., 150 keV) is the usual maximum energy encountered in diagnostic X-ray imaging. Even the gamma rays emitted in radionuclide imaging do not normally exceed 1.02 MeV.

The overall contribution of different attenuation processes is summarised by Fig. 13.6 and by Table 13.5.

TABLE 13.5   Summary of the interaction processes

Process	Description of interactions	Effect of Z, E	Comments
Elastic scattering	Photon interacts with bound atomic electron. Photon energy is less than the electron binding energy. Photon is reradiated from the material with no energy loss.	$\sigma_{coh} \propto Z^2/E$	No energy absorption in the medium. Photon scattered in the forward direction. Effect is negligible in biological tissues because of low Z.
Photoelectric absorption	Photon of energy ≥ the binding energy of an electron interacts with bound electron and ejects it from its shell. Photon disappears as all its energy is absorbed by the electron. Kinetic energy of the electron = E – binding energy. Atom recoils, conserving momentum.	$\tau \propto Z^3/E^3$	Ejected electron loses velocity to surrounding atoms, giving energy to them; i.e., absorption takes place. The electron vacancy created is filled by electrons making quantum jumps and so low-energy characteristic radiation is emitted.
Compton scattering	Photon behaves like a particle and collides with a free electron. Energy of the incident photon is shared between the electron and the scattered photon.	$\sigma \propto$ electron density/E	Energy of the displaced electron is absorbed by the medium, so Compton process produces attenuation and partial absorption. Electron densities of all materials except hydrogen are similar and so σ values are largely independent of the atomic number of the attenuator.
Pair production	Photon of energy ≥1.02 MeV may spontaneously disappear in the vicinity of the nucleus of an attenuator atom, producing an electron and a positron. Positron rapidly annihilated with an electron to form two photons of annihilation radiation, each with energy of 0.511 MeV.	$\pi \propto (E - 1.02)Z$	Probability of pair production increases with E above 1.02 MeV and will not occur at diagnostic imaging X-ray energies.

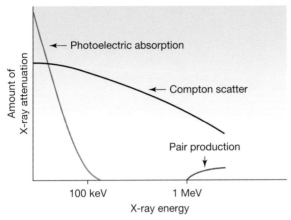

Fig. 13.6 The relative importance of the attenuation processes over a range of X-ray energies

The following important points about the attenuation processes should be noted:
- Photoelectric absorption is important at low X-ray energies, depending on the atomic number of the absorber.
- K-shell absorption edges become more pronounced as the atomic number of the absorber increases.
- Compton scattering dominates over a wide range of energies (≈50 keV to 1 MeV+) in soft tissues.
- Only photoelectric absorption and Compton scattering are important to diagnostic imaging.

13.6   CONCLUSION

As can be seen in this chapter, the attenuation of an X-ray beam as it passes through a patient's tissues is a complicated affair depending on the energy of the photons, the tissue thickness and the atomic number of the tissue through which the beam passes. In medical imaging we are able to alter the photon energy and this has important consequences for the attenuation pattern and the intensity pattern of the X-ray beam emerging from the patient. These issues are discussed in more detail in Chapter 16 where the formation of the radiographic image is considered.

SUMMARY

In this chapter, you should have learnt the following:
- The meaning of the terms, attenuation, absorption and scattering as applied to a beam of radiation passing through matter.
- The factors which control the probability of an interaction taking place between the X-ray photon and an atom of the attenuator.
- The meaning of the terms, total linear attenuation coefficient and total mass attenuation coefficient.
- The mechanism of photoelectric absorption and the factors affecting it.
- The mechanism of Compton scattering and the factors affecting it.
- The relative importance of each of the attenuation processes in radiography.

FURTHER READING

Allisy-Roberts, P.J., & Williams, J. 2007. *Farr's Physics for Medical Imaging*. 2nd edn. Philadelphia: Saunders.

Ball, J.L., Moore, A.D., & Turner, S. 2008. *Ball and Moore's Essential Physics for Radiographers*. 4th edn. London: Blackwell Scientific. (Chapter 17.)

Bushong, S. 2016. *Radiologic Science for Technologists: Physics, Biology, and Protection*. 11th edn. St. Louis: Mosby. (Chapter 9.)

Dendy, P., & Heaton, B. 2011. *Physics for Diagnostic Radiology*, 3rd edn. Boca Raton, FL: CRC Press. (Chapter 3.)

Properties of X-ray beams

CHAPTER CONTENTS

14.1 AIM

The aim of this chapter is to consider the various factors which have an influence on the quantity and/or the quality of the beam of X-ray photons that emanates from the X-ray tube. These factors are relevant both to the characteristics of X-ray images (see Chapter 16) and to radiation doses (see Chapter 21).

14.2 INTRODUCTION

In Chapter 11 we considered the mechanisms by which X-rays were produced in the target of the X-ray tube. In this chapter we will consider the various factors which influence the quantity and/or the quality of the X-ray beam and hence its intensity at a given point. Before we look at this in any more detail, it is first important to ensure that we understand the meaning of the measures "quantity", "quality" and intensity as applied to a beam of X radiation.

DEFINITIONS

The quantity of radiation in an X-ray beam is a measure of the number of X-ray photons in the beam. The terms *quantity* and *exposure* are often interchanged in radiography as the higher the quantity or amount of radiation, the greater the exposure. This is a bit oversimplistic because exposure also relates to beam energy. In fact, probably the simplest method of comparing the quantity of two beams of radiation is to compare the exposure received by an exposure meter. As we shall see in Chapter 21, exposure can be measured quite easily using the unit of air kerma (which means kinetic energy released per unit mass), based on the number of ionisations occurring in a chamber of air that is exposed to an X-ray beam. Dose area product (DAP) meters attached to most X-ray tubes provide a simple way of measuring and comparing X-ray exposures nationally.

The intensity of an X-ray beam is proportional to the quantity of X-ray photons. Strictly, the term intensity refers to the amount of X-ray energy passing through unit cross-sectional area per second and is affected by both the number and energy of the X-ray photons. But it should be noted that in radiography, intensity is often regarded as the number of X-ray photons in an exposure. Within this chapter, several graphs will plot X-ray intensity (in this case the *number* of X-ray photons) on the y-axis and X-ray energy (keV) on the x-axis, because this is a commonly used convention in medical imaging.

The quality of an X-ray beam is a measure of its penetrating power and is therefore related to its average photon energy. Note that the 'quality' of an X-ray beam is a physics concept and should not be confused with the quality of a radiographic image, although the beam will of course affect the image. X-ray beam quality is defined by physical measures such as the peak energy in keV and also by the half-value thickness (HVT), not by terms such as good or satisfactory.

In Chapter 11 we saw that X-ray beams are polychromatic or polyenergetic. This means that they contain X-rays with a broad range of energies caused by the Bremsstrahlung process that results in a continuous X-ray spectrum. However this fact has some disadvantages. Any very low-energy X-rays (sometimes termed *soft rays*) will only produce unnecessary radiation dose in a patient's body without being able to penetrate sufficiently to contribute to an image. Also the wide range of contained X-ray energies has the effect of increasing image noise and reducing image contrast. The quality of an X-ray beam can be increased by removing soft rays, increasing the average beam energy, thereby 'hardening' the beam and making it more 'monochromatic'. This means that the X-ray beam will be more penetrating and will also consist of a narrower range of energies. Various forms of beam filtration can achieve this. However, it is only gamma-ray emissions in radionuclide imaging which are truly monochromatic (i.e., being of a single or several fixed and discrete energies). Fig. 14.1 shows what happens in practice to a polychromatic X-ray beam as it passes through matter.

In Chapter 13 it was mentioned that the linear X-ray attenuation coefficient, which is used to define the X-ray attenuation of matter, is based on the assumption that an X-ray beam is homogeneous, which also means of a single fixed energy, or monochromatic. The real-world situation is that X-ray beams are polychromatic, and hence the term *half-value thickness (HVT)* is used to help define the quality of a beam.

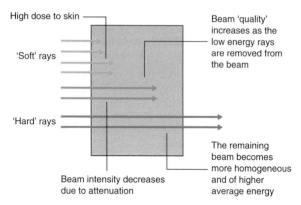

Fig. 14.1 Attenuation of a polychromatic X-ray beam as it passes through matter. Low-energy X-rays are absorbed in the first few centimetres of matter, resulting in an increase in average beam energy as it passes deeper.

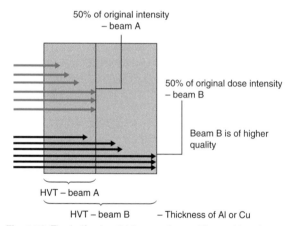

Fig. 14.2 The half-value thickness of two different X-ray beams. It takes a greater thickness of aluminium or copper to reduce the intensity of beam B by 50%, and so beam B is of higher quality than beam A.

DEFINITION

The half-value thickness (HVT) (sometimes called the *half-value layer*) is that thickness of a substance which will transmit one-half of the intensity of radiation incident upon it.

The HVT therefore depends on the attenuating properties of the substance itself and the penetrating power of the beam of X-rays incident upon it. In diagnostic imaging, we might compare the penetrating properties of two beams using thicknesses of a homogeneous material such as aluminium or copper – the higher the HVT, the more penetrating the beam. The concept of HVT is illustrated by Fig. 14.2. For X-ray tube voltages of 70 to 150 kVp, typical HVT figures are 2 to 5 millimetres of aluminium.

Sometimes, first and second half-value layers are defined. The first HVT is that thickness of material which reduces the intensity of the X-ray beam from 100% to 50%. The second HVT is that thickness of material which further reduces the intensity of the X-ray beam from 50% to

25%. For a polychromatic beam, because the beam will harden, acquiring a greater mean energy as it passes deeper into the material, the second HVT will always be thicker than the first HVT.

14.3   THE EFFECT OF mA (AND EXPOSURE TIME) ON THE X-RAY BEAM

If the current through the X-ray tube (mA) is, for example, doubled, the number of electrons flowing across the tube in unit time is doubled. If all the other factors remain unchanged, each electron will have the same chance of

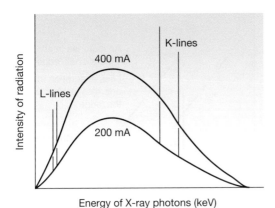

Fig. 14.3 The effect of the mA on the X-ray spectrum. Note that the quantity of the radiation changes (as shown by the alteration of the area under each curve) but the quality of the radiation is unaltered (as shown by the maximum photon energy and the peak photon energy being at the same energy for each graph). Thus we can say that the mA selected for an exposure affects the quantity of the X-ray beam but does not affect the quality of the beam; an increase in the mA will produce an increase in the quantity of radiation from the target.

creating X-ray photons and so the number of photons of each energy produced per unit time will be doubled. If the mA is halved, the same argument can be used to show that the number of X-ray photons of each energy is also halved. Thus we can say that the quantity of the X-ray beam per unit time (or the beam intensity) is directly proportional to the mA through the tube.

$$I \propto mA \qquad \text{Equation 14.1}$$

The effect on the X-ray beam of altering the mA is shown in Fig. 14.3. Note that the area under the graph for 200 mA is half the area under the graph for 400 mA. The maximum photon energy and the minimum photon energy are the same in each case and the average photon energy remains unaltered.

It should be noted that doubling the exposure time will have the effect of doubling the total number of X-rays emitted by an X-ray tube but will not affect the emission of rays per unit time. There is no effect on X-ray photon energies.

14.4 THE EFFECT OF kVp ON THE X-RAY BEAM

The kVp across the X-ray tube influences the force of attraction experienced by an electron released by the fila-

ment as it moves towards the anode. Thus, if the kVp is increased, then the kinetic energy of the electron will be increased. As we saw in Section 14.4, the efficiency of X-ray production by Bremsstrahlung is proportional to E^2, and so this improved efficiency means that:

$$I \propto kVp^2 \qquad \text{Equation 14.2}$$

Thus increasing the kVp across an X-ray tube greatly increases the number of X-rays produced. This is because Bremsstrahlung becomes more efficient as tube voltage increases. Increasing the kVp will also increase the energy of the maximum-energy photons in the beam—if the kVp is 50, then the maximum photon energy is 50 keV, and if the kVp is 100, then the maximum photon energy is 100 keV. As the average photon energy is approximately 30% to 50% of the maximum photon energy, increasing the maximum photon energy will also increase the average photon energy.

It is also possible that increasing the kVp will affect the appearance of the characteristic X-ray spectrum. Characteristic X-rays will not be produced in a tungsten target at a kVp less than 69, because the binding energy of the tungsten K-shell electron is 69 keV. This possibility is shown in Fig. 14.4.

Thus we can say that the kVp selected for an exposure affects both the quantity and the quality of the X-ray beam produced; an increase in kVp will produce an increase in the quantity and the quality of the radiation from the target. Fig. 14.4 illustrates this. A doubling in kVp will increase the total number of X-rays produced by about four times, will double the maximum and average X-ray energies and may affect the characteristic K lines.

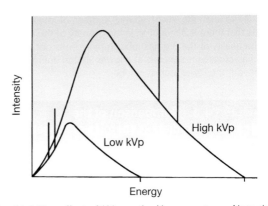

Fig. 14.4 The effect of kVp on the X-ray spectrum. Note that the kVp affects both the quantity and the quality of the radiation beam. Also note that the curve at a lower kVp is unable to produce K-characteristic radiation, although both curves can produce L lines.

14.5 THE EFFECT OF THE X-RAY TUBE TARGET MATERIAL ON THE X-RAY BEAM

As mentioned in Chapter 11, the atomic number of the target material has an effect on the X-ray beam from the tube. The higher the atomic number of the target material, the more positively charged the nucleus of the target atom is and so the more it attracts the negatively charged electrons from the filament which pass close to it. Thus the production of X-rays by the Bremsstrahlung process is more efficient and the intensity of the beam is increased. The maximum and minimum photon energies in the beam are not affected by the target material. This effect is shown in Fig. 14.5, which shows the radiation spectra from a tungsten and a molybdenum target.

The target material also affects the characteristic radiation produced. The energies of the characteristic radiations from a tungsten and a molybdenum target are shown in Table 14.1. Thus, although the target material does not

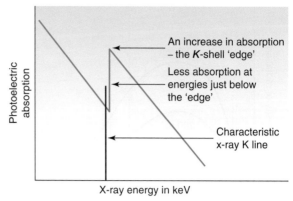

Fig. 14.6 Energies of the K-shell absorption edge and characteristic X-ray K lines for an element—this means that an element is fairly transparent to its own characteristic radiation.

affect the quality of the Bremsstrahlung radiation, it does affect the energy of the characteristic radiation, and this does have some effect on the overall quality of the X-ray beam. This effect may be enhanced by filtering the radiation with a filter made of the same material as the target. This is because an element is relatively transparent to its own characteristic radiation. The reason for this is that the characteristic K-line X-ray energy is slightly below the K-shell absorption edge value (see Fig. 14.6) and thus falls within a trough or low point of X-ray absorption.

14.6 THE EFFECT OF GENERATOR WAVEFORM ON THE X-RAY BEAM

The kilovoltage peak (kVp) refers to the maximum or peak voltage across an X-ray tube during an exposure and is the value which is set when we select the kV during an exposure. In fact, there can be some voltage fluctuation or 'ripple' during an exposure, particularly in the case of older high-voltage generators. This fluctuation may be less when using a three-phase electrical supply (used for most X-ray equipment) than a single-phase supply (which might be used for some very low-powered and portable units). Fig. 14.7 shows the possible effects of voltage fluctuations in a three-phase electrical supply.

When voltage varies during an exposure, the intensity and energy of the X-ray beam will also vary. Thus we can say that the type of X-ray generator waveform affects both the quantity and the quality of the X-ray beam produced. The nearer the voltage across the tube is to a constant potential, the higher the quantity and the quality of the radiation produced at the target. This will result in an X-ray spectrum which is a bit more intense across all energies

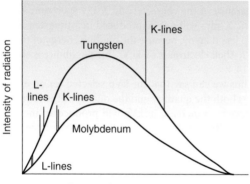

Fig. 14.5 The effect of the target material on the X-ray spectrum. Note that the lower atomic number of molybdenum means that there is a reduction in the quantity of the radiation, but the quality of the Bremsstrahlung radiation is not affected. The characteristic radiation is at a lower photon energy for the target with the lower atomic number.

TABLE 14.1 Comparison of the characteristic radiation energies produced from a tungsten target and a molybdenum target		
	Energy of $K\alpha$ characteristic radiation (keV)	Energy of $L\alpha$ characteristic radiation (keV)
Tungsten $Z = 74$	59.3	8.4
Molybdenum $Z = 42$	17.5	2.2

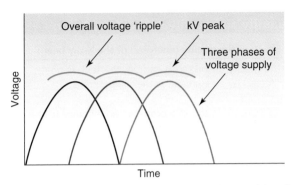

Fig. 14.7 A three-phase X-ray generator waveform and its effect on 'ripple' in the X-ray tube voltage.

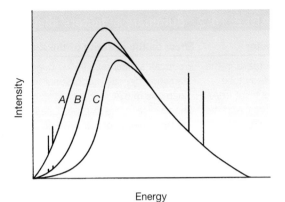

Fig. 14.8 The effect of filtration on the X-ray spectrum. Line *A* represents the spectrum produced at the target of the X-ray tube; line *B* shows how this spectrum is modified because of the inherent filtration of the tube; and line *C* shows how the spectrum is modified because of the total filtration. Note that filtration causes a reduction in the quantity of the radiation but an increase in the quality.

and with a slightly higher average energy. The peak energy will be unchanged. It should be noted, however, that modern high-frequency generators are not affected much by voltage ripple and so this effect is less important than it was previously.

14.7   THE EFFECT OF FILTRATION ON THE X-RAY BEAM

In all the discussion so far we have considered the beam of X radiation produced at the target of the X-ray tube. Before this radiation can be used in radiography, it must first leave the tube. In leaving the tube, the radiation beam must first pass through the glass of the tube insert, the oil in the housing and finally the window of the housing (plus any additional filtration), it is filtered at each stage of this process. Thus to consider the beam which will interact with the patient, we need to consider the effect of filtration on the spectrum of radiation produced at the tube target.

Spectrum *A* in Fig. 14.8 shows the distribution of energies emitted from the tube target. This would be the spectrum of the radiation before it leaves the glass envelope of the tube. As was discussed in Chapter 13, when a beam of radiation passes through any medium, the beam is attenuated by the processes of absorption and scattering. The lower the photon energy, the higher the chance of it being attenuated. So the passage of the X-ray beam through the glass envelope, the oil and the exit window of the shield results in selective attenuation of the lower-energy photons. Because this filtration is inherent to the tube construction, it is known as the *inherent filtration* of the X-ray tube. The spectrum emitted after the inherent filtration is shown as spectrum *B* in Fig. 14.8.

Aluminium has a low atomic number (13) and so can absorb many of the low-energy X-ray photons in a beam of diagnostic energy, by photoelectric absorption (see

Chapter 13). High-energy X-ray photons have a low probability of being absorbed or scattered by the aluminium and so are relatively unaffected by the filtration. This makes aluminium the ideal material for filtration of diagnostic energy X-ray beams. The X-ray beam emerging from the X-ray tube contains a significant number of low-energy photons. If these were allowed to interact with the tissues of a patient, they would be absorbed by superficial tissues and so would contribute to the patient dose but would make no contribution to the image. The amount of low-energy photons in the spectrum can be significantly reduced by incorporating additional filtration into the beam, near the exit port of the tube, before it interacts with the patient's tissues. Such a spectrum is shown as line *C* in Fig. 14.8. The inherent filtration of diagnostic X-ray tubes is usually expressed in millimetres of aluminium equivalent, that is, the inherent filtration is equivalent to the filtration of the beam achieved by the stated number of millimetres of aluminium. The inherent filtration of most diagnostic X-ray tubes is between 0.5 and 1.0 mm of aluminium equivalent. The total filtration in the beam is the sum of the inherent filtration and the additional filtration. This total filtration is between 1.5 and 2.5 mm, depending upon the maximum kVp at which the tube is designed to operate.

As can be seen from Fig. 14.8, filtration affects both the quantity and the quality of the X-ray beam—the greater the thickness of the filtration in the X-ray beam, the less the quantity but the greater the quality of the X-ray beam emerging from the X-ray tube.

TABLE 14.2 Summary of factors affecting the quantity and quality of the X-ray beam

Factor	Effect on the quantity of the X-ray beam	Effect on the quality (energies) of the X-ray beam
Increase in the X-ray tube current (mA)	Produces an increase in the quantity of radiation directly proportional to the increase in mA	The quality of the radiation from the tube is unaffected by an increase in the tube current
Increase in the potential difference (kVp) across the X-ray tube	An increase in the kVp produces an increase in the quantity of radiation produced at the target proportional to the kVp^2	An increase in the kVp produces an increase in the average energy of the photons in the X-ray beam and so produces an increase in the quality of the beam
X-ray tube target material	An increase in the atomic number of the target material will produce an increase in the quantity of radiation produced which is proportional to the increase in the atomic number	A change in the atomic number of the target material will produce no change in the quality of the beam produced by the Bremsstrahlung process. A higher atomic number will produce characteristic radiation of higher energy and, if this is in significant amounts, it will increase the quality of the overall spectrum
Generator waveform	The closer the voltage across the X-ray tube is to a constant potential, the greater the quantity of radiation produced	The closer the voltage across the X-ray tube is to a constant potential, the greater the quality of radiation produced
Filtration	Filtration reduces the quantity of radiation emerging from the X-ray tube. The reduction is related to the thickness and the atomic number of the filter	Filtration improves the quality of the radiation from an X-ray tube by selective removal of the low-energy photons
Focal spot size	No effect	No effect
Exposure time	Increases the total quantity of radiation	No effect on X-ray beam quality
Focus to detector distance (FDD)	Only affects the quantity of radiation received at the detector, not where it outputs at the X-ray tube	No effect on X-ray beam quality

14.8 THE EFFECT OF DISTANCE – THE INVERSE SQUARE LAW

The inverse square law means that the intensity of an X-ray beam decreases according to the square of the distance from the X-ray source. In practice this means that the beam intensity decreases by four times when the distance is doubled. The law is a consequence of the fact that X-rays travel in straight lines and 'fan out' as they travel away from the source, as shown in Fig. 14.9. The law applies only in air and not as an X-ray beam passes through a denser object such as the human body or a filter. This is because there is negligible absorption or scatter of X-rays in air but a lot in denser materials, as described in Chapter 13. The law also requires that the rays arise from a 'point source' (a very small source,

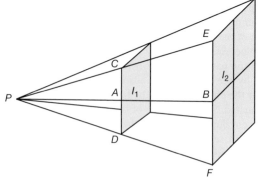

Fig. 14.9 Similar-triangles proof of the inverse square law. Note that the radiation at I_2 is spread over four times the area of I_1 and so the intensity at I_2 is a quarter of the intensity at I_1.

such as an X-ray tube focal spot). The intensity of an X-ray beam in radiography is usually defined as the number of X-rays passing through unit cross-sectional area per second, as mentioned earlier in this chapter. If a radiographer wished to maintain the X-ray intensity at an imaging plate when increasing the focus to detector distance from 100 cm to 200 cm, he or she would need to increase the mAs by a factor of four. The inverse square law also applies to other electromagnetic radiations such as visible light. A light source seems to dim a lot as we move further away from it.

14.9 SUMMARY OF THE FACTORS AFFECTING THE QUANTITY, QUALITY AND INTENSITY OF THE X-RAY BEAM

The factors which affect the quantity and/or quality of the beam of X radiation emerging from an X-ray tube are summarised in Table 14.2. Some factors, such as the generator waveform, X-ray tube target material and added filtration, are generally fixed for a particular X-ray machine and are not within the control of the operator. The kVp and mA can be adjusted by an operator, however. It should be noted that X-ray tube focal spot size does not affect the X-ray spectrum. The X-ray tube focus (or source) to detector distance affects the quantity (but not the quality) of the X-ray beam at the detector via the inverse square law but *not* as it leaves the X-ray tube.

SUMMARY

In this chapter, you should have learnt the following:
- The meaning of the terms quantity and quality as applied to the X-ray beam.
- The effect of the current through the X-ray tube (mA) on the quantity of the X-ray beam produced.
- The effect of the potential difference across the X-ray tube (kVp) on the quantity and the quality of the X-ray beam produced.
- The effect of the atomic number of the target material on the quantity of the radiation produced and on the characteristic radiation from the target.
- The effect of the voltage waveform applied to the X-ray tube (rectification) on the quantity and the quality of the X-ray beam produced.
- The effect of filtration on the quantity and the quality of the radiation beam emerging from the X-ray tube.

FURTHER READING

Ball, J.L., Moore, A.D., & Turner, S. 2008. *Ball and Moore's Essential Physics for Radiographers*. 4th edn. London: Blackwell Scientific. (Chapter 16.)

Bushong, S. 2016. *Radiologic Science for Technologists: Physics, Biology, and Protection*. 11th edn. St. Louis, MO: Mosby. (Chapter 8.)

Dendy, P., & Heaton, B. 2011. *Physics for Diagnostic Radiology*. 3rd ed. Boca Raton, FL: CRC Press. (Chapter 2.)

Digital radiography: computed radiography and digital radiography systems

15.1 AIM

The aim of this chapter is to introduce the reader to the principles of digital radiography (DR). The assumption is made that the reader has read and understood Chapter 11 which dealt with X-ray production.

15.2 THE DIGITAL IMAGE

The traditional method of producing a radiograph using film and intensifying screens is an example of an analogue image. The information contained within the radiograph is represented by a range of continuously varying densities or shades of grey. By contrast, a digital image is divided into a series of very small boxes called *pixels*, arranged in a series of rows and columns called a *matrix* (Fig. 15.1). Within the matrix each pixel has a numerical integer value. If we consider our initial radiograph, we could allocate the value zero to the most-dense value and 255 to the least-dense value, giving a digital scale of 256. Thus any single pixel within the image would have a discrete value between zero and 255. The smaller the image size and the larger the number of pixels in the image matrix, the better the spatial resolution of the image. Most modern digital imaging systems have a matrix of 1024 × 1024 pixels, with the resultant image having a total of 1,048,576 individual pixels.

Digital imaging is used in all imaging modalities in the modern diagnostic radiology department. The pro-cess of converting the analogue radiation image exiting the patient into a digital image differs depending on the imaging modality. However, the principle of changing this analogue signal into a digital one is common to all

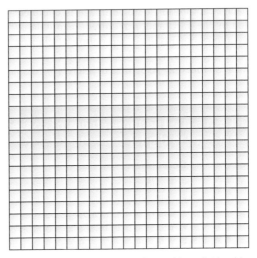

Fig. 15.1 An example of the *matrix* used in a digitised image. Each box of this matrix is called a *pixel* and will have its own density value.

modalities and applications. Advantages of digital imaging include the construction of an image with a high spatial resolution, large dynamic range and good contrast resolution. In addition, imaging data may also be processed by a computer to enhance the diagnostic value of the 'raw' unprocessed image. The data for these images can come from a variety of acquisition modalities and will be received by some form of image receptor (imaging plate, digital array or transducer). The signal then passes through several basic steps before a visible image is produced.

15.3　DIGITAL IMAGE PRODUCTION

If the image is not already in the form of an electrical signal, the first step of the conversion process is to convert the image to an electrical signal. The analogue electrical signal is converted to a digital electrical signal using a device called an *analogue-to-digital converter* (ADC). Within the ADC, the signal undergoes three stages: scanning, quantisation and coding (Table 15.1).

Where any signal is generated from part of a 'moving' image such as during fluoroscopy, it is important to have an ADC with a high sampling rate. This is important so that the ADC can sample and process each individual frame before it is replaced by the next.

Once the data from the ADC is received by the computer, the binary numbers are passed to the computer's central processing unit (CPU). This then directs the data to an area of computer memory called the *frame store*. Once data capture for a single image is complete, it is recalled by the CPU and, if required, manipulated. This facility allows, for instance, the option of altering contrast and brightness, to window on specific values within the image so that only structures of interest are displayed,

to enhance the edges of structures or to subtract one image from another. Having manipulated the images as required, the binary values are recalled from the frame store and, if required, matched to the display capabilities of the computer monitor and passed to an output buffer. Finally, once all data are modified and stored, the CPU monitors the transfer of the data to an appropriate output device (e.g., a computer monitor). This process is illustrated diagrammatically in Fig. 15.2.

15.4　DIGITAL IMAGING IN GENERAL RADIOGRAPHY

Digital imaging systems in general radiography are based on two broad types, computed radiography (CR) and DR. In many instances CR systems are being replaced in favour of DR systems.

15.4.1　Computed radiography

CR image receptors include a cassette that houses a phostostimulable imaging plate (IP). The IP consists of a support layer, a phosphor layer and a protective layer. Radiation exiting from the patient interacts with the phosphor layer which is commonly composed of barium fluorohalide crystals doped with europium ($BaF(BrI):Eu^2$). Some of the photon energies are absorbed by the barium fluorohalide crystals and some are released as visible light through the process of luminescence. A sufficient amount of energy is stored within the phosphor layer to retain a latent image. Barium fluorohalide, referred to as the photostimulable phosphor (PSP), releases visible light when stimulated by a high-intensity laser beam, a process termed *photostimulable luminescence*. A cross-sectional diagram of

---

TABLE 15.1　The three stages of converting an analogue signal into a digital signal using an analogue-to-digital converter

Stage	Description
Scanning	• The incoming signal is scanned as a series of equally spaced horizontal lines. • Each line is divided into a number of equally spaced points producing a series of small 'boxes'. • Each box forms a single pixel. • The scanning frequency controls the horizontal resolution of the image.
Quantisation	• This process allocates a numerical integer to each pixel. On a scale of 1024, for example, each pixel can have an integer value of 0 to 1023. This scale permits the ADC to detect changes in the signal as low as 0.7 mV.
Coding	• This final stage converts the numerical values produced by quantisation into binary numbers. • Binary numbers are the type of number commonly understood by computers. • Once this stage has finished the data is then passed from the ADC to the computer.

ADC, Analogue-to-digital converter.

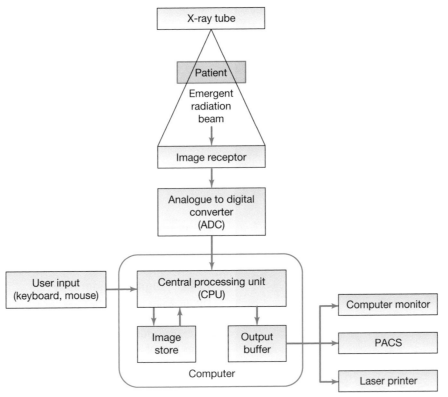

Fig. 15.2 Block diagram of the major components of a digital imaging system. *PACS,* Picture archiving and communications system.

a typical CR IP is shown in Fig. 15.3. An example of a CR IP and a plate reader is shown in Fig. 15.4.

The production of a CR X-ray image is a two-phased process, (1) image capture (latent image) using the IP and (2) image readout. A latent image is formed when the X-ray photons exiting the patient are absorbed by the phos-phor and the europium atoms become ionised by the photoelectric effect. The absorbed energy in the phosphor layer excites the electrons, which are elevated to a higher energy state where they become stored or trapped. The number and distribution of the trapped electrons are proportional to the tissue's differential absorption and form the latent

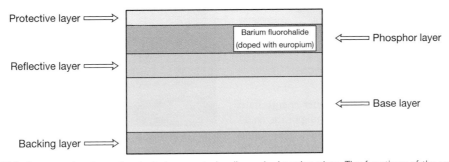

Fig. 15.3 Cross-section through a typical computed radiography imaging plate. The functions of the various layers are discussed in the text.

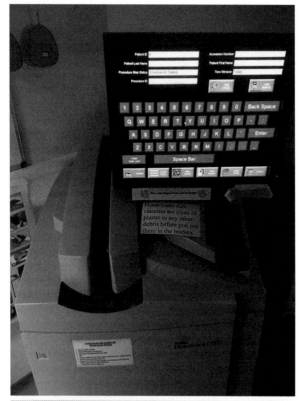

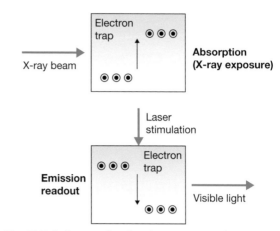

Fig. 15.5 A diagram showing the movement of electrons following X-ray exposure and during image readout.

15.4.2   Digital radiography

DR does not involve the operator taking the IP to a plate reader. Instead the imaging device (flat-panel detector) is either incorporated into the X-ray couch or erect stand or forms part of a mobile cassette sending the image data to a computer as soon as the exposure has been completed (Fig. 15.6). The image is then produced and available on the operator's computer workstation after a few seconds. The technology which forms the flat-panel detectors can be divided into two major types: direct conversion detectors, commonly named *direct digital radiography* (DDR),

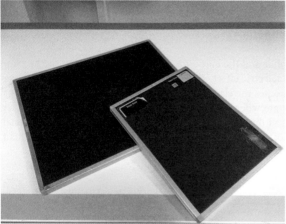

Fig. 15.4 Single plate computed radiography reader (*top*) and two computed radiography imaging plates (*bottom*).

image. These electrons remain in this higher energy state until released during the laser beam scanning of the read-out stage. A diagram illustrating the movement of electrons during X-ray exposure and image readout is shown in Fig. 15.5. Following exposure, the IP should be processed relatively quickly as the latent image dissipates over time.

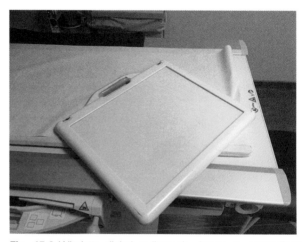

Fig. 15.6 Wireless digital radiography image receptor. The system has the option of including a protective cover (*see in the image*) or replacement with an antiscatter radiation grid (not shown).

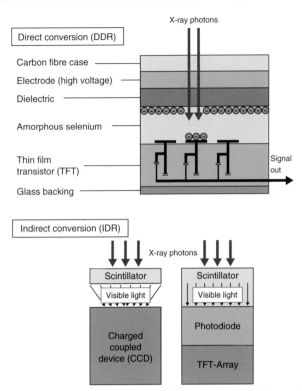

Fig. 15.7 Diagrammatical comparison of direct and indirect conversion digital radiography systems.

and *indirect conversion detectors* or *indirect digital radiography* (IDR) (Fig. 15.7).

15.4.2.1 Direct digital radiography

The outer layer of a DDR plate is a microplated electrode. This allows a charge to be applied via a dielectric layer to an amorphous selenium (a-Se) layer. An amorphous silicon (a-SI) layer absorbs X-ray photons and this results in the liberation of electrons. These electrons are directed by the charge pattern towards the silicon thin-film transistors (TFTs). The TFTs act as switches which send the signal to the processing system where the software converts it to an appropriate greyscale for that pixel.

15.4.2.2 Indirect digital radiography

Indirect conversion flat-panel detectors are similar to DDR detectors except that the conversion is via a two-step process. Within an IDR system the crystals in the caesium iodide layer are struck by the X-ray photons and emit light photons proportional to the energy and intensity of the X-ray photons. Caesium iodine crystals are needle shaped and so emit the spread of light emitted, thus improving

resolution. The light photons fall onto the a-Si layer and cause the emission of electrons within this layer. These electrons are then directed towards the TFTs and the image is produced in a similar way to the DDR method. Because there is potential for the light to diverge before being captured by the a-Se layer, the resolution of this system is not as high as the DDR conversion method.

SUMMARY

In this chapter, you should have learnt the following:
- What is meant by a 'digital image' in radiography.
- The main processes in digital image production.
- The basics of CR and DR in a general setting.

FURTHER READING

Carter, C.E., & Veale, B.L. 2013. *Digital Radiography and PACS*. St. Louis: Mosby Elsevier.

Lanca, L., & Silva, A. 2013. *Digital Imaging Systems for Plain Radiography*. New York: Springer-Verlag.

Exposure factors and the digital radiographic image

CHAPTER CONTENTS

16.1   AIM

The aim of this chapter is to consider the major factors involved in the production of a digital radiographic image. The chapter will first consider the attenuation patterns in a patient that will produce an X-ray image and will then consider how these patterns react with an image receptor to produce an X-ray image. The chapter also summarises how the selection of exposure factors affects the quality of the digital radiographic image produced.

16.2   INTRODUCTION

The quality of the radiographic image is affected by a number of geometrical factors that determine the magnification of the image and the amount of geometrical unsharpness produced, but a digital radiographic image depends on more than simply geometrical considerations. This chapter considers the other factors which contribute to image quality. To understand this, it is necessary to understand the contribution of photoelectric absorption and Compton scattering to the final radiographic image (see Chapter 13).

It is easier to understand the final image quality if we consider image formation as a two-stage process:
1. The production of an X-ray image pattern as the beam of radiation is attenuated by the patient.

2. The production of a radiographic image as this radiation pattern interacts with an image receptor.

Therefore this chapter will consist of two halves, each looking at one of these stages.

16.3   THE X-RAY IMAGE PATTERN

16.3.1   Attenuation of the X-ray beam

We will assume, for simplicity, that the radiation beam from the X-ray tube striking the body is of uniform intensity across the beam. When this beam interacts with the body, different structures will cause different amounts of attenuation and a 'pattern' of radiation intensities is transmitted to the imaging device. If all structures in the beam attenuated the radiation by the same amount, there would be no pattern and no image of any structures would be seen on the X-ray image. A simple example of such differential absorption is shown in Fig. 16.1, where two separate rectangular blocks of bone and soft tissue are shown interacting with the X-ray beam. The profiles of the incident (I_0) and the transmitted (I_T) radiation intensities are also shown.

If again we assume, for simplicity, that the attenuation of the radiation beam is exponential, then:

$$I_B = I_0 e^{-\mu(B)d}$$
$$I_T = I_0 e^{\mu(T)d}$$

Equation 16.1

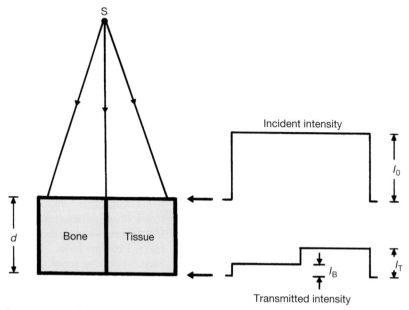

Fig. 16.1 A comparison of the attenuation of an X-ray beam by an equal thickness of bone and soft tissue. Note that the attenuation of X-rays in bone is greater than that by soft tissue.

where I_0 is the intensity of the X-ray beam before it enters the patient, $\mu(B)$ is the total linear attenuation coefficient for bone and $\mu(T)$ is the total linear attenuation coefficient for soft tissue. I_B is the intensity of the radiation transmitted through a thickness d of bone and I_T is the intensity transmitted through a similar thickness of soft tissue. As can be seen from Fig. 16.1, I_B is less than I_T. This is because $\mu(B)$ is greater than $\mu(T)$. There are two physical reasons for this:

1. The density of bone is approximately twice that of soft tissue ($\rho_B = 1.8$; $\rho_T = 1.0$).
2. The average atomic number of bone is approximately twice that of soft tissue ($Z_B = 14$; $Z_T = 7.5$).

The total linear attenuation coefficient is proportional to the number of atoms present in unit volume and the density of the medium. Because the density of bone is twice that of soft tissue, then there must be twice as many atoms in unit volume and so, all other things being equal, the linear attenuation coefficient for bone would be twice that for soft tissue.

To appreciate the importance of the difference in atomic number, we must consider the attenuation process occurring. The equations for each process are summarised here:

$$\tau \propto \rho \times \frac{Z^3}{E^3}$$

$$\sigma \propto \rho \frac{(\text{electron density})}{E}$$

Equation 16.2

where τ is the linear attenuation coefficient for the photoelectric effect, σ is the linear attenuation coefficient for Compton scattering, ρ is the density of the attenuator, Z is its atomic number and E is the photon energy. The higher atomic number of bone means that it will greatly attenuate suitable radiation by the photoelectric effect.

Because the total attenuation is a combination of both the photoelectric effect and Compton scattering, in the diagnostic energy ranges, a given thickness of bone will attenuate radiation approximately 12 times the level of an equal thickness of soft tissue.

The findings are summarised in Table 16.1. The essential points to be taken from the table are that in the diagnostic range of photon energies, the higher atomic number of bone results in photoelectric absorption being the main attenuation process, whereas the lower atomic number of soft tissue means that Compton scattering is the main attenuation process. (In the therapy range of photon energies, the dominant attenuation processes are Compton scattering and pair production, both of which are less dependent on the atomic number of the attenuator.)

A more realistic example of attenuation is given in Fig. 16.2. This simulates the presence of a piece of bone surrounded by soft tissue. A profile of the transmitted radiation intensity is also shown, and it can be seen that its

TABLE 16.1	Comparison of linear attenuation in bone and soft tissue		
Attenuator	Photoelectric $\tau \propto \rho \times Z^3/E^3$	Compton scattering (electron density) $\sigma \propto \rho$ (electron density)/E	Total attenuation $\mu = \tau + \sigma$
Bone $Z = 14$ $\rho = 1.8$	Photoelectric absorption is high when photon energy is low: 12–16 times greater than soft tissue	Predominates at high photon energies 500 keV to 5MeV	Mainly photoelectric absorption at diagnostic energies
Soft tissue $Z = 7.5$ $\rho = 1.0$	Significant at low photon energies <25 keV	Predominates at photon energies >30 keV	Compton scattering is the dominant process if the average photon energy is greater than about 30 keV

minimum corresponds to the maximum thickness of the bone (point A in the figure).

The fraction of the incident radiation transmitted through the thickness $D-d$ of soft tissue is $e^{-\mu(T)(D-d)}$. The total fraction can be found by *adding* the two fractions so that:

$$\frac{I_2}{I_0} = e^{-\mu(B)d} + e^{-\mu(T)(D-d)}$$

$$\text{so } I_2 = I_0 e^{-\mu(B)d} + e^{-\mu(T)(D-d)} \quad \textbf{Equation 16.3}$$

$$\text{or } I_2 = I_0 e^{-\mu(T)D - [-\mu(B)-\mu(t)]d}$$

$$\text{and } I_1 = I_0 e^{-\mu(t)D}$$

The difference between I_2 and I_1 is responsible for the contrast on the X-ray image.

16.3.2 Scatter and the radiographic image

So far, the sections of this chapter have been oversimplified in that the emerging radiation beam is assumed to be composed only of transmitted primary beam. If only photoelectric absorption took place this would be true, but it is not true in the case of Compton scatter where only partial absorption of the photon energy occurs. This scattered radiation may escape from the patient and reach the image recording medium. Unfortunately, such scatter will form an image on the medium, but the image formed by the scatter forms an overall fog and so is not useful. Unless this scatter can be limited, serious image degradation can occur.

Scatter to the X-ray image may be limited in two ways:
1. Limiting the amount of scatter formed.
2. Stopping any scatter formed from reaching the image recording medium.
Each of these will now be considered in turn.

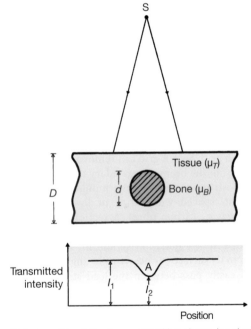

Fig. 16.2 A profile of the transmitted X-ray intensity obtained from a bone embedded in soft tissue.

16.3.2.1 Limiting scattered radiation formation

The amount of scatter formed in the patient depends on the number of atoms involved in scattering interactions. Thus scatter formation is volume dependent, that is, the greater the volume of patient irradiated, the greater the quantity of scatter formed. One of the major ways the operator can limit scatter formation is to reduce the volume of tissue irradiated. This can be done by collimation using a light-beam diaphragm or cones or, in some cases, by tissue displacement. Both these methods will not only produce an improvement in image quality but will also reduce the radiation dose to the patient and others by limiting the scatter formation.

16.3.2.2   Stopping scatter from reaching the image receptor

Once formed, the most common way of stopping scatter from reaching the image receptor is to use a secondary radiation grid. Such a grid can remove about 90% of the scatter from the beam. A secondary radiation grid consists of strips of high-atomic-number material (e.g., lead) interspaced with strips of low-atomic-number material (e.g., carbon fibre). A section through such a grid is shown in Fig. 16.3 where the lead strips are shaded. Primary radiation should hit the grid at right angles to its surface (or nearly right angles to it), so that it will easily pass between the lead strips (see ray 2).

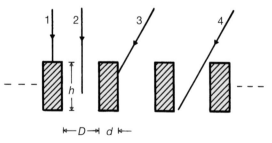

Fig. 16.3 The principle action of a secondary radiation grid. Scattered rays (3 & 4 in the diagram) are more likely to strike the lead slats and be absorbed than the primary rays (1 & 2 in the diagram).

Primary radiation (ray 1) may strike a lead strip and be absorbed. Because scatter (rays 3 and 4) are at an oblique angle to the primary beam, these rays have an increased probability of striking a lead strip and being absorbed. If the angle is very small (see ray 4) such scatter may 'miss' the lead strip and strike the image receptor, but such rays do not contribute to image degradation as the more oblique rays. The fraction of the primary beam stopped is given by the ratio $d/(D + d)$ because this is the fraction of the grid covered by lead; in practice this means the exposure must be increased when using a grid.

Various factors of grid design may be chosen to optimise the performance of a secondary radiation grid for a particular application:

- The *grid ratio* (r) is the height of the strips (h) to the width between them (D):

$$r = \frac{h}{D} \qquad \textbf{Equation 16.4}$$

It can be appreciated from Fig. 16.3 that increasing the height of the lead strips or reducing the space between them (i.e., increasing the grid ratio) will increase the efficiency of the grid in absorbing scattered radiation with a relatively small scatter angle.

- The grid lattice or lattice density is a measure of the number of lines of absorber per centimetre. If we consider that the space between each strip is controlled by the grid ratio, then the number of lines per centimetre will affect the thickness of the individual lines. Grids with a high lattice density (i.e., 30–40 lines per centimetre) will have very fine lines and so do not degrade the image. If grid lattice density is low, the grid lines are visible and detract from image quality. A solution to this problem is to move the grid during the exposure so that the grid lines are blurred out. Such a device is known as a *Potter–Bucky diaphragm* or, more commonly, as a *bucky*.

- As mentioned earlier, the grid will absorb some of the primary radiation and so it is necessary to increase the exposure when using a grid to compensate for this. The amount by which the exposure must be increased is known as the *grid factor*.

$$\text{grid factor} = \frac{\text{exposure with grid}}{\text{exposure without grid}} \qquad \textbf{Equation 16.5}$$

Note that this equation is accurate only if the kVp used for the exposure remains constant. A change of kVp will result in a change in the amount and type of scatter produced (see Insight, Section 16.3.2.1). It will also change the contrast range of the image (see Section 16.3.3). For most grids encountered in a diagnostic department, the grid factor will be between 2 and 6.

16.3.3 Effect of kVp on the X-ray image

The effect of a change of kVp on the spectrum of radiation produced by the X-ray tube will be discussed in Section 16.4 and, as can be seen from Fig. 16.2, the average energy for a single-phase two-pulse generator is about one-third to one-half of the maximum photon energy. This means that if 90 kVp was applied across the X-ray tube, the maximum photon energy would be 90 keV, but the average photon energy would be approximately 40 keV. We can apply the various scattering and attenuation coefficients to a beam of radiation generated at 90 kVp that we would apply to a monoenergetic beam of photon energy of 40 keV. The effect of increasing kVp is to increase the average photon energy and reduce the linear attenuation coefficients of both bone and soft tissue. The radiation beam is more penetrating.

From Equation 16.2, it can be seen that increasing photon energy will reduce the amount of photoelectric absorption (τ) more than it will reduce Compton scattering (σ) because the photoelectric effect is proportional to I/E^3. Because of less photoelectric absorption, there is less differentiation in absorption between bone and soft tissue— there is less contrast between the densities in the radiographic image. As already mentioned, an increase in kVp will also result in more scatter reaching the image receptor, further reducing contrast. Increasing kVp degrades image contrast in the ways mentioned earlier. There are practical advantages in using a high kVp. These are:

- It increases the intensity of the radiation beam, allowing a reduction in exposure time.
- It results in a higher percentage of the radiation beam being transmitted through the patient, again allowing a reduction in the exposure time.
- Because a higher percentage of the incident beam is transmitted through the patient, the absorbed radiation dose received by the patient is reduced.

INSIGHT

The 'best' image is the one that most clearly demonstrates the structures we wish to see! There are some situations in which a low kVp is used to produce a high contrast between tissues of almost the same density (e.g., mammography) and others where we may wish to use a high kVp to demonstrate structures of very different radiopacity in the same image (e.g., high kV chest radiography).

16.4 THE RADIOGRAPHIC IMAGE PATTERN

The X-ray image pattern discussed so far in this chapter may be used to form an image on a number of different image receptors, for instance on a visual display unit (VDU), a photostimulable imaging plate (PSP) or even a film-intensifying screen combination, although the latter is very rarely used today.

When the image is displayed on a VDU, the light intensity is directly proportional to the radiation intensity, whereas a PSP has a similar linear response. This is not so when the radiation image is transferred to a photographic emulsion using intensifying screens. The intensifying screen produces light in proportion to the intensity of the X-ray image pattern. This light produces a latent image in the film. Processing then converts the invisible latent image into a permanent one. This blackening effect is not linear. An instrument called a *densitometer*, which is calibrated to measure optical density, can be used to assess the density or amount of blackening produced. Density is defined as $\log_{10}(I_0/I_t)$, where I_0 is the intensity of the light on the processed film and I_t is the intensity of the light transmitted through it. Examination of a processed image will show that the darker the image, the less light transmitted through it and the higher the optical density. When plotting the density of the film at different exposures, it is usual to plot density against the logarithm of the relative exposure to accommodate the wide range of exposures to which the emulsion can respond. A graph of these densities can be produced; this is known as the *characteristic curve* of that emulsion. Fig. 16.4 shows a typical characteristic curve for

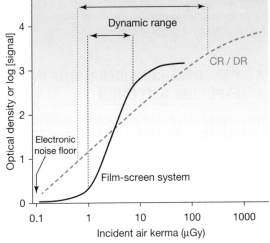

Fig. 16.4 Typical characteristic curves of both film-screen and computed radiography/digital radiography systems.

both film-screen and computed radiography/digital radiography (CR/DR) systems.

Features of this graph will now be discussed (see Fig. 16.4):

- Even when the relative exposure is zero, the film-screen emulsion will show some density. This is referred to as *base plus fog*. It results from the small amount of fog produced by the chemical activity of the developing process and any tint that may be present in the base material of the film. The density of this region is normally less than 0.2.
- There follows an initial horizontal portion where an increase in exposure produces no increase in density. This is often referred to as the *threshold* of the curve.
- The toe of the curve is the point at which the emulsion is becoming increasingly responsive to differences in exposure.
- There follows a region where an increase in exposure produces a linear increase in density. We aim to set X-ray exposure factors so that the exposure to the film falls in this part of the characteristic curve.
- The linear increase 'flattens' off at the shoulder. This usually occurs at densities between 3 and 4. We can only see contrasts between densities of just over two with the unaided eye; densities above this are seen as black. Industrial radiography makes use of this region.

In contrast, a CR/DR system has a linear response almost over the entire exposure range, giving it a very high bit depth (see Chapter 15). Image processing software permits the selection of the range of the bit depth of the displayed image and also compensates for both over- and underexposure, although with gross underexposure, image is more noticeable. For most systems there is a plateauing point at extreme exposures where there is no increase in signal (as a result of receptor saturation).

16.5   PRACTICAL CONSIDERATIONS IN EXPOSURE SELECTION

Where anatomical exposure selection in not available, the interrelationships between the various factors that affect image quality are complex and require considerable skill to master. There is a strong subjective element in selecting the 'best' image but no absolute rules can be laid down for exposure factors. The wide degree of variability in shape and size of the patients themselves, together with other practical difficulties (e.g., patients who are unable to keep still during the exposure), would provide so many exceptions that it is impossible to adhere to a strict set of rules. The operator's experience is therefore critical in producing images of consistently high quality under all conditions. The

following paragraphs should be considered with these general comments in mind.

In the chapter on X-ray beam properties we saw that, broadly speaking, the quality of the radiation in an X-ray beam depends on the kVp across the X-ray tube and the quantity of radiation produced on the mAs that flows through the X-ray tube during the exposure. If the kVp selected is too low, denser body structures (e.g., the bony skeleton) will not be penetrated by the X-ray beam, resulting in excessive contrast and an increase in radiation dose to the patient. However, too high a kV reduces the contrast between structures and can produce significant amounts of scattered radiation. Unless this scatter is prevented from reaching the image receptor by the use of a secondary grid, image degradation can occur.

Image manipulation software can compensate for excessive density if too high an mAs is selected, but the operator may not be aware of their error and the patient will receive an excessive dose of radiation as a result. The exposure index shown on the monitor screen is an indicator of this. If the mAs selected is excessively low, image manipulation software can often produce an acceptable image, although pixellation may be present.

16.6   EXPOSURE FACTORS AND SELECTION PRINCIPLES

The fundamental principles surrounding the correct selection of radiographic exposure factors by a practitioner do not change simply because of change in image receptor (film-screen, CR cassette or DR flat-panel). When undertaking radiographic examinations, practitioners must determine the radiation exposure needed to produce an image of sufficient quality to meet the diagnostic purpose of the examination. Defining a sufficient image quality level for diagnostic purposes is in itself a difficult task; the requirements from any given examination are likely to vary between different clinical indications and also on a patient-by-patient basis. Image quality guidelines do exist within the literature, but they are often unvalidated or were developed in an era of film-screen systems. It is accepted that a sufficient or adequate quality image should have sufficient density/brightness to display the key anatomical structures, an appropriate level of contrast to allow the differentiation between adjacent structures together with sufficient spatial resolution and minimum image distortion (see Table 16.2).

16.6.1   Kilovoltage peak (kVp)

Image quality is dependent on the sufficient quantity and energy of X-ray photons reaching the image receptor. Tube potential (kVp) is responsible for ensuring adequate penetration of the anatomical part and is needed to generate

TABLE 16.2 Definition of common image quality terminology

Property	Definition
Density	The degree of image darkening; sufficient quality images require 'optimum' density.
Contrast	The ability of an imaging system to discriminate objects with small differences in density.
Spatial resolution	Refers to the ability of an imaging system to detect and discriminate small objects that are close together.
Magnification	An increase in the dimension of an object on an X-ray image when compared with its life size.
Distortion	The misrepresentation of the shape (length or width) of an object.

differences in the X-ray photon energies leaving the patient. Differences in the X-ray photon energies are essential to produce an acceptable level of image contrast. In modern digital radiographic practice, kVp selection cannot simply follow the practices observed when using film-screen systems. Within digital imaging (CR and DR) many practitioners would opt for higher tube potentials when compared with those used on film-screen systems. There are, however, exceptions and these would include chest radiography and studies involving children. Digital systems are different in that image processing allows the contrast and density of an image to be optimised independently. A point worthy of consideration is that kVp selection should also consider the specific composition of the image receptor. All digital detector mediums have, to some extent, depending on their absorption characteristics, a higher dose efficiency at lower kVps.

16.6.2 Additional beam filtration

The use of additional beam filtration, such as thin layers of copper or aluminium, can help reduce the entrance surface dose for certain body parts. Most national regulators currently require that all X-ray tubes have inherent beam filtration of at least 2.5 mm of aluminium equivalent. Additional filtration provides further opportunities for removing the lower energy part of the X-ray tube spectrum; such energies are completely absorbed by the patient and do not contribute to the resultant image. Additional filtration of 1 mm aluminium combined with 0.1 or 0.2 mm of copper have been suggested and are used routinely in paediatric radiography in many countries. The use of additional filtration does carry limitations for adult imaging where it would typically require an increase in exposure time; this has negative consequences for tube life and also when attempting to minimise motion artefacts.

16.6.3 Antiscatter radiation grids

Antiscatter radiation grids are typically used for locations where there is high absorption and a high level of scattered radiation, for example, when imaging the abdomen, pelvis or lumbar spine. This leads to a reduction in image quality with respect to the signal-to-noise ratio and also contrast. Use of an antiscatter radiation grid provides the opportunity for optimising image quality but is associated with the need for a higher radiation dose (two or three times higher than acquisitions without a grid). CR and DR technologies are more sensitive to scattered radiation; the incorporation of an antiscatter radiation grid should follow similar principles to those used in film-screen radiography. The lower K-absorption edge of CR and DR detector materials makes it more sensitive to the effects of lower energy scattered radiation when compared with film-screen systems. The requirement for an increase in exposure factors (radiation dose) when including a grid has been a universally accepted disadvantage. Several researchers have evaluated the removal of a grid for a number of examinations when using CR/DR systems. Such investigations have had limited success but the recent introduction of a 'virtual grid' has reinvigorated interest in nongrid techniques. Virtual grid technology uses advanced computer-based postprocessing algorithms to electronically remove image noise (from scattered radiation). Early experiences of this technique have demonstrated improvements in image quality together with substantial reductions in radiation dose. Further studies are necessary to fully evaluate the potential of this technology.

16.6.4 Image noise

For DR, image noise is inversely proportional to the radiation dose reaching the image receptor. A visual assessment of image noise by the practitioner is a routine quality assurance step within clinical practice. The human visual system is both highly subjective and relatively insensitive to changes in noise. Identification in changes to the noise levels on X-ray images requires significant changes to the radiation dose incident on the detector. Physical measures of noise, for example, signal-to-noise ratios (SNRs), are more sensitive to changes in exposure factors (detector dose) but are of limited value in routine clinical practice because of the steps needed for their calculations. SNR values are also constrained by the anatomy and pathology contained within an image and are often considered to be more suitable when evaluating the imaging appearances of test objects.

16.6.5 Speed-class system

Radiographic speed is defined as the inverse of the radiation exposure necessary to produce a net film optical density equal to 1. This classification system is not useful in DR because the densities of CR and DR images are arbitrary and are dependent on the computer processing and not simply radiation dose. Within film-screen systems, speed is determined by the thickness and composition of the intensifying screen and this also provides a description of the spatial resolution. For CR systems, the phosphor thickness and the laser spot size are determinants of spatial resolution. For both CR and DR technologies, the pixel size is also an important factor.

Within DR, the quality of an image is no longer governed by the signal strength alone (X-ray flux) but by the image SNR. Characterising the SNR performance of a DR system in terms of how efficiently it uses the number of incident X-ray photons during image formation has resulted in the metric termed detective quantum efficiency (DQE). DQE is sometimes used as a surrogate measure for the radiation dose efficiency of a detector because the required radiation dose to a patient decreases as the DQE increases for the same image SNR and exposure factors. DQE is dependent on the radiation exposure, spatial frequency, modulation-transfer function (MTF) and detector material. High DQE values indicate that less radiation is needed to achieve identical image quality; increasing the DQE and leaving the radiation dose constant will result in improved image quality. The ideal digital detector would have a DQE of 1, or 100%; this would mean that all radiation energy is absorbed by the detector and converted into an image (see Fig. 16.5).

16.6.6 Exposure index

In an attempt to give the practitioner feedback about the actual detector dose for a clinical image, digital systems now provide an 'exposure indicator'. A definition of an exposure indicator and how it can be used within radiography has only recently been standardised but has been extensively debated amongst the medical imaging community. Despite this, exposure indicator values presented by manufacturers on commercially available CR and DR systems vary between vendors. As such it is difficult to make comparisons between imaging systems, and it is also difficult to fully understand what modifications are required to radiographic technique to make improvements based simply on these values.

For DR systems, exposure indicators provide a feedback mechanism for the radiographer regarding the radiation dose delivered to the image receptor. Over- or under-

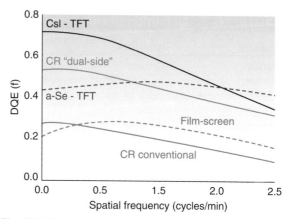

Fig. 16.5 Detective quantum efficiency (*DQE*) as a function of spatial frequency for different image receptor systems. Note the Cesium Iodide a-Se amorphous Selenium (CsI) detector has superior DQE when compared with an a-Se detector (the worst being film-screen).

exposure of an image will deliver an incorrect exposure indicator, whereas a correct exposure will provide a value within a specified target range. The indicator is typically a vendor-specific value that provides the radiographer with an indication of their exposure accuracy for a specific examination. Exposure indicators have many different names, depending on the vendor, and may include S-number, REG, IgM, ExI and Exposure Index (see Table 16.3, Fig. 16.6). Carestream currently references its exposure indicator as an exposure index or EI for both CR and DR systems. Within these systems, the EI is a representation of the average pixel value for the image in a predefined region of interest (ROI). With each vendor having its own method and terminology, this has created confusion amongst radiographers who have equipment from multiple vendors within their institution. As a result, the International Electrotechnical Commission (IEC) and the American Association of Physicists in Medicine (AAPM), in cooperation with manufacturers, developed an international standard for EI. The IEC EI is unique to the receptor type being used and the examination being performed. Within this work three default target exposure index (TEI) values are preloaded onto the system and represent target exposures for bucky, nonbucky and paediatric examinations. Following exposure, the system will determine and present the IEC EI and the deviation index (DI). The DI quantifies the difference between the actual EI and the target E; this feedback allows the radiographer to track and adjust his or her own exposures (see Table 16.4). When the actual EI is equal to the target EI, the DI will be zero. A positive or negative DI indicates the amount of exposure greater or lesser than the target.

TABLE 16.3 Manufacturer and exposure index parameters for a range of digital radiography systems

Manufacturer	Exposure indicator name	Symbol	Units	Exposure dependence, X
Fujifilm	S value	S	Unitless	$200/S \propto X$ (mR)
Carestream	Exposure index	EI	Mbels	$EI + 300 = 2X$
Agfa	Log of median of histogram	lgM	Bels	$lgM + 0.3 = 2X$
Konica	Sensitivity number	S	Unitless	For QR = k, $200/S \propto X$ (mR)
GE	Uncompensated detector exposure	UDExp	µGy air kerma	$UDExp \propto X$ (mR)
	Compensated detector exposure	CDExp	µGy air kerma	$CDExp \propto X$ (mR)
	Detector exposure index	DEI	Unitless	DEI ~ ratio of actual exposure to expected exposure scaled by technique and system parameters
Philips	Exposure index	EI	Unitless	$1000/X$ (µGy)
Siemens	Exposure index	EXI	µGy air kerma	X (µGy) = EI/100

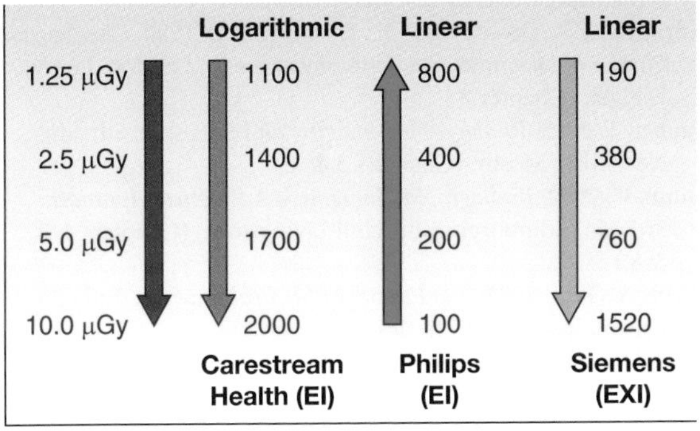

	Logarithmic	Linear	Linear
1.25 µGy	1100	800	190
2.5 µGy	1400	400	380
5.0 µGy	1700	200	760
10.0 µGy	2000	100	1520
	Carestream Health (EI)	Philips (EI)	Siemens (EXI)

Fig. 16.6 Sample of exposure indicator scales used by different vendors.

TABLE 16.4 The relationship between deviation index and the % difference from the target exposure index

Deviation index (DI)	% of target
3	~100% too high
2	~58% too high
1	~26% too high
0	Correct
−1	~21% too low
−2	~37% too low
−3	~50% too low

16.7 FACTORS AFFECTING IMAGE QUALITY

16.7.1 Detection efficiency

For CR and DR systems, the efficiency in which the X-ray photons exiting the patient are absorbed is determined by the absorber density, thickness and composition. The detection efficiency can be increased by increasing the density of the material or the absorber thickness; this is usually with a trade-off in spatial resolution.

16.7.2 Dynamic range

In digital chest radiography, the ratio of the maximum to minimum X-ray exposures incident on the detector surface can be greater than 100:1. To facilitate high-quality DR, the image receptor must be able to maintain a good contrast resolution over this wide dynamic range. The dynamic range of an X-ray system is the ratio between the largest and smallest X-ray intensities that can be imaged. The smallest useful X-ray intensity is determined by the intrinsic system noise; the X-ray signal must be large enough to exceed this noise, combined with the X-ray quantum noise. The largest intensity is determined by the receptor saturation. The dynamic range of a digital imaging system is often referred to as the latitude.

16.7.3 Spatial sampling

All digital detectors sample the continuously varying X-ray fluence at their input at discrete locations separated by an interval called the sampling pitch. For CR systems, the sampling pitch is the distance between the adjacent laser beam positions during the readout phase. For DR systems, the sampling pitch is the centre-to-centre distance between charge-collecting detector elements.

16.7.4   Spatial resolution

Spatial resolution is the ability of an imaging system to allow two adjacent structures to be visualised as being separate. Spatial resolution losses occur because of geometric factors, for example, size of the X-ray focal spot and light diffusion within the image receptor. In CR imaging, the primary source of spatial resolution loss is the scattering of laser light during readout. Spatial resolution in DR depends primarily on two factors: (1) for indirect systems, the spread of light photons in the X-ray-to-light conversion process and (2) the size of the detector elements.

SUMMARY

In this chapter, you should have learnt the following:

- How the X-ray beam is attenuated by bone and soft tissue (Section 16.3.1).
- The effect of scattered radiation on the X-ray image and subsequently on the X-ray image (Section 16.3.2).
- Methods of limiting the amount of scattered radiation formed (Section 16.3.2.1).
- Methods of reducing the amount of scatter reaching the image receptor, including factors that affect the efficiency of a secondary radiation grid (Section 16.3.2.2).

- The effect of a change of kVp on the X-ray image pattern (Section 16.3.3).
- How the X-ray image pattern is changed into the radiographic image (Section 16.4).
- What is meant by the characteristic curve of an emulsion (Section 16.4).
- Practical considerations in the choice of exposure factors (Section 16.5).
- The contribution of individual exposure factors and their selection principles (Section 16.6).
- Factors affecting radiographic image quality (Section 16.7).

FURTHER READING

Ball, J.L., Moore, A.D., & Turner, S. 2008. *Ball and Moore's Essential Physics for Radiographers*. 4th edn. London: Blackwell Scientific. (Chapter 16.)

Carter, C.E., & Veale, B.L. 2010. *Digital Radiography and PACS*. Philadelphia: Mosby Elsevier. (Chapters 6 & 7.)

Curry III, T.S., Dowdey Jr., J.E., & Murry, R.C. 1990. *Christensen's Physics of Diagnostic Radiography*. 4th edn. London: Lee & Febiger. (Chapter 2.)

Fauber, T. 2013. *Radiographic Imaging and Exposure*. 5th edn. New York: Mosby. (Chapters 3 & 4.)

Gunn, C. 2002. *Radiographic Imaging – A Practical Approach*. 3rd edn. Edinburgh: Churchill Livingstone. (Chapters 4, 5 & 8.)

Webb, S. (Ed.). 2002. *The Physics of Medical Imaging*. 2nd edn. Bristol: Institute of Physics. (Chapter 2.)

Mobile, portable and dental X-ray systems

CHAPTER CONTENTS

17.1   AIM

The aim of this chapter is to introduce the reader to the principles of radiography using mobile, portable and dental X-ray systems. The assumption is that the reader has read and understood Chapter 11 which dealt with X-ray production.

17.2   INTRODUCTION

Mobile and portable X-ray units have been developed to accommodate patients who are unable to be moved to the radiology department for their radiographic examination. Such patients may be bed-bound or living in a remote location from the nearest hospital. Alternatively, patients within healthcare settings may be too unwell to attend the radiology department, and an X-ray examination at their bedside may be more appropriate. Whether these examinations are performed within formal healthcare settings or as domiciliary examinations will influence the type of equipment that is used.

17.3   MOBILE X-RAY SYSTEMS

A mobile X-ray unit has a means of being moved. It is mounted on wheels and usually has a drive motor and a motion brake. These systems are larger and heavier than portable X-ray units and as such need to be motorised or pushed by human power. Traditionally, they are confined to a single location and are used in conjunction with computed radiography (CR) or digital radiography (DR) image receptors.

There are distinctively two types of mobile X-ray unit:

Battery-powered units: These units use rechargeable batteries for both X-ray production and motor power. Such systems provide a high-frequency direct-current pulsed power supply which is equivalent to the 3-phase 12-pulse supply in a standard X-ray room. These systems are heavier and more bulky than the capacitor-discharge units and require frequent charging. Several systems have automatic exposure paddles incorporated into the design to provide greater exposure accuracy. Battery-powered units have, approximately, a 4% ripple. Newer battery-powered mobile X-ray units have been combined with wireless digital-imaging receptors to provide a totally independent X-ray unit (see Fig. 17.1). The ability to see almost instantaneous X-ray imaging at the point of care has provided a novel way for managing acutely ill patients. Changes to the position of lines and tubes can be undertaken without the need to move the image receptor, and this makes care more efficient at the bedside.

Capacitor-discharge unit: These systems require access to a wall power outlet (230 V). Within the units, a capacitor stores charge which is then released during the exposure. Movement of the X-ray unit is by human muscle power and as such these systems are lighter and smaller than the battery-powered units. Such systems are required to be plugged into mains electricity during X-ray production and therefore cannot be used for some situations (e.g., during power outages). Capacitor-discharge units have a smaller ripple of around 1%. These systems are typically encountered on neonatal intensive care units where exposures tend to be relatively small and significant movement of the unit around the healthcare institution is not re-

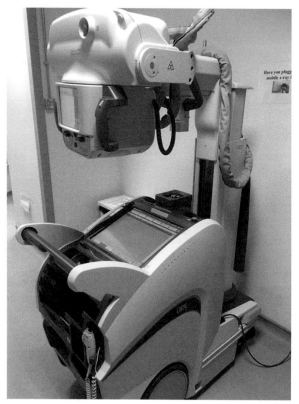

Fig. 17.1 An example of a modern digital mobile X-ray unit with a wireless digital radiography image receptor incorporated into the design. (From Warrington & Halton Hospital NHS Foundation Trust.)

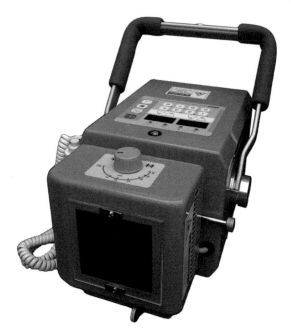

Fig. 17.2 An example of a portable X-ray unit. (Courtesy of EcoRay.)

quired. An absence of batteries within a capacitor-discharge unit limits some of the faults that can occur with mobile systems and also reduces the costs for maintenance. Capacitor-discharge units are less common that battery-powered units because their versatility around a healthcare institution is somewhat reduced.

17.4   PORTABLE X-RAY SYSTEMS

A portable X-ray unit is distinct from a mobile X-ray unit in that it can be carried by a single able-bodied person (see Fig. 17.2). In some instances, it can be taken around the hospital; however, its more common application is in the provision of radiographic services outside of the healthcare environment, (e.g., a patient's home or nursing home). Performing clinical radiography outside of the healthcare setting has been universally given the term *domiciliary visit*. Domiciliary visits have traditionally had limited value in that the image quality and opportunities for repeat imaging imposed limitations on the service. More recently, there has been increased interest in domiciliary examina-

tion as a method for reducing the potential to spread infection and to reduce the logistical requirements for patient transfers to a formal healthcare facility, that is, hospital. Such systems, because of the nature of their design, pose restrictions in the range of examinations available and the types of patients who can be imaged.

17.5   DENTAL X-RAY SYSTEMS

There are two main types of dental X-rays: intraoral (where the image receptor is located inside of the oral cavity) and extraoral (where the image receptor is located outside of the mouth). Intraoral X-rays are the most common type of dental X-ray examination and, perhaps unsurprisingly, there are a number of different intraoral dental X-ray examinations.

Common intraoral X-ray examinations: Periapical (PA) X-rays are designed to show the whole tooth, from the crown to beyond the root. PAs are used to detect unusual changes in the root and surrounding bone structures. Bite-wing (BW) X-rays provide an overview of the upper and lower teeth in one area of the mouth. Each BW shows the tooth from the crown to the level of supporting bone. BW X-rays are commonly used to detect decay between teeth (interproximal caries) and changes in the thickness of the bone (bone loss). Occlusal X-rays follow the development and placement of an entire arch of teeth in either the lower or upper jaw.

Common extraoral X-ray examinations: Orthopantomograms (OPGs) show the entire mouth area—all of the

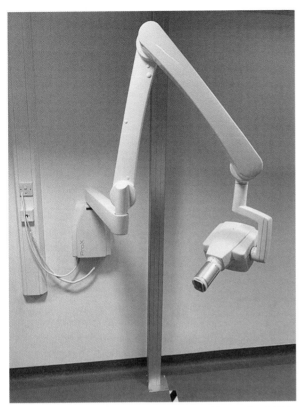

Fig. 17.3 An example of an intraoral dental X-ray unit which is wall mounted. (From University of Salford.)

teeth in both the upper and lower jaw on a single image. This image uses a tomography technique to show a particular layer/slice through the mouth while blurring out nonessential structures. A lateral cephalogram (lateral ceph) is a side view (X-ray) profile of the face and mouth and is useful when planning the realignment of teeth and/or the facial bones. This technique provides clear visualisation of bony structures and soft tissues. Cone-beam computed tomography is a relatively new X-ray technique which creates a three-dimensional image of dental structures, soft tissues, nerves and bone. It is useful for guiding implant placement and for evaluating cysts and tumours in the face and mouth.

17.5.1 Intraoral dental X-ray units

There are numerous conventional dental X-ray units available from a wide variety of manufacturers. Each of these systems will vary in terms of appearance, functionality and cost but will all have three main components (a tube head, positioning arm and control panel). Such dental units can either be fixed (wall, floor or ceiling mounted; see Fig. 17.3) or mobile (attached to a frame on wheels). In the literature there are also descriptions of hand-held dental X-ray units that can have benefit in veterinary practice and for forensic applications.

There are a number of differences between standard X-ray tubes and those found on dental X-ray units (see Fig. 17.4). The tube head for dental units contains a glass X-ray tube, including a filament, copper block and X-ray target (made from tungsten). Transformers are present to step-up the mains voltage to a high kV; a step-down transformer is required to produce a low voltage for heating the filament. The glass X-ray tube or envelope is surrounded by a lead shield to

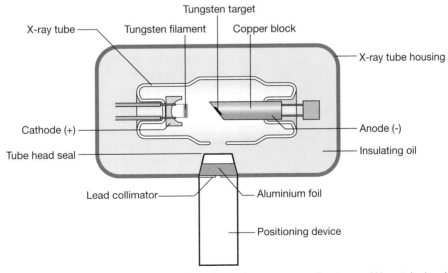

Fig. 17.4 A schematic outlining the configuration and components of an intraoral X-ray tube head.

minimise leakage and is surrounded by an oil reservoir to facilitate heat removal. Aluminium filtration is present at the exit port to remove the low-energy (soft) radiation. Fixed to the tube head is a collimator. This is either a metal disc or a cylinder with a central aperture and is designed to shape and limit the beam size to the intraoral image receptor. Unlike in conventional X-ray systems, the field size and centring point are not defined with the aid of a light beam. Dental X-ray systems rely on the collimator/cone for accurately positioning the tube relative to the sensor and for minimising the beam to the relevant structures (radiation protection).

17.5.2   Extraoral dental X-ray units

An OPG is produced by a combination of rotational movement of an X-ray tube and the detector/film around the head of the patient. There are several OPG units available, which all work on the same principle but differ in how they achieve rotational movement to visualise the dental arch. The dental arch, although curved, is not the shape of a circle. To produce the required elliptical horseshoe-shaped focal trough, the OPG system employs the principle of narrow-beam rotational tomography. The focal trough or corridor on an OPG image is three-dimensional; all structures within the trough/corridor, including the mandible and teeth, will be in focus on the final X-ray image. OPG equipment typically includes an X-ray tube head, either a cassette/cassette carriage assembly or integrated digital detector, and patient positioning apparatus. OPG machines are often combined with specialist apparatus to provide the option for cephalometry (see Fig. 17.5). Such systems make use of a single X-ray tube and image receptor and are of a lower cost than two separate systems.

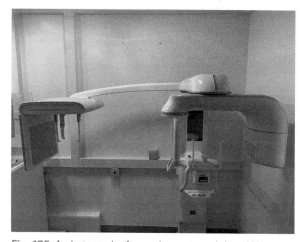

Fig. 17.5 A photograph of a modern extraoral dental X-ray machine. The equipment used in this example is capable of acquiring orthopantomogram and lateral cephalostat images. Acquisition is facilitated by an in-built digital radiography detector. (From Warrington & Halton Hospital NHS Foundation Trust.)

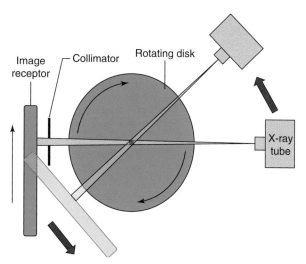

Fig. 17.6 Schematic diagram of the functionality of an orthopantomogram machine.

During the OPG examination, the X-ray tube and image receptor orbits the patient (see Fig. 17.6) and the right and left sides of the mandible are exposed to radiation using multiple different centres of rotation. The apparent alteration of the centre of rotation achieves a U-shaped focal layer. This focal layer is three-dimensional and reflects the shape of the mandible in a 'typical' patient but can vary by equipment vendor. The thickness of the layer is generally narrower anteriorly and thicker posteriorly to reflect anatomical differences. OPG images are typically magnified by between 10 and 30% and acquisitions typically take between 10 and 20 seconds.

A lateral cephalostat (see Fig. 17.7) is an X-ray taken of the side of the face using very precise positioning. Precise positioning and a dedicated imaging unit allow various measurements of faciomaxillary structures to be made to determine the current and future relationship of the maxilla and mandible and therefore assess the nature of a patient's bite. Such imaging is particularly useful when planning orthodontic treatment. It is essential for a cephalostat machine to have in-built head positioning and stabilising apparatus and the availability of a moveable aluminium wedge filter. This filter is positioned between the patient and the anterior part of the image receptor. This is designed to attenuate the X-ray beam selectively in this region because the facial soft tissues are not dense enough on their own to produce a radiographic shadow. Increasing the attenuation in the anterior soft tissues of the face allows them to be visualised on the final X-ray image. The examination is undertaken using a 200-cm source-to-image distance to reduce image magnification. A calibrated radiopaque ruler is placed on the nasion to provide a reference for actual anatomical dimensions in median sagittal plane.

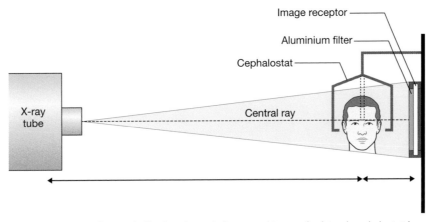

Fig. 17.7 A schematic diagram indicating the technique used to acquire lateral cephalostat images.

The goal of lateral cephalometry is to provide accurate and reproducible measurements of faciomaxillary structures over a period of time/treatment.

SUMMARY

In this chapter, you should have learnt the following:
- The different types of mobile X-ray systems available (Section 17.3).
- The types of equipment used to conduct domiciliary radiography examinations, using portable X-ray equipment (Section 17.4).
- The different types of dental X-ray systems (Section 17.5).
- The components and options for intraoral dental X-ray units (Section 17.5.1).
- The requirements for extraoral dental X-ray units (Section 17.5.2).

FURTHER READING

Whaites, E., & Drage, N. 2013. *Essentials of Dental Radiography and Radiology*. 5th edn. London: Churchill Livingstone. (Chapters 2 & 3.)

Mammography

CHAPTER CONTENTS

18.1   AIM

The aim of this chapter is to explore the modifications to standard X-ray equipment that are specifically designed to image breast tissues. The physics of X-ray beams consisting of a narrow range of low-energy photons is described, because these beams emphasise photoelectric absorption differences between soft tissues and are particularly useful in breast imaging.

18.2   INTRODUCTION

X-ray mammography depends upon the ability to display small density and atomic number differences between soft tissues. This particularly applies to the microcalcifications which can be an early sign of breast cancer. Thousands of symptomatic women and those participating in breast screening programmes (asymptomatic) rely upon X-ray physics to provide an accurate diagnosis. Conventional radiography, which uses X-ray tubes with tungsten targets (see Chapter 12) and tube kilovoltages of 40 and upwards, has difficulty in showing small soft tissue differences. This situation has been somewhat improved with the advent of high-resolution digital-imaging methods which provide a wide 'dynamic range' of signal intensities, but despite this advancement, alternative techniques must be employed to demonstrate breast pathologies. These consist of microcalcifications and altered soft tissue densities in glandular, lactiferous and fatty structures. Mammography X-ray units must be compact and manoeuvrable to image all parts of the breast, including the axillary tail.

18.3   TISSUE X-RAY ATTENUATION CHALLENGES FOR BREAST IMAGING

Atomic number differences (calcification ≈ 14, water ≈ 7, fat ≈ 6) can be accentuated using photoelectric attenuation of X-ray (see Chapter 13) which predominates at low X-ray photon energies, and is directly proportional to atomic number cubed ($\propto Z^3$). It is also known that photoelectric absorption is inversely proportional to X-ray energy cubed ($\propto 1/E^3$). Thus the keV values (energy values) of X-ray photons must be very small if they are to experience high photoelectric attenuation in the low atomic number soft tissues of the breast. A good source of low keV X-ray photons is required, without producing rays that are of such very low energy that they will be absorbed in the skin and increase radiation dose. Although it will never be possible to produce a purely monoenergetic (single-energy) X-ray beam because the Bremsstrahlung process of X-ray production provides a continuous X-ray spectrum (see Chapter 11), it would be ideal if we could produce a 'narrow band' X-ray spectrum, with the bulk of X-rays being found across a small range of energies. This would reduce radiation dose to the breast and also enhance X-ray absorption differences between tissues, increasing image contrast.

18.4   X-RAY BEAM ADAPTATIONS FOR BREAST IMAGING

The requirements for a narrow and low-beam energy range for mammography can be met in part by using molybdenum rather than tungsten as an X-ray tube target material.

TABLE 18.1   Features of tungsten and molybdenum targets for X-ray production

Element (symbol)	Tungsten (W)	Molybdenum (Mo)
Atomic number, Z	74	42
Characteristic K lines	~59 & 69 keV	~17.5 & 19.5 keV
K-shell absorption edge	69.5 keV	20 keV

Some of the key properties of tungsten and molybdenum are summarised in Table 18.1.

The intensity of the 'continuous X-ray spectrum' (see Chapter 11) which results from Bremsstrahlung in the X-ray tube target is proportional to the target atomic number Z. Thus there will be fewer continuous-spectrum X-ray from a molybdenum target than from one made of tungsten.

INSIGHT

Bremsstrahlung is a more effective process in high atomic number X-ray tube targets because the electrostatic attraction between unlike charges is proportional to their magnitude. An electron passing through the X-ray tube target has a charge of −1 and will experience a greater attraction to a tungsten nucleus of charge +74 than to a molybdenum nucleus of charge +42. The nuclear charge, of course, is determined by the number of protons. The greater attraction will result in more 'braking' of the electrons and thus more loss of energy in the form of X-ray photons.

X-ray spectra that could be expected from tungsten and molybdenum targets operating at a tube voltage of 30 kVp are shown in Fig. 18.1.

It can be seen that molybdenum provides a spectrum in which the characteristic K lines of 17.5 to 19.5 keV

are important relative to a minor continuous component. The tungsten spectrum mostly consists of continuous X-ray and the characteristic K lines are absent at a tube kVp of only 30 (because tungsten K lines occur only at 59 keV and up). However, there is a small characteristic L line from tungsten at about 11 keV. For mammography, we want a narrow spectrum of useful X-ray of about 17 to 25 keV and thus the molybdenum output is best.

The X-ray spectrum from a molybdenum target can be further improved by inserting a molybdenum filter into the X-ray beam exiting the tube. This is because a filter made of an element is relatively transparent to the characteristic X radiation emitted from an X-ray tube target made of that same element. This principle is illustrated in Fig. 18.2.

In Fig. 18.2, it can be seen that the use of a molybdenum filter further suppresses the continuous spectrum but preserves the characteristic K-line X-ray emissions. Note that the energies of the K lines in keV correspond to a 'low point' in the absorption curve for molybdenum. Little X-ray absorption takes place in molybdenum at these energies and thus the characteristic X-rays from a molybdenum target can pass through easily. But just above the energy of these characteristic lines there is a sudden jump in X-ray absorption at 20 keV, which is the K-shell 'absorption edge' for molybdenum.

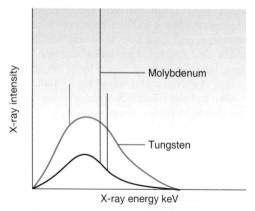

Fig. 18.1 X-ray spectra from tungsten and molybdenum targets operating at 30 kVp.

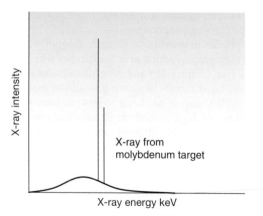

Fig. 18.2 An X-ray spectrum (*in black*) from a molybdenum target, after passing through the molybdenum filter.

An 'absorption edge' occurs when the energy of X-ray photons is just equal to the binding energy of an electron in a shell orbiting the nucleus of an atom. At this energy, the X-rays can ionise an electron from the shell (for example, from the *K*-shell) and a lot of X-ray absorption takes place. At just below this energy level, relatively little absorption takes place because the X-rays do not have enough energy to ionise the electron. The binding energy is that energy that must be put in to overcome the attractive force from the atomic nucleus that holds an electron in place in a shell. It is always greatest for inner (*K*-) shell electrons and increases with the atomic number of the atom. The characteristic K-line X-ray energy is equal to the energy difference between an electron in the *K*-shell and an electron in an outer (usually *L*- or *M*-) shell. Remember that in characteristic X-ray production an electron transfers between shells. The energy difference between the *K*- and *L*-shells is slightly less than the *K*-shell binding energy.

Rhodium, with an atomic number of 45 and K-line emissions of about 20 keV, has been used as an alternative X-ray tube target material for mammography, with a rhodium filter. Tungsten targets can be used in conjunction with a rhodium or palladium filter which effectively removes X-ray photons of about 24 keV and upwards.

18.5 IMAGE QUALITY CONSIDERATIONS

In mammography, a very small X-ray tube focal spot is necessary to reduce geometric unsharpness and maximise resolution. The use of relatively low tube kVp values helps to permit focal spots of small physical size because heating stresses on the target material are small at low tube voltages. An additional tactic is to tilt the anode angle (see Fig. 18.3) to obtain a small effective focal spot, using the 'line focus' principle (see Chapter 12). Use of a large source-to-image distance (SID) further reduces geometric unsharpness. Positioning of the anode end of the X-ray tube towards the nipple permits a slightly larger X-ray intensity towards the chest wall, using the 'anode heel effect'.

Effective compression of the breast is one of the essential elements of mammography but is also associated with patient discomfort and concern. The potential benefits of compression include:
- A more uniform breast thickness resulting in a better fit of the radiation exposure into the detector's dynamic range.
- Reduction in blurring from patient motion.
- A reduction in scattered radiation and an improved contrast sensitivity.

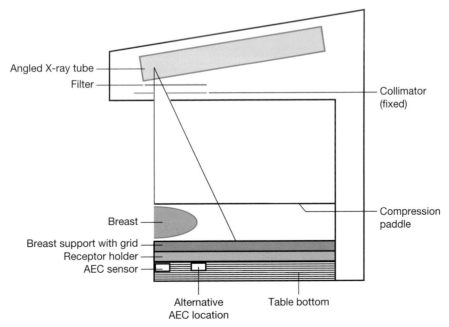

Fig. 18.3 An illustration of the main components of a full-field digital mammography (FFDM) system. *AEC,* Automatic exposure control.

- Reduction in the radiation dose from the examination.
- Improved visualisation of the tissues near the anterior chest wall.

Improvements in digital imaging technology have allowed high-resolution images with an extended greyscale to be obtained. Digital imaging provides a wide dynamic range, thereby enabling a range of image densities to be recorded on a single image. This, when coupled with post-processing capabilities such as subtraction and edge enhancement, increases the visibility of breast lesions.

Although digital mammography promises radiation dose reductions, it must be remembered that too low an X-ray tube mA value might increase image noise and reduce breast lesion detection capabilities. Breast screening programmes provide an interesting example of the 'risk–benefit' relationship that must be considered when delivering ionising radiation. Screening of asymptomatic younger women is undesirable as it would detect relatively few cancers and carry a relatively high risk of cancer induction from ionising radiation.

A grid is used in mammography (as in other X-ray examinations) to absorb scattered radiation and improve contrast sensitivity. Contrast sensitivity is the characteristic of an imaging process that determines the visibility of objects in the body that have low physical contrast. When compared with grids for conventional radiography, grids for mammography have a lower grid ratio and the material between the strips has a low X-ray absorption. Within the mammography machine the grid is located within a bucky device that moves during X-ray exposure to blur and reduce the visibility of grid lines.

Image quality depends on an appropriate exposure being delivered to the imaging receptor. The photon energy spectrum of the X-ray beam is one of the most critical factors in optimising the procedure with respect to contrast sensitivity and radiation dose. The X-ray beam spectrum depends on the anode material, selected filter and the kV range (24–32 kV). These factors are either set by considering the thickness of the breast and density or by the automatic exposure control (AEC) function, if available. In mammography, the AEC typically makes a brief exposure to measure penetration through the breast and from that calculates the most appropriate technical factors for imaging. When using the automatic exposure device to determine the X-ray beam spectrum, the operator must prioritise either the contrast sensitivity or the radiation dose from the examination. When undertaking mammography using film-screen, the aim is to use enough radiation exposure to produce the necessary film density which gives maximum contrast. With digital receptors, the aim is to optimise image noise and radiation dose to the breast. When managing the main mammography exposure, the

AEC requires the involvement of the operator. AEC sensors must be correctly selected and positioned in relation to the relevant anatomy and breast conditions and the 'Density' or exposure control set accordingly. Because the AEC system is key to delivering effective image quality, it should be periodically evaluated by both the manufacturer and local medical physicists.

As previously stated, within mammography systems, the automatic selection of kV is a design feature of some systems. Selecting the tube potential is often based on a short, low-level 'preexposure' that is used to measure the penetration characteristics of the breast. From this a kV value is determined and set automatically for the procedure. Selection of tube potential is also combined with the automatic determination of the target-filter combination.

The use of digital receptors in mammography offers several advantages over film. Three of these advantages are now detailed:

- Dynamic range. A valuable characteristic for digital mammography receptors is the ability to provide a constant sensitivity over a wide range of exposures. The full range of exposures can be covered by the wide dynamic range of the system and as a result considerable variation in exposure to the receptor (error) can be tolerated without loss of contrast.
- Image processing. A variety of processing parameters can be applied to an image to change the image characteristics. Contrast processing is common and is used to make digital acquisitions more like conventional film-screen images. Within digital mammography a wide variety of processing options are available to improve quality and visibility.
- Windowing. As used in the display and viewing of most digital medical images, windowing is the last phase in optimising the contrast and visibility of specific objects and structures within an image.

It is difficult to provide a precise estimate of the radiation dose to the breast during mammography. This problem is hampered by variations in breast anatomy, not being able to insert dosimeters into or onto the breast. To overcome this, the usual process is to make dose measurements at the surface of the breast and to use data from within the literature (dose factors) to calculate the mean glandular dose (MGD).

18.6   FUTURE DEVELOPMENTS IN MAMMOGRAPHY

Digital breast tomosynthesis (DBT) is a relatively new technique which acquires multiple low-dose mammographic projections throughout the breast (see Fig. 18.4).

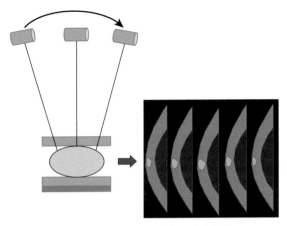

Fig. 18.4 An illustration of the principles of digital breast tomosynthesis (DBT). Within DBT, the tube rotates relative to the detector acquiring images in slices.

Recent research has shown that DBT can reduce the number of false-positive findings and improve the detector rate of invasive cancers.

Contrast mammography (CM) uses standard iodinated contrast agents together with mammography units to answer physiological questions about a breast lesion in a similar manner to magnetic resonance imaging (MRI). Published studies have demonstrated that CM can have an equal or nearly equal sensitivity to MRI, but with a higher specificity.

SUMMARY

In this chapter, you should have learnt the following:
- Breast pathology is best imaged making use of photo-electric absorption at low X-ray tube kVp (Section 18.2).
- X-ray mammography employs a number of adaptations of conventional X-ray tubes, especially the use of molybdenum targets and low-beam energies (Section 18.3).
- These are designed to increase image contrast between breast lesions and normal tissues, by emphasising the X-ray attenuation differences that occur because of photoelectric absorption.
- DBT and CM are potential new imaging methods for evaluating breast pathologies (Section 18.6).

FURTHER READING

Aminololama-Shakeri, S., & Khatri, V.P. Emerging modalities in breast cancer imaging. *Surg Oncol Clin N Am*. 2014: 23(4): 735–749.

Bushong, S.C. 2008. *Radiologic Science for Technologists*. 9th edn. New York: Mosby.

Dendy, P.P., & Heaton, B. 1999. *Physics for Diagnostic Radiology*. 2nd edn. London: Taylor and Francis.

Hogg, P., Kelly, J., & Mercer, C. 2015. *Digital Mammography*. London: Springer.

Fluoroscopy

CHAPTER CONTENTS

19.1 AIM

Fluoroscopy is a technique that is widely used in radiography to produce images of moving structures. These can be used for real-time diagnostic imaging and the guidance of treatments. The aim of this chapter is to explain how fluoroscopic images are formed, concluding with a consideration of image quality and radiation dose issues.

19.2 FLUOROSCOPIC PRINCIPLES

Materials called *phosphors* absorb high-energy photons such as X-rays and in turn emit short bursts of visible light photons. This overarching process of phosphors emitting light in this way is termed *fluorescence* and the monitoring of this light produced during radiological procedures is termed *fluoroscopy*.

Phosphor materials are very widely used in radiography and need to have two characteristics, (1) the ability to strongly absorb X-rays and (2) the ability to convert a proportion of this absorbed energy into visible light. X-ray absorption (by the photoelectric absorption process) is improved by the presence of high atomic number elements such as caesium, barium and iodine. These all typically have K-shell absorption edges at about 30 to 35 keV, which are well placed to absorb X-ray photons produced at about 70 to 100 kVp (diagnostic energy range). The overall conversion rate of X-ray energy to light energy (luminescent radiant efficiency) is normally about 10% to 20% for phosphor materials. This means that considerable X-ray beam intensities are required to produce enough light for a glowing fluoroscopic image to be viewed directly (without amplification). Such a system is not practical and would expose staff members to large doses of radiation in the process. A device capable of improving the brightness of the fluoroscopic images is required (image intensifier). Image intensifiers have been available since the 1950s and have revolutionised real-time X-ray imaging procedures.

19.3 THE IMAGE INTENSIFIER

In radiography, an image intensifier is simply a device which amplifies the visible light resulting from the fluoroscopic process. This section will describe a typical image intensifier, which is based around a cylindrical evacuated tube designed to accelerate and focus electrons. These devices have been partly replaced by more modern 'solid-state' devices or 'flat-panel' fluoroscopy units, but are still widely used in radiography (see Fig. 19.1).

The common X-ray image intensifier involves various energy changes between the input and output phosphors of the device, as shown in Fig. 19.2.

The key components of an image intensifier are shown in Fig. 19.3. The input phosphor typically contains caesium iodide (CsI). CsI crystals are usually needle shaped and transmit the emitted light effectively down 'light channels' to the photocathode. CsI is a high atomic number material which encourages the absorption of X-ray photons. The photocathode contains caesium antimony compounds which emit electrons (photoelectrons) from their surface when light is absorbed. It should be noted that light photons from the CsI crystals are not converted into photoelectrons. Within the photocathode, light energy (from the

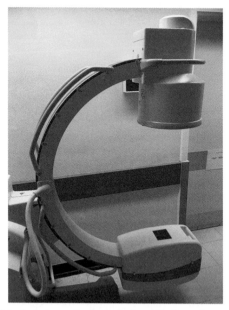

Fig. 19.1 A photograph of a typical mobile C-arm image intensifier which would be commonly used in the operating theatre environment for providing X-ray guidance during surgical procedures. (From Warrington & Halton Hospital NHS Foundation Trust. With permission.)

CsI crystals) is used to promote the energy of existing electrons within the photocathode material so that they are emitted from it.

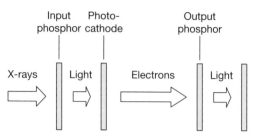

Fig. 19.2 An illustration of the conversion processes that take place within an image intensifier.

From Fig. 19.3, it is evident that the electrons emitted from a large photocathode are focused down onto a small output phosphor. This size difference contributes to the increase in brightness, or brightness gain, which is obtained at the output phosphor relative to the input phosphor. A further method for intensifying the image is through flux gain. This refers to the relative numbers of incident X-ray photons striking the input phosphor to emitted light photons leaving the output phosphor. This ratio is generally in the region of 1:10^4 to 10^5, that is, a single X-ray photon would subsequently produce 10,000 visible light photons. To achieve this, energy is put into the system, largely by accelerating electrons from the photocathode through a vacuum across a potential difference of around 25 kV towards an anode. The speeding electrons have a lot of kinetic energy when they strike the output phosphor, which responds by emitting many light photons.

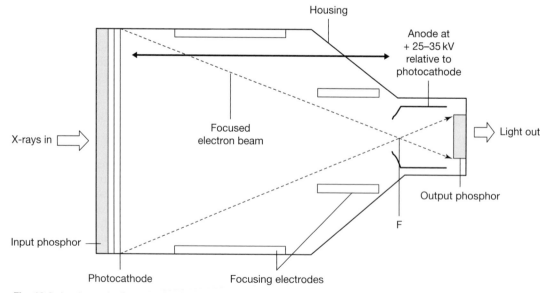

Fig. 19.3 A schematic diagram of an image intensifier. F is the focal spot of the electron beam. In reality, the input phosphor, photocathode and output phosphor are slightly curved, and each is circular when seen 'face on'. The housing contains a vacuum.

When considering the photocathode, the size difference when compared with the output phosphor contributes to the increase in brightness, or brightness gain. This refers to the gain that occurs from the input phosphor relative to the output phosphor and as previously specified is in the region of $1:10^4$. If the charge of the focusing electrodes is adjusted, this will affect the position of the electron beam focal spot (F) and can produce magnification of the fluoroscopic image.

The output phosphor is typically made of zinc-cadmium sulphide with the addition of silver. This phosphor emits light when struck by electrons. The light from the output phosphor is fed into components-linked viewing monitors and image recording devices. The latter are now based on digital technology.

The conversion of an input of a relatively few X-ray photons to an output of many light photons can result in image noise, owing to the phenomenon of quantum mottle. If individual X-ray photons are very efficient at producing an amplified signal and as such the number of X-ray photons can be reduced, any random variations in X-ray density can become visible and produce noisy appearances on an image.

19.4 FLAT-PANEL (SOLID-STATE) FLUOROSCOPY SYSTEMS

Modern image intensification devices are increasingly based on solid-state 'flat-panel' components, rather than on evacuated image intensifier tubes. X-ray photons incident on a detector array are converted into an electronic output signal. There are two main types of detector:

1. Indirect systems include a layer of phosphor material such as CsI, coated on top of an amorphous silicon photodiode. They permit low radiation doses, because of the image amplification of the phosphor layer, but incur possible losses in image resolution because of the light spreading that occurs.
2. Direct systems use an amorphous selenium photoconductor to absorb X-rays directly and convert them into an electronic signal. Such systems have a very high image resolution, with a slight radiation dose penalty relative to indirect systems.

A simplified diagram of an indirect X-ray detector is shown in Fig. 19.4. Each cell has a top layer of scintillation crystal made of CsI activated with thallium, which produces light when struck by X-ray photons. The atomic numbers of Cs and I are 55 and 53, respectively, and this results in good X-ray absorption. Each absorbed X-ray photon produces around 10^3 light photons. Below this, an amorphous silicon photodiode (see Fig. 19.5) converts about 50% of the light into an electrical charge. This pattern of charge is stored and converted into an electrical signal within a two-dimensional pixel array. Self-scanning of a two-dimensional array of electrodes containing switching elements in a thin film transistor (TFT) reads the stored charge distribution.

In the direct X-ray detector, there is no intermediate phosphor layer. X-ray absorption in the selenium produces negative charges (electrons) and positive charges (electron 'holes'—essentially the absence of electrons) that migrate to the electrodes. Selenium has a relatively low atomic number of 34 and thus its X-ray absorption efficiency decreases at higher X-ray energies.

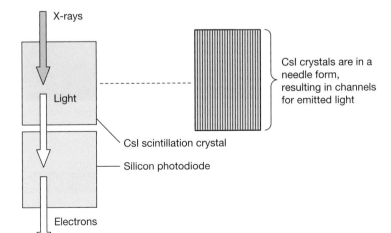

Fig. 19.4 Key components of an indirect detector cell for digital X-ray imaging. A two-dimensional matrix of such cells produces the signal for a pixel display. *CsI*, Caesium iodide.

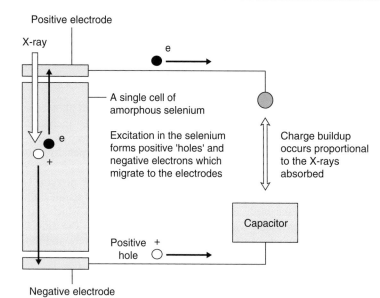

Positive electrode

X-ray

e

A single cell of amorphous selenium

e

+

Excitation in the selenium forms positive 'holes' and negative electrons which migrate to the electrodes

Charge buildup occurs proportional to the X-rays absorbed

Capacitor

Positive + hole ○

Negative electrode

Fig. 19.5 Key parts of a direct detector cell for digital X-ray imaging. A two-dimensional matrix of such cells produces the signal for a pixel display.

19.5 FLUOROSCOPIC IMAGE QUALITY

Traditional image intensifiers suffer from some effects that are a feature of their geometry. Because the photocathode is curved, the image may appear more magnified towards the edges; this effect is known as *pincushion distortion* and is illustrated in Fig. 19.6. Additionally, the *geometry of the system* may result in a characteristic where the centre of the image field appears brighter than the periphery (*vignetting*; see Fig. 19.7). *Blooming* (excessive brightness) of the resultant image, typically occurs when a region of gas or air is present within the field of view; this occurs as a result of the limitations in the ability of the system to record a wide dynamic range of intensities. Flat-panel fluoroscopy systems are not affected by pincushion distortion, vignetting or blooming, because of their flat geometry and wide dynamic range.

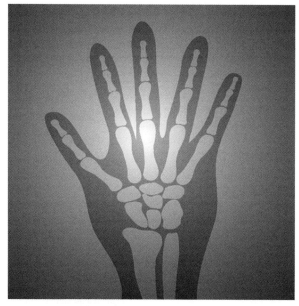

Fig. 19.7 A simple example of vignetting on a traditional fluoroscopy image. Note that the periphery of the image is darker than the central region.

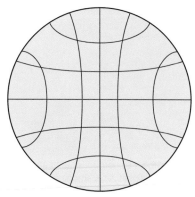

Fig. 19.6 Pincushion image distortion (exaggerated here).

Both image intensifiers and flat-panel fluoroscopy systems can be prone to ghosting artefacts. These show up as residual image brightness when an object was present in a previous X-ray exposure (but has now left). Previous exposures can alter the performance of detector elements. Lag refers to a motion blurring that can occur during fluoroscopy of a moving object, because of time delays in the response of the phosphors and amorphous Si or Se. The image resolution of image intensifiers is affected by magnification and by the dimensions of individual digital detector elements or phosphor grains. The performance of the display screen monitor will also greatly affect image resolution.

Image noise can occur in all X-ray detectors and consists of random statistical and electronic fluctuations in the size of signal across the surface of the image. The signal-to-noise ratio (SNR) is important in imaging because it defines the relative sizes of useful signal (based on real features in a patient or test object) to random signal fluctuations. Detector quantum efficiency (DQE) is an important measure of imaging performance and is defined as the SNR2 in the image output divided by the SNR2 in the X-ray photons at the input of the device. A value of 1 would indicate perfect performance with no loss of SNR, but this is never achieved. Typical DQEs for flat-panel fluoroscopy devices are in the region of 0.5 to 0.8, with direct digital detectors being more prone to electronic noise than indirect digital detectors.

19.6 DOSE REDUCTION IN FLUOROSCOPY

Fluoroscopic procedures can result in a high radiation dose to patients, especially in long procedures such as interventions (treatments) undertaken with fluoroscopic guidance. Deterministic radiation effects such as radiation erythema (skin reddening) are not normally encountered in diagnostic imaging but can result from prolonged fluoroscopy, especially in a high X-ray tube output mode.

Automatic brightness control (ABC) monitors light output from image intensifiers and increases X-ray output if light levels fall. This feature can increase radiation doses if light output levels fall from any of the following causes:
- Image magnification.
- Ageing and inefficient image intensifiers.
- Large distance between the patient and the image intensifier input.

Solid-state image intensifiers tend to be more efficient than traditional devices and should provide dose reductions. Pulsed mode operation provides a periodic 'blipped' X-ray tube output and is a useful means of reducing radiation dose when maximal image quality is not required using traditional image intensifiers. This mode is also standard practice for solid-state image intensifiers. There is a legal requirement for manufacturers to provide dose-reduction measures such as ABC and pulsed fluoroscopy.

Fluoroscopic doses can also be reduced by:
- increasing X-ray tube kVp.
- reducing X-ray tube mA.
- reducing screening time.
- avoiding small X-ray tube to patient distances.
- making use of 'undercouch' X-ray tubes and lead-impregnated plastic curtains.

See Chapter 21 for further discussion of dose-reduction methods in radiography.

SUMMARY

In this chapter, you should have learnt the following:
- Fluoroscopic imaging converts an X-ray input to a visible light or electrical output (Section 19.2).
- Phosphor materials absorb X-ray and produce visible light emissions (Section 19.2).
- Image intensifiers amplify the output signal and result in large radiation dose reductions to patients and staff (Section 19.3).

FURTHER READING

Allisy-Roberts, P.J., & Williams, J. 2007. *Farr's Physics for Medical Imaging*, 2nd edn. Edinburgh: WB Saunders.

Bushong, S.C. 2008. *Radiologic Science for Technologists*. 9th edn. St Louis: Mosby.

Dendy, P.P., & Heaton, B. 1999. *Physics for Diagnostic Radiology*. 2nd edn. London: Taylor and Francis.

Computed tomography scanning

CHAPTER CONTENTS

20.1   AIM

The aim of this chapter is to provide its readers with an overview that will enable them to understand the basics of contemporary computed tomography (CT) scanning processes.

20.2   INTRODUCTION

It is difficult for today's radiographers and radiologists to imagine working in an imaging department without a CT scanner, which was first demonstrated in the 1970s by its inventor, Sir Godfrey Hounsfield. It revolutionised many imaging procedures, making dangerous diagnostic techniques unnecessary. It also provided improved demonstration of other body parts, especially soft tissue and overlying structures, which are difficult to demonstrate using conventional techniques. The physics and mathematics of CT imaging is a complex topic. This chapter provides the reader with an overview that will enable them to understand the fundamental basics of the process.

20.3   THE DEVELOPMENT OF THE CT SCANNER

The evolution of CT technology has been principally described in terms of the progression through a series of successive 'generations' (Fig. 20.1). The first generation of CT scanners was of the translate–rotate type. A single source consisting of a finely collimated pencil beam was focused on a single detector that moved on a frame in a transverse direction across the body, the gantry on which the source and detector was mounted then rotated through 1 degree and another transverse movement was made. As can be imagined, this was a very slow process requiring approximately 5 minutes to produce a single slice. This restricted scanning to the demonstration of bony skeletal structures and soft tissues in which movement did not take place (i.e., brain).

The second-generation scanners were still of the translate–rotate type. These used a fan-shaped beam and an arc of about 30 detectors. To compensate for the reduced beam attenuation at the periphery of the body, a 'bow tie' filter was placed between the source and the patient. The increased area covered in each translation and by the arc of detectors permitted rotation of 10 degrees on each rotation, producing a substantial reduction in the time per slice. However, because of the complexities of the translation–rotation movement, and owing to the large mass of equipment to be moved in the gantry, imaging times were still in the order of several seconds per slice.

The third-generation scanners were known as the *rotate–rotate design*. The width of the radiation beam and the arc of

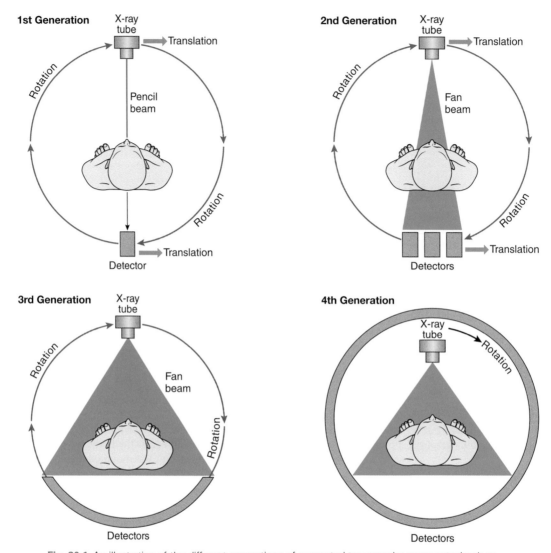

Fig. 20.1 An illustration of the different generations of computed tomography scanner technology.

the detectors were increased to 60 degrees. The geometry of the detector arc produced a constant source-to-detector distance, an advantage in image reconstruction, and also permitted better beam collimation reducing scatter formation. The increased detector arc had the effect of reducing time per slice to the order of approximately 1 second, substantially reducing the risk of motion artefacts. One major disadvantage with this system was that the failure of a single detector would result in the production of a 'ring' artefact. Nowadays this is corrected by image processing software.

Fourth-generation scanners have what is sometimes termed a stationary–rotate geometry, in which the X-ray

tube rotates within a stationary circle of detectors. The earlier sodium iodide scintillation detector linked to a photomultiplier tube has been replaced by ceramic scintillation detectors. These detectors have a better response to radiation of the energy range used in CT. The photomultipliers have been replaced by solid-state photodiodes. The photodiode is far smaller than the photomultiplier tube and requires considerably less power to operate.

The reduction in size has permitted the detectors to be arranged in a continuous circular array containing as many as 40,000 individual detectors while the X-ray tube rotates around the patient within the circle of detectors.

Fourth-generation systems are free from the ring artefact problem associated with third-generation scanners and are capable of sub-second slice production times.

The medium-frequency generator has permitted the development of 'slip ring' technology. The low-tension supply is supplied to a stationary ring of contacts, while the high-tension (HT) transformer, rectification system and X-ray tube are mounted on a second ring which rotates about the stationary ring. This innovation has eliminated the need for the X-ray tube to return to its starting position before commencing another rotation and was a forerunner to helical CT scanning.

20.4   SCANNER SUBSYSTEMS

20.4.1   The patient support couch

This is about 1.5 metres long: the end nearest the gantry is often narrowed to pass through the aperture (bore) of the gantry. Before the scan, couch position height and longitudinal movement can be adjusted by the user; good radiographic practice necessitates that the couch is positioned to place the patient at the isocentre of the scanner bore. Such practices promote optimum image quality whilst delivering examinations with lower radiation doses. During the CT examination the couch is computer controlled to ensure that CT slices are acquired at the right location and table speed.

20.4.2   The gantry

The gantry (Fig. 20.2) consists of a large box-like structure with a central aperture (bore) through which the patient is passed during the scan. Within the gantry are the X-ray tube, HT transformer, rectification system, collimators, detectors and the motor drive and control system to move the X-ray tube

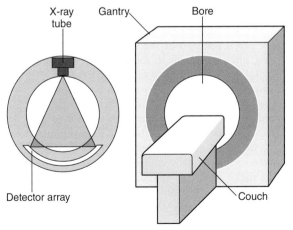

Fig. 20.2 Typical arrangement of the components of a computed tomography scanner.

during the scan. Such systems are mechanically complex in that they must be able to allow sub-second (~0.5 seconds) rotation of the X-ray tube and detector array around the patient.

20.4.3   The X-ray generator

X-ray generators used in current CT scanners are of the order of over 80 kW. They typically use a three-phase mains supply collected from the slip ring and have a medium-frequency output. Radiation output is often pulsed, with each pulse lasting for about 3 milliseconds. Pulsing permits the cooling of the X-ray tube between pulses and permits a higher generator rating. Generator output is monitored and controlled by an onboard microprocessor.

20.4.4   The X-ray tube

The X-ray tube is very different in design from the tube used in conventional radiography. It has a much larger and thicker anode and a higher heat capacity in the order of 6000 kilojoules with a cooling rate of 1000 kilojoule per minute. The heat load on the focal spot is calculated by a computer algorithm which automatically adjusts the mA to prevent overloading. In early CT scanners tube cooling issues often restricted the selection of acquisition parameters and the maximum permissible scan length. Modern advances in X-ray tube design and tube cooling have almost eradicated such tube cooling issues.

20.4.5   The computer subsystem

The computer subsystem is possibly the most important part of the scanner and has many different functions (Fig. 20.3). The monitoring part of the system accepts input from input devices on the operator console and controls exposure and movement of the scanner during the scan. The main part of the system is concerned with data collection and manipulation. It collects the incoming data from the detector system and processes it. This requires the capacity to solve 25,000 simultaneous equations per second. It then passes the data to short-term storage and also displays the data as an image on the operator and reporting workstations. These data can be passed back to the image manipulation section to be reformatted to produce a different image on the workstations before the image is passed to long-term image storage. Ultimately, in the majority of imaging departments CT images are stored within institutional picture archiving and communication system (PACS).

20.5   ADVANCES IN COMPUTED TOMOGRAPHY TECHNOLOGY

Slip ring and developments in computer technology have made the development of helical and multislice techniques possible. These will now be examined in more detail.

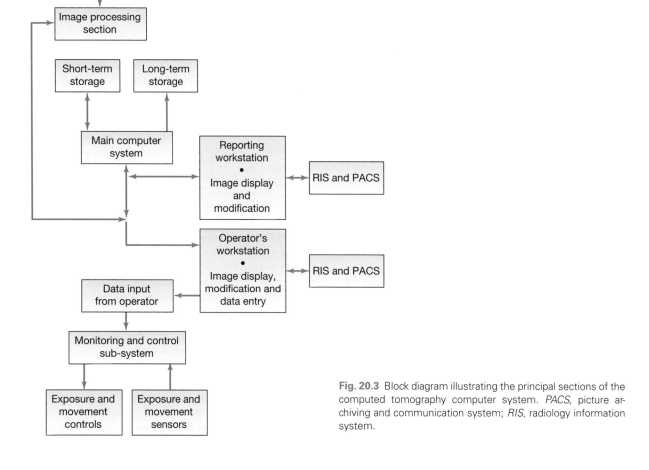

Fig. 20.3 Block diagram illustrating the principal sections of the computed tomography computer system. *PACS,* picture archiving and communication system; *RIS,* radiology information system.

20.5.1 Helical or spiral computed tomography

Helical, or spiral, CT was first introduced in the early 1990s following the development of slip ring technology. This meant there was no longer a need for tube rotation to stop and return to its original starting point and advance the patient table into the gantry before commencing another rotation, effectively ending the necessity for the 'shoot-move' or 'start-stop' sequence followed with conventional CT. In conventional CT, slice width was determined by the collimation of the beam. This is not possible with helical CT in which the data are produced as a continuous spiral of information (Fig. 20.4).

With helical CT, the slice width is determined by two factors: beam collimation and pitch. Pitch is the rate of longitudinal movement of the table through the

gantry per revolution of the X-ray tube. The effect of varying pitch is shown in Fig. 20.5. As with conventional CT, collimation and pitch are fixed for a given examination.

The apparent slice width is determined by a factor termed *index* used in the image reconstruction process. As index is a software function it is variable and an image can be reconstructed using different index values, producing separate, contiguous or even overlapping slices.

The major advantage of spiral CT is speed. A large patient volume can be scanned in a short period of time, typically 6 to 20 seconds. The patient can hold their breath for the entire exposure, and artefacts caused by motion blur are eliminated. With contrast studies, it is possible to demonstrate high density contrast flow through a complete

Sequential

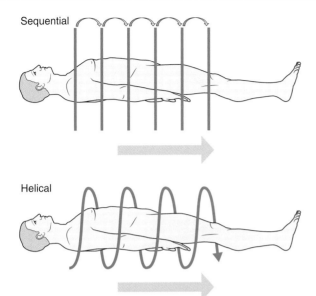

Helical

Fig. 20.4 An illustration of the differences between sequential and helical computed tomography scanning.

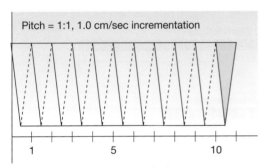

Pitch = 1:1, 1.0 cm/sec incrementation

Scan location on the Z axis (cm)

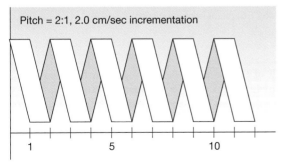

Pitch = 2:1, 2.0 cm/sec incrementation

Scan location on the Z axis (cm)

Fig. 20.5 Effect of pitch (speed of couch movement) for a given examination.

system, and this has also introduced the option for multi-phase scanning.

The major disadvantage of spiral scanning is loss of image resolution on the z-axis resulting from the continual couch movement. Higher resolution can be obtained by slowing down the rate of couch movement (reduced pitch), but this prolongs scanning time and increases patient dose.

20.5.2   Multislice computed tomography

The first multislice CT scanner, called the Elsinct TWIN, was developed in 1993 and, as the name implies, it employed a double ring of solid-state detectors, separated by an annular ring of tungsten to prevent cross-scatter between each ring of detectors.

This was rapidly followed by scanners using 4, 8, 18 and up to 64 rings of detectors (Figs. 20.6 and Fig. 20.7). Instead of acquiring data from all the rings in multislice array, improved technology makes it possible to select the rings that are activated, effectively producing different slice widths as well as using all the elements in the detector array, producing separate, contiguous or even overlapping slices. Multislice CT has been of particular benefit in CT angiography, which relies on precise timing to ensure good opacification of the arteries.

Other improvements in CT technology have resulted in reduction in component weight, with faster rotation times of up to three rotations per second. Software improvements mean that it is now possible to resolve 0.35-mm voxels at a transverse speed of 19 cm per second on the z-axis.

The most recent innovations are multislice scanners capable of producing 640 slices per rotation. Detector arrays of this size enable cardiac CT angiograms and whole-brain perfusion studies to be carried out in a single exposure. Manufacturers have also even produced mobile CT scanners for use on hospital wards which can be integrated into the back of emergency response vehicles (ambulances). The latter are a consideration when evaluating patients suspected of acute stroke living in remote locations.

All these improvements have resulted in the benefits of reduction in radiation dose to the patient and improved image resolution.

Improved software technology has resulted in the introduction of three-dimensional imaging and the use of colour in the resultant image.

20.5.3   Dual-output computed tomography

The pulsing of the X-ray tube output has meant that is has been possible to develop dual-output CT scanners using the output of the X-ray tube in which one exposure is made at 150 kVp followed by an exposure at 90 kVp. The resulting data from the detectors are merged. This technique

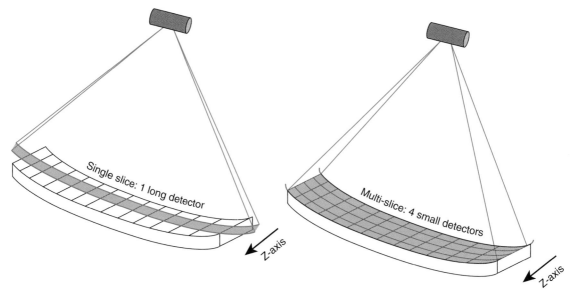

Fig. 20.6 Illustration of the differences between single and multislice computed tomography (MSCT) detector arrays.

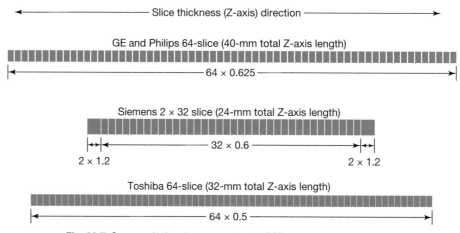

Fig. 20.7 Symmetrical and asymmetrical MSCT detector configurations.

results in increased emphasis of the differences in the absorption edges between tissue and contrast agents and differing tissues.

The latest generation of dual-energy scanners makes use of two X-ray tubes (Fig. 20.8) operating at different energies and two banks of detectors, resulting in a better-balanced arrangement on the rotating ring. This has permitted increased rotation speeds of 0.28 seconds per rotation. As a result, couch movement in the z-axis can be increased by up to 43 cm per second. The combined result of this is much shorter scanning times so that a complete thorax can be scanned in 0.6 seconds (less than a heartbeat) and a whole body scanned in less than 5 seconds.

Spectral CT, or dual-source or dual-energy, has the potential to have a major impact on medical imaging practices. Spectral CT is based on viewing the same anatomy but at two different energy (kV) levels. Different energy levels, as previously stated, can be achieved using two X-ray tubes, fixed at 90 degrees to each other within the

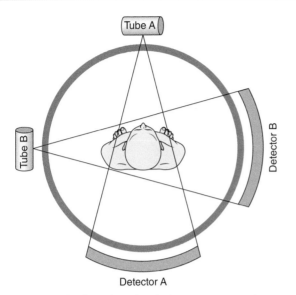

Fig. 20.8 Configuration of a dual-source computed tomography scanner.

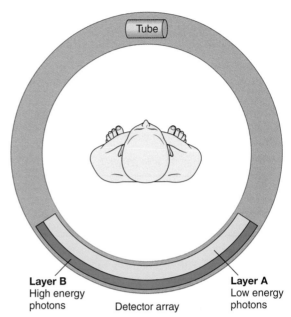

Fig. 20.10 Spectral imaging is also possible without any modification of the X-ray tube; new detector technology permits selection of different energy X-ray photons.

80−140 kVp fast switching

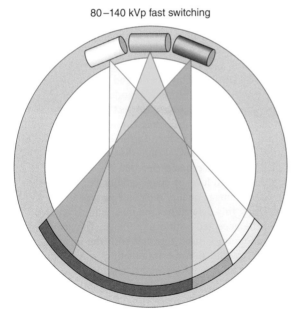

Fig. 20.9 An illustration of spectral imaging opportunities using the rapid switching (80–140 kVp) of an X-ray tube.

gantry or fast kV switching of a single X-ray tube during the scan (Fig. 20.9). More recent advances in detector technology have produced detectors that can record different kV levels during a scan (Fig. 20.10).

The advantage of spectral imaging is that different anatomical features are enhanced at different energy (kV) levels. This removes the need to scan a patient multiple times, at different energy levels, to achieve various tissue enhancements. Additionally, the spectral software can highlight or eliminate chemical compounds based on their atomic number, including iodine, calcium and metals. This provides an option for achieving a virtual unenhanced CT scan from a scan acquired using an iodine-based contrast agent.

20.5.4   Dose-reduction technologies

Historically, all CT systems reconstructed images based on filtered back projection (FBP) because it was fast and could be achieved using the available computer technology. Major advances in computer processing power together with reductions in the price of computer systems has led to all major CT vendors offering iterative reconstruction (IR). IR works by revisiting an image over and over with multiple iterations to clean up artefacts and clarify the image pixel by pixel. This enables CT scanning at much lower doses than previously available. For example, cardiac CT scans performed over 10 years ago would have produced radiation doses of 20 to 30 mSv. Today, with a combination IR and new detector technology it is possible to acquire a scan of the heart with doses less than 1 mSv.

TABLE 20.1   Comparison of chest computed tomography lesion conspicuity between filtered back projection and iterative reconstruction

	FBP		ASIR 50%	MBIR
	Standard dose	Low dose	Low dose	Lose dose
Consolidation or mass	4.9 ± 0.2	4.7 ± 0.6	4.8 ± 0.4	4.9 ± 0.2
Ground-glass attenuation	5.0 ± 0.2	4.8 ± 0.4	4.8 ± 0.4	4.8 ± 0.4
Reticular opacity	5.0 ± 0	4.9 ± 0.4	5.0 ± 0	5.0 ± 0
Bulla, emphysema or cyst.	4.9 ± 0.2	4.5 ± 0.6	4.6 ± 0.5	4.6 ± 0.5
Mediastinal lymph node enlargement	4.8 ± 0.4	3.0 ± 0.5	4.0 ± 0.5	4.7 ± 0.5

ASIR, Adaptive statistical iterative reconstruction; *FBP*, filtered back protection; *MBIR*, model-based iterative reconstruction. (Modified from Ichikawa Y, Kitagawa K, Nagasawa N, Murashima S, Sakuma H. CT of the chest with model-based, fully iterative reconstruction: comparison with adaptive statistical iterative reconstruction. BMC Medical Imaging 2003:13: https://doi.org/10.1186/1471-2342-13-27.)

The traditional FBP algorithm is based on several assumptions, which simplifies CT geometry to make a compromise between image reconstruction speed and image noise. Recent changes to reconstruction processes have allowed more complex assumptions to be made about the CT geometry. This when combined with multiple iterations of image reconstruction has resulted in slightly longer reconstruction times but less image noise. This new approach of IR has allowed lower dose CT acquisitions to be performed with relatively similar image quality. IR has been shown, when compared with FBP, to reduce the quantum noise without any effect on spatial or contrast resolution. With further advances in computer processing technology it is now possible to have faster image reconstructions with even more complex algorithms. A newer approach, termed *model-based IR (MBIR)*, uses detailed models of a number of the key characteristics of radiation and CT equipment. MBIR uses both forward and backward projections to match the reconstructed image to the acquired data iteratively and as such requires a longer reconstruction time. For example, if a CT scanner is capable of reconstructing using FBP 15 images per second, this would reduce to 10 per second for IR and only 1 per second for MBIR. MBIR images would have substantially less noise than both the FBP and IR images and could, therefore, be acquired at a much lower dose. An example, within clinical practice, an example of MBIR would be an abdominal CT examination acquired using a similar radiation dose to conventional abdominal X-ray imaging (Table 20.1).

As with CT-based automatic exposure control or mA modulation there is now the ability to use information obtained from the scout/topogram/scanogram to select an appropriate tube potential (*kV assist*) for the subsequent CT examination. Selection is based on the attenuation data received during the scout projections and also takes into consideration the patient size and the diagnostic task. The use of kV assist or automatic tube potential selection is intended to decrease the $CTDI_{vol}$ while still achieving a defined level of image quality. CT dose index (CTDI) is a standardized measure of radiation dose output of a CT scanner. The suffix vol is often added to acknowledge the contribution of the CT protocol pitch factor. Unlike mA modulation, the kV is determined from the scout views and then fixed for the remainder of the CT acquisitions. Tube potential does not vary in either an angular or longitudinal direction as with mA modulation.

Almost all commercially available CT scanners provide the option for automatically adjusting the mA (and as a result the $CTDI_{vol}$) to achieve a desired level of image quality. The precise mechanisms for modulating the mA will vary between manufacturers. Correct functioning of the automatic exposure control (AEC) system requires that the patient is correctly positioned in the isocentre of the CT scanner. Within any AEC system the user specifies an image quality reference parameter that the scanner uses to define the desired level of image quality. For many manufacturers, the image quality reference parameter is a noise index. Using this determines the maximum level of noise that can be accepted within any image. The scout/topogram/scanogram is used together with the image quality parameter to plan the mA modulation. mA modulation can occur in all three dimensions, and for the x–y-axes is deemed angular modulation (Fig. 20.11) and in the z-axis it is termed longitudinal modulation (Fig. 20.12).

Additional algorithms have been built into modern CT scanners which automatically reduce the dose for superficial tissues such as the eyes and the anterior chest, creating a virtual shield for radiosensitive anatomy (organ dose modulation). To maintain image quality, the tube current may need to be increased for the other projectional angles; as such, this technology can reduce the dose to organs at the surface of the body but may increase the absorbed dose to other organs.

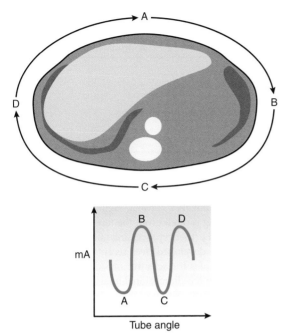

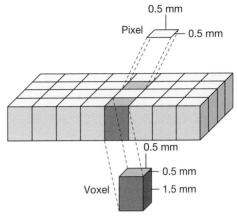

Fig. 20.13 Diagram showing the relationship between pixels and voxels.

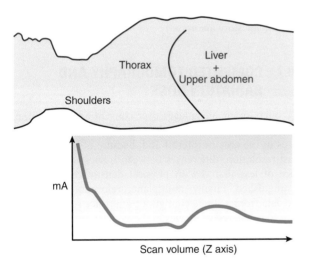

Fig. 20.11 Principles of *x*–*y*-axis (angulation) mA modulation; note that the mA is higher for the wider portions of anatomy.

Fig. 20.12 Principles of *z*-axis (longitudinal) mA modulation; note that the mA is higher for the denser/thicker parts of anatomy.

20.6   FORMATION OF THE COMPUTED TOMOGRAPHY IMAGE

The CT image differs from the image produced by other imaging modalities, in that the image is reconstructed from the attenuation data received by the image detectors in the image-processing section of the computer system. The image-processing section receives the data from the detectors as a continuous data stream. The first task it carries out is to convert these data into picture elements or *pixels*; this is commonly done using a complex mathematical function called *convoluted back projection*. The value of each pixel is in turn the summation of the attenuation of the X-ray beam by the tissues in the volume element or *voxel* to which the pixel relates (Fig. 20.13). Each pixel is then allotted a CT number based on the attenuation of the X-ray beam of the voxel. CT numbers range from −1000, which corresponds to air, to +4000, which corresponds to dense compact bone. Water has a CT number of zero. Equation 20.1 indicates the relationship between tissues and CT number. The exact CT number for a given substance or tissue can be calculated using the formula:

$$CT\,k\,number = \frac{(\mu_t - \mu_w)}{\mu_w}$$ **Equation 20.1**

where μ_t is the attenuation coefficient of the substance or tissue, μ_w the attenuation coefficient of water and k a constant that determines the scaling factor of the range of CT number. The linear attenuation of a substance or tissue is, in turn, dependent on the kVp used for the examination.

The result of this process, which requires considerable computer processing power, is a slice of data in which the bit depth of the image is approximately 2^{12}. This is beyond the range of shades of grey that can be displayed on the monitor screen (~256) and also the range of grey that can be perceived by the human eye (~64).

Once this task is completed, the data pass out of the image processing section into a short-term image store where they are stored as a 'stack' of individual slices and the bit

TABL   0.2   An example of a series of typical window width and level values

Examination	Window width (WW)	Window level (WL)
Brain (soft tissue)	80	40
Temporal bones	2800	600
Chest (lungs)	1500	−600
Chest (mediastinum)	350	50
Abdomen (soft tissue)	400	50
Spine (bone)	1800	400

depth is reduced to one within the display limitations of the monitor. The data are then copied to the operator's console where they are displayed according to the window selected.

Two factors are used in windowing: the window level which selects the CT number that will occupy the midpoint of the window, and window width which determines the total range of CT numbers displayed on the monitor (Table 20.2). A wide window produces a low-contrast image with little difference between adjacent CT values, whereas a narrow window produces a high-contrast image. CT numbers above and below the selected window depth are displayed as black or white respectively (Fig. 20.14).

In addition to windowing operations, further data processing operations can be performed. Additional software options permit the viewing of the images in the stack as a series of projections in a coronal, sagittal or oblique plane. Such reprocessing is often given the term *multiplanar reformatting* (MPR). Further reprocessing options exist and have been extensively developed over recent years (Table 20.3). One option includes the selective masking of CT values to produce virtual three-dimensional images.

For these operations to take place, the data in the short-term image store is copied back into the image processing system where the required algorithms are applied, and the modified data are copied back to the console. Once the operator has completed their part of the examination, the modified data are transferred in the final format to the long-term image store (PACS) and the data in the short-term image store are erased.

20.7   COMPUTED TOMOGRAPHY AND RADIATION DOSE

CT offers many advantages over conventional projection radiography. It eliminates the superimposition of structures in the area of interest and, because of its high-contrast resolution, differences between tissues with a difference of less than 1% in physical density can easily be distinguished. Finally, multiplanar reformatting permits the data from a single contiguous multislice scan or spiral scan to be viewed as images in the axial, coronal or sagittal planes, or even to perform three-dimensional reconstructions from the data acquired. This has made examinations such as virtual colonoscopy possible, which is of particular value because it delivers a lower radiation dose than a conventional barium enema.

Angiograms, including cerebral, cardiac, abdominal and peripheral, are also procedures which have become far less invasive through the use of CT. Pulmonary angiography in particular has proved very useful in ruling out pulmonary embolism because of its high sensitivity (>90%). These factors have resulted in CT becoming the modality of choice for these procedures. CT is also a sensitive

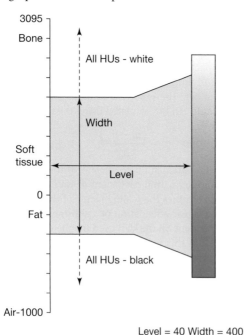

Fig. 20.14 An illustration of the concept of applying window width and levels to a computed tomography image.

TABLE 20.3 Postprocessing options available on modern computed tomography scanners/workstations

Postprocessing option	Description
Multiplanar reformats (MPRs)	Provides the ability to visualise axial computed tomography (CT) images in multiple planes (coronal, sagittal, oblique and curved). A common feature on all CT platforms.
Three-dimensional (3D) object reconstructions	Allows CT anatomy to be viewed in true 3D. Such systems provide visualisation of anatomy and pathology as a surface-shaded display or volume rendered image.
RaySum reconstructions	Provides the opportunity to post-process CT datasets and conventional radiography style images.
Virtual endoscopy	This algorithm allows the observer to visual contrast filled lumen as a virtual endoscopy projection. This technology has applied for studies of the colon, urinary tract and vascular tree.
Computer-aided detection (CAD)	Such algorithms can help improve efficiency and help reduce interobserver variability. CAD technologies currently have a role in the detection of polyps within the colon and lung nodules. Within the development of artificial intelligence and machine learning it is likely that there will be a greater contribution of CAD to CT diagnosis.
Computer-aided nodule analysis and risk yield (CANARY)	This is a software solution which segments lung nodules from the surrounding parenchyma. It also facilitates the evaluation of density features and can be used as a biomarker to characterise lung nodules and assign a risk of adenocarcinoma.
Computer-aided lung informatics for pathology evaluation and rating (CALIPER)	This is a software algorithm that classifies and quantifies features of lung parenchyma on high-resolution chest CT scans. It automatically characterises diffuse lung diseases such as emphysema.
Respiratory-induced motion analysis	Such systems provide an opportunity to analyse and characterise respiratory-induced motion which can help make radiotherapy planning more precise.
Enhanced colonic visualisation	An efficient reading workflow solution for detecting colonic lesions. Provides visualisation of the colon in two-dimensional, 3D and 360-degree dissection views.
Bone removal and vessel analysis	Fast routine analyses of CT angiography studies. Also includes the option to standardise vascular reporting.
Cardiac analysis	Dedicated software for cardiac visualisation, analysis and reporting. Ability to fuse cardiac physiological and anatomical information. Focus on anatomical, functional and perfusion information.
CT neuro perfusion analysis	Software providing the automatic tissue assessment of perfusion changes. Can be used for both stroke and tumour angiogenesis assessments.
Integrated registration	Multimodality image management. The ability to fuse and register multimodality datasets.
Calcium scoring	Advanced imaging software that detects, quantifies and scores cardiac calcium plaque burden.
Device planning	Integrated software for using CT datasets to plan valve placements and endovascular aortic aneurysm repair procedures.

method for diagnosis of abdominal disease. It is used frequently in the staging of cancer and the follow up of its progress.

It is also a useful test to investigate acute abdominal pain (especially of the investigation of suspected aortic aneurysm and bowel obstruction). Other non-ionising modalities such as magnetic resonance imaging (MRI) and ultrasound are used for investigations of the liver and kidneys. Unfortunately, despite improvements, CT remains a relatively high-dose modality; although the latest dose-reduction software can result in significantly lower doses so that the dose from a CT of the chest can be reduced to below 1 mSv, this software is still not yet available on all scanners.

The greatly increased availability of CT, together with its value for an increasing number of conditions, has been responsible for a large rise in its popularity. So large has this rise been that the comprehensive 2000/2005 survey of medical radiation dose in the United Kingdom revealed that, although CT scans constituted only 7% of all radiological examinations, they contributed 47% of the total collective dose from medical X-ray examinations. Thus, increased CT usage has led to an overall rise in the total amount of medical radiation used, despite reductions in other areas.

This trend is no restricted to just the United Kingdom. In the United States, for example, in 1980 there were about 3 million CT scans per performed compared with 62 million scans in 2006.

As with all examinations involving the use of ionising radiation, a major problem is the reduction of radiation dose. This can be achieved by the following:

- Where practicable, new software technologies should be used to reduce random noise and enhance structures. These can reduce dose by as much as 70% while still producing high-quality images.
- All CT examinations should observe the diagnostic reference levels (DRLs) recommended by the Department of Health.
- The clinical benefit to the patient should be evaluated carefully against modalities such as ultrasound and MRI that do not use ionising radiation.

SUMMARY

In this chapter, you should have learnt the following:
- The differences among the first-, second-, third- and fourth-generation CT scanners (Section 20.3).
- The contents of the scanner gantry (Section 20.4.2).
- The functions of the computer system (Section 20.4.3).
- What is meant by 'slip ring technology' (Section 20.5.1).
- How helical CT differs from conventional CT (Section 20.5.1).
- What is meant by 'multislice CT scanning' (Section 20.7).
- The advantages of dual-energy CT scanning (Section 20.5.3).
- The process of the formation of the CT image (Section 20.5.6).
- The advanced image postprocessing features on modern CT scanners (Section 20.5.4).
- What additional image reconstruction options are available (Section 20.6).
- The link between attenuation of the X-ray beam and CT number (Section 20.6).

FURTHER READING

Bushong, S.C. 2008. *Radiologic Science for Technologists: Physics, Radiobiology and Protection*. St. Louis: Mosby. (Chapter 23.)

Seeram, S. 2015. *Computed Tomography, Physical Principles, Clinical Applications and Quality Control*. 4th edn. London: Elsevier.

Radiation dosimetry and protection

CHAPTER CONTENTS

21.1   AIM

The aim of this chapter is to introduce the reader to the concepts of exposure, absorbed dose and dose equivalent. It then goes on to consider methods of absolute measurement of radiation dose and different relative methods of dose measurement. The purpose is also to introduce the reader to the basic legal requirements for the safe use of ionising radiation. This will cover the key documents involved in the United Kingdom and the basic organisation of radiation safety in healthcare institutions. This chapter will also examine the practical ways in which radiation safety is implemented in radiology or radiotherapy departments.

21.2   INTRODUCTION

We live in an environment where we are continuously subjected to ionising radiation from natural causes such as cosmic rays and naturally occurring radionuclides. In fact, about 90% of the average UK radiation dose comes from natural sources. In addition, there are artificial contributions to the radiation dose because of fallout from nuclear weapons testing, leakage from nuclear power plants, manufacture of radionuclides and medical exposure to radiation. All ionising radiations, whether natural or artificial, constitute a hazard. It is assumed that the greater the radiation dose to which the population is exposed, the greater the hazard. The accurate measurement of radiation dose received by the population is therefore important in trying to quantify the hazard. Medical radiation constitutes the largest single contribution of artificial radiation exposure to the population in the United Kingdom and so it is important to minimise this radiation dose and hence the total population dose. However, the hazards associated with medical irradiation must be considered against the benefits from diagnosis and treatment. This risk–benefit concept will be discussed later in this chapter.

21.3 UNITS OF EXPOSURE AND DOSE

When an X-ray beam passes through air, it produces excitation and ionisation of the air molecules. The electrons ejected in this first interaction (e.g., during photoelectric absorption) can have sufficient energy to ionise other atoms and so produce more electrons—delta rays. Delta rays are responsible for the great majority of ionisations, often referred to as secondary ionisations. The net effect on the air is:

- the formation of electrical charges in the air by ionisation
- the absorption of energy by the air as the electrical charges are slowed down by collision with the air molecules (thus producing further ionisation)
- the consequent production of heat energy because of the transfer of energy to the air molecules.

The traditional measure of exposure concerns the first of these effects only and is a measure of the amount of ionisation that occurs in air. The unit of exposure is defined as:

> **DEFINITION**
>
> The exposure at a particular point in a beam of X or gamma radiation is the ratio Q/m, where Q is the total electrical charge of one sign produced in a small volume of air of mass m.

The units of exposure are coulombs per kilogram ($C.kg^{-1}$) of air. Remember that exposure can be defined only for air and only for X or gamma radiation.

Exposure rate ($C.kg^{-1}.s^{-1}$) is a measure of the intensity of a beam of given quality because the greater the number of photons at a given energy passing through unit area, the greater the amount of ionisation of air in unit time.

In air, the proportions of ionisation and heat produced by the absorption of radiation are approximately constant and therefore do not depend on the energy of the radiation. The total amount of ionisation produced in air is proportional to the energy absorbed from the beam, for example, the average energy required to produce ionisation in air is about 33 eV, so an X-ray photon of energy 33 keV which is fully absorbed in air produces about 1000 primary ionisations.

The atomic number of air is 7.64, which is close to that of muscle at 7.42. For this reason, the mass absorption coefficients of air and muscle are very similar. This means that the energy absorbed from an X-ray beam by a given mass of air is very similar to the energy absorbed from the beam by the same mass of muscle. The energy absorbed by both air and muscle is thus proportional to the exposure measured in air.

This is the main reason for the importance of air as a medium in radiation dosimetry as it allows the dose in tissue to be calculated from knowledge of the air exposure.

21.3.1 Exposure and air kerma

In recent years, the term 'exposure' has fallen out of common usage and has been replaced by absorbed dose in air or air kerma (the initials of kerma stand for <u>k</u>inetic <u>e</u>nergy <u>r</u>eleased per unit <u>m</u>ass of <u>a</u>bsorber); for instance, the maximum permissible radiation leakage rate from the X-ray tube is now quoted in air kerma. The main reason is that it is much easier to calculate the absorbed dose in a structure from the air kerma.

21.3.2 Absorbed dose and kerma

The measurement of the quantity of electrical charge produced in air by ionisation is not the same as the measurement of the energy actually absorbed, although the two quantities are proportional to each other. The energy absorbed by a unit mass of the medium is stated as the absorbed dose and is defined as:

> **DEFINITION**
>
> The absorbed dose in a medium is in the ratio E/m, where E is the energy absorbed by the medium because of a beam of ionising radiation being directed at a small mass m.

The unit of absorbed dose is the *Gray* (Gy) and so we can say that 1 Gray = 1 joule per kilogram (1 Gy = 1 J.kg^{-1}).

Note that exposure is defined in terms of X or gamma radiation only, whereas absorbed dose is defined in terms of any ionising radiation. Therefore the absorbed dose from alpha-particles, beta-particles and neutrons are all measured in Grays. However, ultraviolet radiation is only capable of excitation rather than ionisation of the atoms of the medium and so is outside the scope of the definition of absorbed dose.

If all the electrons produced by the primary and secondary ionisations within a medium are stopped within it, then it can be seen that the energy removed from the beam of ionising radiation is the same as the energy absorbed by the medium (this makes the assumption that all the fluorescent or characteristic radiation is absorbed, as is the case in body tissues). This does not necessarily apply to a very small volume within the medium—such a volume may be removing energy from the beam but the absorbed energy may be deposited outside the volume (but still within the body) owing to the distance travelled by the electrons before coming to rest. Electrons with an energy of 1 MeV travel for about 5 mm in tissue before coming to rest.

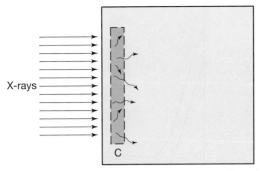

Fig. 21.1 X-rays interacting with atoms in volume *C* produce electrons which may travel outside of *C*.

This effect is illustrated in Fig. 21.1. Here an incoming X-ray beam of high energy interacts with a volume element *C* within the medium. Because of the high energy of the beam, the electrons produced by Compton scatter are scattered in a forward direction, so much of their energy is absorbed outside the volume *C*. There will also be secondary ionisations resulting in the production of delta rays, but for simplicity these are not shown in the figure. In general, if the secondary electrons produced within the volume deposit a total energy E within the medium, and E_{IN} and E_{OUT} are the total energies of the electrons entering and escaping from the volume, then the absorbed dose in Grays is given by:

$$\text{absorbed dose} = \frac{(E + E_{IN} - E_{OUT})}{m} \quad \textbf{Equation 21.1}$$

where m is the mass of the particular small volume considered. If a larger volume is considered, then this formula can be used to calculate the average absorbed dose in that volume.

Electronic equilibrium is said to occur if $E_{IN} = E_{OUT}$ because there is no net loss or gain of the electrons over the small volume being considered. If $E_{IN} = E_{OUT}$ is a constant value not equal to zero, there is said to be quasielectronic equilibrium. If the intensity of the radiation is varied, the net loss or gain of electrons will vary in proportion. An example of electronic equilibrium occurs in the free-air ionisation chamber, which will be discussed later in Section 21.5.2.

The absorbed dose expresses the quantity of energy absorbed in the medium owing to a beam of ionising radiation passing through it. As stated at the beginning of this section, the site of the attenuating events (e.g., photoelectric absorption) may be at some distance from the absorption process because of the distance travelled by the ejected electrons before coming to rest. The quantity which measures the amount of attenuation in a small volume is called the kerma (see Section 21.3.1).

Kerma is also measured in Grays and may differ significantly from the absorbed dose at any particular position within the medium.

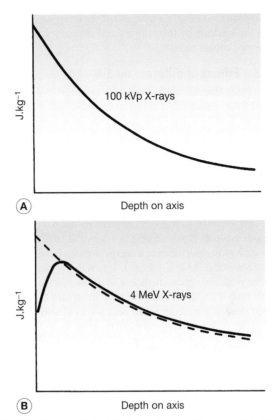

Fig. 21.2 Kerma (*dashed line*) and absorbed dose (*solid line*) for (A) 100 kVp diagnostic X-ray beam and (B) 4 MeV therapy beam. In (A) the two curves are coincident, but they are different in (B) because of the increased energy and hence range of the secondary photons produced.

The absorbed dose and kerma along the axis of a beam of X radiation are shown in Fig. 21.2. Fig. 21.2A shows the case where an X-ray beam generated at 100 kVp is incident upon soft tissue; this type of situation might occur in diagnostic radiography. The electrons released in the primary and secondary ionisations are of relatively low energy and so are absorbed close to the site of the initial attenuating interactions. The kerma and absorbed dose at any particular point along the beam axis are essentially the same and the curves are coincident in the figure. This is not the case if the X-ray beam has high photon energy because electrons produced by the initial ionisation have considerable energy and so deposit their energy some distance from the point of the original attenuation process. As can be seen in Fig. 21.2B, the kerma and the absorbed dose resulting from 4 MeV X-rays interacting with tissue are not the same. It may be easier to understand these curves if it is remembered that:

- the kerma is a measure of the attenuation—the number of photoelectric and Compton events

• the absorbed dose is a measure of the energy deposited in the medium by the primary and secondary electrons being brought to rest.

21.3.3   Effects of different media

Instruments that are used to measure absorbed dose or absorbed dose rate are called *dosimeters* and *dose-rate meters*, respectively. Some of these instruments are described in more detail in later sections of this chapter (see Section 21.5 onwards). It is common practice to calibrate these meters to read the absorbed dose or dose rate in air through which the X-rays or gamma rays are passing. Such a dosimeter may read 0.5 mGy as the total absorbed dose in air at a point within an X-ray beam. It must not be inferred, however, that this is the absorbed dose that would be received by any other medium if placed in the same position. For two media to receive the same absorbed dose, each must absorb the same energy from the beam per unit mass (remember, 1 Gy = 1 J.kg^{-1}). This is the same as saying that the mass absorption coefficient of the two media must be equal. Thus if D_{air} is the absorbed dose in air and D_m the absorbed dose in a medium when both are irradiated with the same beam of X-rays, it follows that if the mass absorption coefficients are not equal, this equation may by drawn up:

$$\frac{D_m}{D_{air}} = \frac{(\mu_a / \rho)_m}{(\mu_a / \rho)_{air}}$$

$$\text{or } D_m = D_{air} \times \frac{(\mu_a / \rho)_m}{(\mu_a / \rho)_{air}}$$

Equation 21.2

If the mass absorption coefficient of air and the given medium are known at the energy of the X-ray quanta, the absorbed dose in the medium may be calculated using Equation 21.2. In practice, this allows us to measure the absorbed dose in air at a certain point and then calculate the absorbed dose in the patient at the same point without subjecting the patient to a great degree of discomfort.

The mass absorption coefficients of both air and bone vary with photon energy. These variations of the two coefficients are shown in Fig. 21.3A and the variations in the ratio of the two coefficients are shown in Fig. 21.3B. As can be seen from the graphs, at low photon energies (50 keV is shown with the broken line in Fig. 21.3A), the mass absorption coefficient of bone is considerably higher than that of air. This is because at low energies the photoelectric effect predominates ($\tau/\rho \propto Z^3/E^3$) and the atomic number of bone ($Z = 14$) is approximately double that of air ($Z = 7.64$). For this reason and because of the large difference in density, we get a high level of contrast between bone and air on an X-ray image (this can be seen on a chest X-ray image or on radiography of the paranasal sinuses). At an energy of about 1 MeV, however, the two graphs are

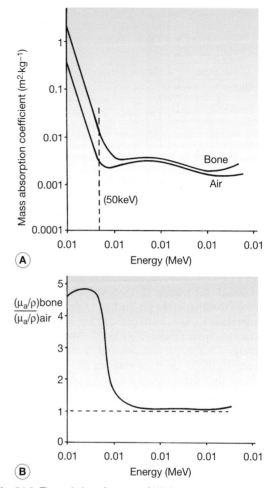

Fig. 21.3 The variation of energy of (A) the mass attenuation coefficients of air and bone and (B) the ratio of the two coefficients.

very close and the ratio of the two coefficients approaches 1. This is because of the dominance of Compton scatter in this region ($\sigma/\rho \propto$ electron density and the electron density for bone and air is approximately the same). This means that there would be a low level of contrast between the two if they were radiographed using 1 MeV photons. At above about 10 MeV the curves again diverge owing to the greater amount of pair production in bone compared with air ($\pi/\rho \propto Z$). Thus it is clear that an instrument calibrated to read absorbed dose in air must be used with caution when calculating the absorbed dose in another medium as the relationships between the absorption coefficients vary with the photon energies. This is particularly the case in the diagnostic range of energies where absorption is principally by the photoelectric effect, which is very sensitive to both atomic number and photon energy.

21.4   QUALITY FACTOR AND DOSE EQUIVALENT

As described in the previous section, the absorbed dose measures the energy absorbed per unit mass of the medium when it is subjected to any type of ionising radiation. The biological effects of the radiation on tissue, for instance, do not depend solely on the absorbed dose, but also on the type of radiation and on the absorbed dose rate. It is found that alpha-particles will cause considerably more damage (about 20 times as much) in a biological specimen compared with the same absorbed dose of X-rays. It is also found that radiation delivered as a single large dose will generally cause more biological damage than the same dose fractionated into multiple small doses and delivered over a period of time.

The differences in biological effects of different types of ionising radiations are the result of the different densities of ionisations they produce in a sample. Radiation, which causes large numbers of ionisation per unit length of track through a material, will cause large amounts of biological damage. You may remember, when an atom is ionised (e.g., by a photoelectric interaction), an electron (negative ion) is released and the atom now becomes a positive ion. An ion pair has been formed. X-rays and beta-particles do not produce ion pairs as close together as do the more massive protons or alpha-particles of the same energy. Protons or alpha-particles are brought to rest quickly within the medium by losing their kinetic energy in the production of many ions over a short distance—an alpha particle of energy 1 MeV will travel only 5×10^{-3} mm in tissue, protons will travel 3×10^{-2} mm and beta-particles will travel 5 mm before being brought to rest. Because of this, the larger particles break chemical bonds, which are very close together, and so the chance of repair is reduced. This means that they have a greater biological effect on the specimen. It is also found that neutrons will produce dense ionisation by the ejection of protons from the nuclei or by nuclear recoil. The absorbed dose in Grays is thus not an accurate measure of the biological effects of different types of radiation owing to the very different patterns of ionisation produced. The unit used to measure the overall biological effects of different types of radiation is called the *unit of dose equivalent* and is measured in sieverts (Sv). The absorbed dose in Grays and the dose equivalent in sieverts are related to each other, as shown in Equation 21.3:

$$\text{dose equivalent (Sv)} = Q \times \text{absorbed dose (Gy)} \times N$$

Equation 21.3

where Q is known as the *quality factor* for the radiation and is related to the number of ion pairs produced per unit length by the radiation. N includes other factors that may affect the biological process, such as the *dose rate*. In many

TABLE 21.1   Quality factors for different ionising radiations

Type of ionising radiation	Quality factor
X-rays or gamma rays	1
Electrons or beta-particles	1
Thermal neutrons	2/3
Fast neutrons (neutrons of high energy)	10
Protons	10
Alpha-particles	20
Recoil nuclei (e.g., alpha decay)	20
Fission fragments	20

cases, the value of N is 1 and so the equation is frequently quoted without the factor N appearing.

Table 21.1 shows the value of the quality factor for different types of radiation. Note that Q is unity for X-rays and gamma rays so the absorbed dose is the same as the dose equivalent for these radiations. The biological effect of particulate radiations is therefore compared with that of X-rays or gamma rays by means of the value of Q. As can be seen from Table 21.1, electrons also have a quality factor of unity. This is because an external beam of electrons will produce secondary electrons with the same election density as X-rays and gamma rays. However, alpha-particles have a Q of 20, indicating that the same absorbed dose will produce 20 times as much biological damage as the same absorbed dose of X-rays.

Because Q is a comparative number, the sievert has the same units as the Gray (J.kg^{-1}). The quality factor may be considered a scaling factor relating the biological effect of absorbed dose to the same dose of X-rays or gamma rays.

Dose equivalent in sieverts has a vital role to play in radiation protection, where it is required to consider the sum of the effects of exposure to different types of radiation.

INSIGHT

The dose equivalent is too crude a unit for use in radiobiology because it considers the average effect(s) on a group of cells. In radiobiology, we wish to look more precisely at individual effects on cells (e.g., impairment of cell reproduction). For this, we use a more precise scaling factor—the relative biological effectiveness (RBE). The RBE compares the absorbed doses of different ionising radiations required to produce the same biological effect. As with the quality factor (Q), these are usually compared with the same dose of X or gamma radiation.

The remainder of this chapter is concerned with a brief overview of some of the methods used to measure exposure and absorbed doses.

21.5   ABSOLUTE MEASUREMENT OF ABSORBED DOSE

The absolute measurement of absorbed dose in air resulting from a beam of X-rays requires very careful techniques and very specialised equipment. It is more suited to a specialised laboratory than to a hospital or university department environment. In the United Kingdom, the National Physics Laboratory and in the United States, the National Bureau of Standards calibrate and check specialised dosimeters under carefully controlled conditions. Such dosimeters are termed *absolute standards*. Dosimeters used in hospitals and universities are sent to such centres on a regular basis to be calibrated against the absolute standards; such dosimeters are then known as *secondary standards*. Further dosimeters are calibrated against these secondary standards. Such dosimeters are known as *substandards*. This initial section considers the way an absolute measurement of absorbed dose may be made, and the following section (Section 21.6) is an overview of the most common of the relative methods of assessing absorbed dose.

21.5.1   Calorimetry

A beam of X-rays or gamma rays will be attenuated as it passes through a medium, and the attenuation processes (see Chapter 13) will produce many ionisations within the medium. The atoms of the medium eventually absorb the kinetic energy of the electron ejected from their atoms. This results in these atoms having an increase in their kinetic energy—heat will be produced in the medium. The

medium will experience a temperature rise that is proportional to the heat energy absorbed by the medium and therefore the absorbed dose. It is known that:

$$Q = mc\left(T_2 - T_1\right)$$

where Q is the heat energy, m is the mass of the body, c is its specific heat capacity and $(T_2 - T_1)$ is the temperature rise experienced by the body.

We also know from the earlier sections of this chapter (see Section 21.3.2) that absorbed dose (D) is energy per unit mass of the medium and so:

$$D = \frac{Q}{m}$$

Thus, we can produce the equation:

$$D = c\left(T_2 - T_1\right) \qquad \textbf{Equation 21.4}$$

Using this equation, if we know the specific heat capacity of the medium, the absorbed dose may be calculated from the temperature rise produced in an irradiated medium. This is known as the *calorimetric method of absorbed dose measurement*. However, the temperature rise produced is very small: 1 Gy will produce a temperature rise of about $2 \times 10^{-4}\,°C$ and so the process needs very controlled conditions and is most appropriate when measuring very large absorbed doses of radiation. A more sensitive method is to collect the charge produced in an ionisation chamber; this is described later.

21.5.2   The free-air ionisation chamber

The free-air ionisation chamber shown in Fig. 21.4 uses ions produced by the absorption of an X-ray beam in air collected by oppositely charged plates situated in the air.

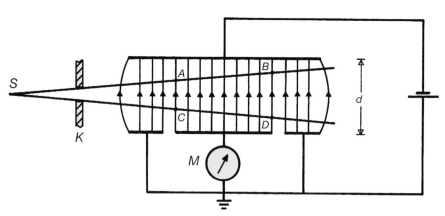

Fig. 21.4 A diagrammatic vertical section through a free-air ionisation chamber. S is the radiation source, K is a collimator and d is the separation distance between plates AB and CD. The electrons resulting from the ionisation that takes place in the area ABCD are collected on the collecting plate CD which is connected to the meter M. This measures the negative charge produced as a result of the radiation.

The liberated electrons are attracted towards the positive plate and the positive ions are attracted towards the negative plate. Thus charge, whose magnitude is proportional to the exposure in coulombs per kilogram and the absorbed dose in Grays, flows through the chamber. Certain precautions are necessary, however, to achieve accurate results:

- As shown in Fig. 21.4, the central lower disc is surrounded by an annulus which is at earth potential. Because Fig. 21.4 is a vertical section through such a chamber, the annulus appears as if it were two separate plates. This construction enables an accurate estimation of the volume of air from which the ion pairs are collected because it ensures that the lines of electrical force are at right angles to both the collecting plates. Note that this is not the case at the outer edge of the annulus, where the lines of electrical force are bowed outwards, thus including an unknown quantity of air beyond the edge of the plates. The volume of air from which the ion pairs are collected may be calculated by knowing the geometry of *ABCD*. Ion pairs produced outside this volume are still collected by the annulus but do not pass through the meter *M* and its associated electronic amplifier and do not contribute to the current indicated by the meter.
- Some electrons produced by ionisation in the region *ABCD* will escape and produce further ionisations over the annulus rather than the central disc. This suggests that the current measured by the meter, *M*, is too low, but this is not the case because on average the same number of electrons are gained by the volume under consideration. This is a case of electron equilibrium, described earlier (Section 21.3.2).
- The potential difference across the plates must be sufficiently high to collect all the ion pairs produced in the air. If we irradiate a free-air ionisation chamber with a steady beam of radiation, the current flowing through the chamber will vary with the potential difference across the plates, as shown in Fig. 21.5.
- Below the saturation voltage, some of the positive and negative ions recombine by mutual attraction (or germinal recombination) and so not all ions are collected. Above saturation voltage, the electrical field strength between the plates is large enough to ensure that all the ions move to the appropriately charged plate for collection. The actual voltage depends on the separation on the plates, but typically this is in the region of a few hundred volts.
- The separation of the plates, *d*, shown in Fig. 21.4, must be sufficiently large to enable the production of all the secondary ionisations in air. No electron produced during the ionisation process must reach the plates before it produces all the ion pairs of which it is capable. If *d* is too

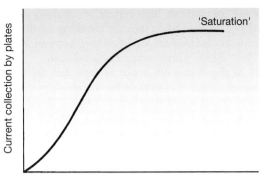

Fig. 21.5 The variation of current flowing through the meter, *M*, in Fig. 21.4 with the applied potential across the plates.

small, then the current measured by the meter, *M*, will be too low because there are too few ion pairs produced in the air volume and hence the estimate of the exposure or absorbed dose will be too low. The required plate separation depends on the energy of the x- or gamma-ray beam because photons with high energies will produce electrons with correspondingly high energies that will travel further in air. Typical values vary from about 20 cm for photon energies up to 250 keV to several metres for photons of energy above 1 MeV. From this it can be seen that the greater the energy of the beam, the more cumbersome the measurement, caused by the necessity for greater separation of the plates.

- The total charge in coulombs measured by the free-air ionisation chamber is a direct measure of the exposure in C.kg^{-1} and is proportional to the absorbed dose in Grays (J.kg^{-1}). The mass of the air irradiated depends on the temperature and the pressure of air and must be corrected for the effects of these variations. If ρ_0 is the density of air at a known temperature and pressure, then the mass of the air m_0 in the irradiated volume, v, can be calculated as $m_0 = \rho_0 v$. At a new temperature and pressure (T_1 and P_1), the density changes to $\rho_0 T_0 P_1 / T_1 P_0$ so the mass of the air, m', being irradiated is given by:

$$m' = m_0 \times \frac{T_0}{T_1} \times \frac{P_1}{P_0} \qquad \textbf{Equation 21.5}$$

The exposure (in C.kg^{-1}) is the ratio of the total charge collected to the mass of air irradiated (m'). The absorbed dose (in Grays) is calculated from the energy absorbed divided by m'—the energy absorbed can be calculated from the charge collected because it takes about 33 eV to produce one ion pair in air.

The ionisation method is not suitable for use with liquids owing to the very rapid germinal recombination of the ions and the relatively high current which flows through many liquids, even when they are not being irradiated. A semiconductor (see Section 21.6.6) may, however, be used to collect the ion pairs produced by irradiation.

From the discussion, it can be seen that the free-air ionisation chamber is suitable for the absolute measurement of exposure and absorbed dose in air. The absorbed dose, which would have occurred in another medium, placed in the same beam of radiation may be calculated from the mass absorption coefficients, as explained earlier in Section 21.3.3.

21.5.3   Chemical methods of dose measurement

We have already established that radiation affects the chemical bonds between atoms of a material through which it passes by both ionisation and excitation of electrons. Research has shown that ionising radiation is able to transform a dilute solution of ferrous sulphate, $FeSO_4$, to ferric sulphate, $Fe_2(SO_4)_3$, by rearrangement of the chemical bonds. The number of ferric ions so produced is proportional to the absorbed dose; 100 eV of absorbed dose will produce about 15 ferric ions. A chemical measurement of the concentration of the ferric ions produced at a given energy of a given radiation beam may be used as a measure of the absorbed dose in water.

Such a chemical dosimeter may be calibrated against either of the two preceding methods of absorbed dose measure. It is included in this section on absolute methods of dose measurement because once the conversion factor between quantity of ferric ions is known, no further calibration is necessary. The process of calibration is similar to the calculation of absorbed dose in the free-air ionisation chamber from the knowledge of the energy required to produce an ion pair in air.

This method of dose measurement is known as the *Fricke dosimeter*, but it is only suitable for the estimation of very large doses, in excess of 20 Gy. This is because of chemical impurities present in the solution, the rapid rate of germinal recombination of the ions produced and relatively insensitive methods of chemical estimation of the quantity of ferric produced. However, it is particularly suitable for use with high-energy radiation beams and for irregular shapes of irradiated volumes. The advent of conformational radiotherapy treatment and the requirement under the Ionising Radiations (Medical Exposure) Regulations (IR(ME)R) to optimise radiation dose to the patient have resulted in the development of a number of polymer gels. These are tissue equivalent with a density of 0.99 g.cm^{-1} and show a linear response to high-energy photons from 300 keV to in excess of 8 MeV. Ionising radiation also has a polymerisation effect on the gel supporting the ferrous sulphate atoms; this reduces germinal recombination

and prevents migration of the ferric sulphate atoms formed outside the beam area. Magnetic resonance spectrometry is used to estimate the number of ferric sulphate atoms present. If placed (in a suitable container) in a phantom, such dosimeters may be used to confirm the steep dose gradients that are an essential feature of conformational therapy treatments.

21.6   TYPES OF DETECTORS AND DOSIMETERS

So far in this chapter we have considered the measurement of absorbed dose by absolute methods. These form a standard against which other types of dosimeter can be compared or calibrated. There are many such relative methods by which absorbed dose may be estimated, each with some advantages and disadvantages. The most common of these methods are briefly outlined in the following pages.

21.6.1   The thimble ionisation chamber

The size and configuration of the free-air ionisation chamber discussed so far make it a suitable instrument for the standardisation of radiation dose measurement but totally unsuitable for routine dose measurement in a hospital environment—a plate separation of 5 metres would be required if we needed to measure the dose rate at a patient's skin from a cobalt-60 source!

The thimble ionisation chamber shown in Fig. 21.6 circumvents some of these difficulties by, as it were, 'condensing' the air into a solid medium surrounding the central electrode. The cap of the thimble chamber is said to be *air equivalent*, that is, it is made of a material that has the same atomic number as air (e.g., graphite, bakelite, plastic) and so its absorption properties are the same as the same mass of air. The central aluminium electrode has a fixed amount of positive charge put on it from an external source. When the chamber is irradiated, some of the more energetic electrons liberated in the cap will penetrate into the air of the chamber and be attracted to the central electrode. Thus the central electrode will lose some of its positive charge. By the choice of suitable materials, the thimble chamber can be made to have the same absorbing properties as the same mass of air. Such a device is calibrated for several photon energies against a standard chamber, such as the free-air

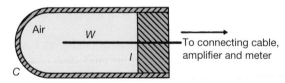

Fig. 21.6 Construction of a thimble ionisation chamber. *C*, Cap; *I*, insulator; *W*, central wire.

chamber described earlier in this chapter, and a correction factor is used to convert the indicated loss of charge from the central electrode to true absorbed dose. The choice of wall thickness of the cap is one of the factors that influence the applied correction because a thin cap may not produce sufficient electrons entering the chamber, whereas too thick a cap will absorb more radiation than it needs to. Note that the vast majority of the electrons used to measure the change in charge or the current through the chamber are produced in the wall of the chamber and not in the air cavity of the chamber, but it is the passage of such electrons into the air cavity that enables the change in charge or the current to be measured. Corrections for variations in the temperature and pressure of the air must be made, as is the case for the free-air chamber.

Thimble-type chambers are still extensively used in radiation measurements in hospitals. For example, the calibration of the radiation output from a radiotherapy machine is usually accomplished using a thimble chamber connected to an electronic amplification system, which measures and displays the charge produced in the chamber during irradiation. However, to relate the reading obtained because of a given exposure to the radiation output of the machine (usually expressed in cGy.min^{-1}), certain correction factors need to be applied. These include the following:

- The reading must be corrected for temperature and pressure.
- The reading must be corrected by a factor which relates the reading of this substandard unit to a secondary standard unit calibrated by a national body (e.g., the Health Protection Agency)—this correction factor depends on the energy of the radiation.

- The correction which requires to be applied to the secondary standard to compare it with the absolute standard—this is again related to the energy of the radiation and a factor to convert exposure to absorbed dose at the appropriate radiation energy.

In addition, there may be some machine-dependent correction factors, such as correction for 'switch-on' and 'switch-off' errors.

21.6.2 The Geiger–Müller counter

The thimble chamber described in the previous section is an example of an ionisation chamber where the charge collected on the electrodes is proportional to the energy absorbed from the X-ray beam. The Geiger–Müller counter works on the principle of gas multiplication and gives the same magnitude of electrical pulse per absorption event whatever the energy of the absorbed radiation. The structure of a typical Geiger–Müller tube is shown in Fig. 21.7A.

The glass envelope contains an inert gas (argon) at low pressure and two electrodes—a positively charged central electrode and a negatively charged mesh cylinder. Ionisation is caused in the gas by the entry of a photon or by the entry of particulate radiation (if the window is sufficiently thin to allow particles to enter the envelope). The ions are attracted to the appropriate electrode and, as they pass through the gas, they gain sufficient energy to eject electrons from the gas atoms if the potential difference between the electrodes is sufficiently great. The electrons so produced continue this process and rapid gas multiplication takes place, especially near the central electrode because the field strength is great in this region. The effect of gas multiplication is such that well in excess of 1 million electrons are collected by the

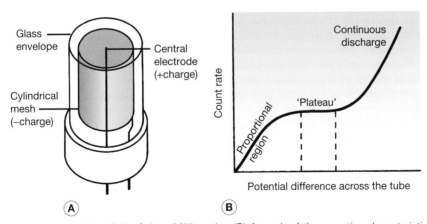

Fig. 21.7 (A) Basic construction of the Geiger–Müller tube. (B) A graph of the operating characteristics of such a tube, which is operated on its plateau region.

central electrode for every single ion produced in the primary absorption process. These 'electron avalanches' form the pulses, which allow the system to count the number of initial ionisation events. The presence of a small quantity of alcohol vapour in the gas helps to quench the gas multiplication process so that it does not become continuous. It does this by absorbing the kinetic energy of the positive ions in the gas so that they are prevented from striking the mesh with sufficient energy to release further electrons and so keep the process going indefinitely. Alternatively, the potential difference between the electrodes may be momentarily reduced after an electron avalanche, thus terminating the gas multiplication. In either case, there is a dead time after each pulse, where another absorption event, if present, is not recorded. A typical dead time is 5 μs and so the differences between the observed count rates and the real count rates are negligible except at high count rates—at an observed count rate of 1000 per second, the true count rate is 1005, whereas at an observed count rate of 100,000 per second, the true count rate is 200,000! The correct potential difference to be applied to a Geiger–Müller tube is determined in practice by plotting a graph of the count rate obtained when a small radioactive source is placed near the tube against the applied voltage. Such a graph is shown in Fig. 21.7B. Three distinct regions of such a graph exist:

1. The proportional region, where some gas multiplication takes place and the sizes of the electrical pulses are proportional to the energy deposited in the gas by the radiation.
2. The plateau region, where maximum gas amplification takes place and all electrical pulses have the same size, irrespective of the energy of the radiation.
3. The continuous-discharge region, where the electrical field strength is sufficient to ionise the gas atoms and so produce continuous unwanted gas multiplication. The plateau is usually between 100 and 1500 V, depending on the size of the Geiger–Müller tube.

As can be seen, the Geiger–Müller tube is suitable for detecting the presence of radiation rather than for an accurate estimation of absorbed doses because the pulses bear no relationship to the energy of the radiation causing them. For this reason, it is often used as a contamination monitor for radioactive spillage or as a method of determining whether radiation is present in a specific area.

21.6.3 Scintillation detectors

The operation of a scintillation detector employing a sodium iodide crystal and a photomultiplier tube is described in Section 22.3.3, which considers radionuclide imaging and nuclear medicine in more detail.

Any suitable scintillating material can be used, whether solid or liquid, and the principle of operation is that the size of the electrical pulse produced by the photomultiplier is proportional to the energy deposited in the scintillator. Scintillation plastics have been produced which have an atomic number close to that of air and tissue. These can be termed as being *air equivalent* and so have similar variations of absorption to air, with variations in photon energy. They are useful in estimating absorbed dose in air. Sodium iodide has a much higher atomic number than air and will show a marked variation in absorption with photon energy, especially near its absorption edges. This requires correction factors to be applied for different photon energies if an accurate estimation of the absorbed dose in air is to be made. This is particularly so for thin crystals, which show a more marked variation in absorption with photon energy compared with thick crystals.

Scintillation counters are very sensitive devices and are used in many applications in radiography and radionuclide imaging, for example, for the detection of radioactive contamination, for estimation of in-vitro radioactivity, as radiation detectors on computed tomography and osteoporosis scanners and as the detection mechanism in gamma cameras.

21.6.4 Thermoluminescent dosimetry

The basic physics of thermoluminesce has already been described. Thermoluminescence may be used to estimate radiation doses using lithium fluoride in the form of powder, extruded chips or impregnated Teflon discs or rods. The impurities in the lithium fluoride generate electron traps, and the number of electrons which are 'stuck' in these traps is proportional to the absorbed dose in the lithium fluoride. The average atomic number of lithium fluoride is 8.2 so it is close to soft tissue ($Z = 7.5$). Both have similar absorption variations with photon energy. The small discs do not show up on X-ray images and so may be strapped to the part of the body where we wish to measure the absorbed dose. After irradiation, the discs are heated, and the amount of light emitted is compared with a standard dosimeter to which a known dose has been given. The dose to the disc can then be calculated by direct proportion. The discs are then annealed and may be reused.

The fact that the discs have radiolucency similar to tissue allows us to use them to estimate radiation dose without interfering with the X-ray image or radiotherapy treatment. The discs are small, measuring only a few millimetres across, and so may be used to estimate the dose to different structures in the body during a diagnostic or therapeutic procedure. An additional advantage is that they can be used to monitor radiation dose ranging from 1 μGy to 1 kGy.

The role of thermoluminescent dosimetry (TLD) in personnel monitoring will be considered later in this chapter.

21.6.5   Photographic film

Photographic film will produce an increase in optical density when it is irradiated and processed. The response, however, is not in linear proportion to the absorbed dose of the emulsion. A calibration graph for the particular film at known radiation doses and specific processing conditions must be produced. This is a major disadvantage if it is to be used as a method of dose estimation. It is also true that the film emulsion has a higher atomic number than tissue (AgBr has an average atomic number of 41) and so has significantly higher photoelectric absorption at low energies. For these reasons, the use of photographic film has largely been replaced by TLD.

21.6.6   Semiconductor detectors

As we saw in Section 7.10 electrons in a semiconductor can readily have their energy raised to that of the conduction band and so can take part in electrical conduction. The absorption of energy from an X-ray photon (by either photoelectric absorption or Compton scattering) can raise an electron to the conduction band energies. This electron causes secondary electrons from the atoms of the material to be raised to the conduction band, by imparting some of its energy to them. If a potential difference is placed across the semiconductor, then these electrons are collected before they have time to recombine. Thus there is a current pulse whose magnitude is proportional to the number of electrons and hence the absorbed dose within the semiconductor. This is similar to the current through an irradiated ionisation chamber and the semiconductor detector can be thought of as a solid-state ionisation chamber. It has the great advantage over the air ionisation chamber that it produces 10 times as many ion pairs for a given dose of radiation and so is much more sensitive to small doses. This is because only 3 eV is required to produce an ion pair in a semiconductor, compared with 33 eV to produce an ion pair in air. The electrical signal obtained from the semiconductor device is more accurate (it has a smaller statistical uncertainty) and may, for example, be used to produce very accurate gamma-ray spectra.

Semiconductor detectors may be calibrated against a thimble chamber, such as for a given energy of radiation.

Semiconductor detectors tend to be used for more specialised forms of radiation detection (e.g., a small semiconductor detector may be inserted into the rectum to measure rectal dose). Metal Oxide Semiconductor Field Effect Transistors (MOSFETs) are types of semiconductor that can generate dose estimates immediately following irradiation. Fig. 21.8 illustrates the mobile MOSFET system distributed by Best Medical.

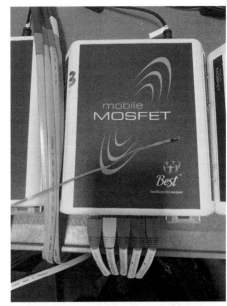

Fig. 21.8 Photograph of the Mobile MOSFET dosimetry system supplied by Best Medical. This wireless system has the option of receiving data from up to five dosimeters (centre).

21.7   PURPOSE AND SCOPE OF RADIATION PROTECTION

One of the basic tasks of radiation protection is to establish levels of risk to the population resulting from this source and then to take steps to keep these levels of risk from this source as low as possible.

The purpose of radiation protection in medicine is to produce and maintain an environment, both at work and in the outside world, where the levels of ionising radiation from this source pose a minimal acceptable risk for human beings. Before beginning any discussion on radiation protection, understand that our environment can only be described as *relatively safe* from the effects of radiation from artificial sources.

Once the levels of risk from such radiation have been determined, appropriate dose-equivalent limits (see Section 21.9) may be set so that the risk associated with such radiations is no greater (and frequently is much less) than other aspects of life (e.g., the risk of injury resulting from a traffic accident). Establishing such dose-equivalent limits, and ensuring that staff work within these limits, helps to prevent harm.

These ionizing radiation risks may be divided into two categories: (i) stochastic (chance) effects which can occur at any dose level but are unlikely at low doses. These effects include cancer as well as genetic changes and exhibit a long time lag (latent period) before they become manifest. (ii) deterministic effects which only appear above a dose

TABLE 21.2   Core of knowledge

1   Nature of ionizing radiation and its interaction with tissue
2   Genetic and somatic effects of ionizing radiation and how to assess these risks
3   The ranges of radiation dose given to a patient during the course of a particular procedure, the main factors affecting dose and methods of measuring dose
4   Principles of dose limitation and optimisation
5   Principles of quality assurance applied to equipment and techniques
6   Specific requirements of children and of women who are or may be pregnant
7   Precautions necessary when handling sealed and unsealed radioactive sources
8   Organizational aspects of radiation protection and the procedure for suspected overexposure
9   Statutory responsibilities
10 Knowledge of the clinical value of the procedure requested, in relation to other available techniques
11 Importance of using radiological information, e.g. reports and images from a previous investigation

threshold and are unlikely to occur in routine diagnostic imaging. These effects include radiation erythema (skin reddening) and cataract.

A full study of radiation protection would need to cover:
- radiobiology
- genetics
- statistical analysis of risk
- the fate and decay patterns of radioactivity released into the environment
- the absorbing power of different materials to different radiations.

Such a vast scope of study cannot be covered in a single chapter, or even in one book. Only a simplified review of practical methods of reducing radiation doses to radiation workers and their patients from the medical use of ionising radiation will be considered here. These points are covered in the core of knowledge which all radiographic staff are expected to learn as part of their education. This consists of 11 key items as summarised in Table 21.2. Items 1 to 9 are of particular importance to the operator, whereas items 10 and 11 have particular reference to the role of the practitioner.

21.8   LEGAL ASPECTS

The legislation governing radiation is often confusing to the student. The International Commission for Radiation Protection (ICRP) has produced recommendations on ra-

diation protection. These recommendations do not have the force of law. Laws based on these recommendations are then produced by the nations of the world.

In the European Union (EU), this is attained through directives (i.e., 2013/59/EURATOM), and all member states in the EU are required to implement these directives. In the United Kingdom, the following acts and regulations are concerned with radiation safety:
- Health and Safety at Work Act [HSW 1974]
- Ionising Radiation Regulations [IRR 2017] Statutory Instrument 2017/1075
- Radioactive Substances Act 1993 [RSA 1993]
- Ionising Radiation (Medical Exposure) Regulations 2017 [IR(ME)R 2017] Statutory Instrument 2017/1322
- Radioactive Substances (Hospitals) Exemption (Amendment) Order [RS(H)EO 1995] Statutory Instrument 1995/2395.

The inspectorate of the Health and Safety Executive (HSE) is responsible for ensuring that employers and employees comply with the above regulations. IRR 2017 applies to all radiation work and radiation workers in both the private and public sectors of the nuclear industry and those who may be affected by such work activities. In contrast, IR(ME)R 2017 applies whenever humans are irradiated for diagnostic, therapeutic, research or other medical or dental purposes, and where in-vitro medical tests are conducted, and is enforced by the Care Quality Commission (CQC). These regulations apply to staff, students, patients and their friends and relatives who are acting as comforters or carers, and to volunteers in research projects and members of the public. The above are all legal documents, and are often difficult for the layperson to understand. 'User friendly' methods of meeting the requirements of these laws have been published as the *Approved Codes of Practice* and *Guidance Notes*. These do not have the force of law, but in a prosecution the defendant must be able to prove that their method of work is as good as, or better than, that recommended in the code or guidance notes.

21.8.1   Organisation of radiation safety

The employer (e.g., the hospital trust) is ultimately responsible for maintaining radiation safety for staff, patients and others who may be affected by their work activities. They have specific obligations under the regulations and meet these through a number of radiation safety experts:
- The Radiation Protection Adviser (RPA): an accredited, medically qualified physicist who is appointed by the employer to advise the employer on radiation safety and compliance with the regulations. This includes the production of local rules and written systems of work, the designation of work areas, the supervision of quality assurance programmes and acceptance testing of new equipment.

- The Radiation Protection Supervisor (RPS): every area of the institution in which ionising radiation is used must have an RPS appointed by the employer. Each RPS must understand the specific requirements of radiation safety as applied to their area of work. Because the RPS is responsible to the employer for ensuring the safety measures are implemented and maintained, such individuals are usually departmental leads as they have the authority necessary to do this.
- The Radiation Safety Committee (RSC): this committee oversees all radiation safety issues, including research, and ensures that the reports of the RPA are implemented, and radiation safety standards are maintained.

21.8.2 Responsibilities of the manufacturer

The manufacturers have obligations that are designed to improve the radiation protection offered by their equipment. These include such features as limiting radiation leakage from the X-ray tube so that it does not exceed 1 mSv.h^{-1} at a distance of 1 metre in any direction from the focus of the tube, the provision of suitable antiscatter protection, the use of low-absorption interspacing material in secondary radiation grids, the use of a high-output rectification system, provision of an automatic (preferably anatomically programmable) timer and 'dead-man operation' of exposure switching so that releasing the exposure switch during an exposure automatically terminates the exposure. If the equipment is capable of fluoroscopy, a pulsed fluoroscopy system must be used.

21.9 DOSE-EQUIVALENT LIMITS

Table 21.3 summarises the dose-equivalent limits specified by the Ionising Radiation Regulations 2017. Note that these limits exclude any dose received from natural radiation sources or medical treatment of the individual concerned.

21.9.1 Designated radiation workers

If an employee is likely to receive a whole-body dose equivalent of ionising radiation exceeding 6 mSv per annum, then that person must be designated as a classified radiation worker by the employer. A person who is a classified radia-

tion worker must be subject to medical surveillance, with periodic reviews of health at least every 12 months.

It is not sufficient to rely on an individual's history of doses received if they are less than the three-tenths limit. The potential doses which may be received in a set of circumstances must be assessed. The reason for designation may be that the individual works in controlled areas (see Section 21.5.1) but this is not, on its own, sufficient reason for designation. Even if the local rules (see Section 21.5), when strictly obeyed, indicate that doses in excess of the three-tenths limit will not occur, persons who work with radiation sources capable of producing an overdose in a few minutes will need to be classified.

The radiation dose which the classified person receives should be measured using a suitable personal dosimeter—the doses must be assessed by an approved dosimetry service based on accepted national standards.

This discussion does not mean that radiation workers who are not classified should not be monitored, but monitoring is a precaution and one which may be used to justify nonclassified status, although there is no legal requirement for this.

21.9.2 Personnel dosimetry

The monitoring of radiation dose to staff is carried out by the use of TLDs.

Fig. 21.9 shows the plastic Harshaw card, which has a number for identification purposes stamped on the outside. The outer wrapping (white) protects the lithium fluoride/polytetrafluoroethylene (PTFE) TLD inserts on the card from light and alpha radiations, as well as providing chemical protection and a measure of physical protection. The card contains two discs of thermoluminescent material. One disc is positioned behind the open window of the badge whereas the other disc is behind the plastic dome. Note that the card is designed so that it can only be inserted into the holder in the correct way. Each card is identified by a unique barcode strip used in the automated dose-reading process.

The cardholder has two windows (Fig. 21.9): a long rectangular window along the top edge to display the wearer's identity number and a circular open window that lies directly over one of the TLDs on the card. This TLD records all weak and strongly penetrating radiations, including beta

TABLE 21.3 Summary of the dose limits specified by the Ionising Radiation Regulations 2017			
	Employees & trainees (18+ years)	Trainees (<18 years)	Other persons
Whole body—effective dose	20 mSv	6 mSv	1 mSv
Eye lens	20 mSv	15 mSv	15 mSv
Skin	500 mSv	150 mSv	50 mSv
Hands, forearms, feet & ankles	500 mSv	150 mSv	50 mSv

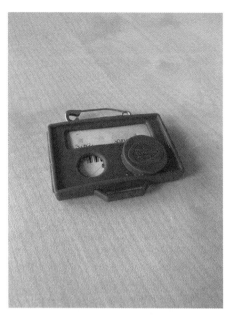

Fig. 21.9 An example of a thermoluminescent dosimetry badge and holder used for monitoring purposes. A safety pin is seen attached to the badge and provides a method of attachment to clothing.

radiation. This dose-reading produces the Hp0.7 or whole-body dose. The other TLD lies under the dome, which is made of thick (90 mg.cm^{-2}) plastic. This TLD is used to record the more penetrating and gamma radiations producing the Hp10 dose or depth received by the wearer.

Thermoluminescent materials may also be used to measure doses to specific organs, for example, they can be wrapped round a finger to measure the dose to that finger or incorporated into a headband for eye lens dosimetry. The major disadvantage of TLDs is that they are retrospective monitors and are processed and read after exposure.

'Real-time' dosimeters (often called pocket dosimeters, because they can be worn in pockets of laboratory coats) can give an instant readout on a digital display. Some can provide additional data, such as a breakdown of the rate at which the dose was received, or even sound an audible alarm to indicate that radiation is being detected. Such systems, when integrated with computer systems, are being used to monitor occupational exposure in interventional radiology.

21.9.3   Employees who have been overexposed

If an employee's annual whole-body dose exceeds 20 mSv, the RPA must notify the HSE who will conduct an investigation to see if the working practices involved are in keeping with the *as low as reasonably achievable* (ALARA) principle (or whether improvements may be made which would lead to a reduction in the dose).

21.10   LOCAL RULES

Under IRR 2017, the employer has a legal responsibility to ensure that written local rules are produced for all departments (or areas) where employees are involved in work with ionising radiation. These rules must be brought to the attention of all employees working in these departments. In practice, the RPA advises the employer on the formulation of these rules and it is the task of the RPS to ensure that the rules are known and put into practice by colleagues in their respective departments.

The local rules for a department should be displayed in a prominent position, or positions, within the department concerned, and should contain the following information:

- The names and contact details of the RPA and RPS for the department (or area).
- A description of each designated area in the department (see Section 21.5.1).
- Details of restrictions of access to such areas.
- Written systems of work detailing the procedures and protocols for the department.
- Details of any contingency plans.

21.10.1   Designated areas

There are two types of designated area (see Table 21.4) — controlled and supervised areas. All designated areas must be delineated by physical boundaries (i.e., walls). However, in the case of radiography involving the use of mobile X-ray units, this requirement is dropped, provided that an area of at least 1.5 metres from the X-ray tube is under the continual supervision of the operator at all times. Warning signs must be posted at all entrances to the areas, preferably at eye level, and include a warning light to indicate if an X-ray unit is activated or an exposure is being made.

21.10.1.1 Design of designated areas

The function of the X-ray room is to provide an enclosure for the X-ray examination or treatment unit and limit access to the radiation area. It should also provide adequate shielding to the rest of the environment from the radiation produced, so that individuals outside the room do not receive a radiation dose that would exceed the annual effective dose limit to a member of the public. In diagnostic radiography, provision is made for a barrier inside the room behind which staff may be protected from the radiation while they operate the unit, while viewing the patient through a protective window.

TABLE 21.4 Description of designated areas

Type of designation	Requirements for designation	Permitted access
Controlled area	An area where any person is likely to receive an effective dose greater than 6 µSv per year or three-tenths of any relevant dose limit	• Classified radiation workers • Radiation workers who follow a written system of work, designed to restrict significant radiation exposure in that area • Patients undergoing medical diagnostic or therapeutic exposures
Supervised area	• An area where any person is likely to receive an effective dose greater than 1 mSv per year or one-tenth of any relevant dose limit • An area under review for upgrading to a controlled area Note that a supervised area cannot be situated inside of a controlled area	Persons whose presence is necessary during a radiation exposure

If there is more than one X-ray tube operating from the generator in a diagnostic room, there must be a visual indication (usually a warning light) to indicate which tube is in circuit and capable of producing radiation if energised. With radiotherapy treatment rooms, because of the much higher radiation energies used, the equipment is operated from outside the treatment room and the patient viewed through a closed-circuit TV system. Entry to the treatment area is through a maze and the entry of an individual into the maze during treatment automatically terminates the treatment through a system of interlocks.

The level of radiation protection given by barriers and walls is usually stated in terms of their lead-equivalent. The lead-equivalent gives a basis for comparing one barrier with another at a given beam energy.

DEFINITION

The lead-equivalent of an absorbing material is the thickness of lead which would absorb the same amount of radiation as the given material when exposed to radiation of the same type and quality.

In the diagnostic range of beam energies (up to 150 keV), the photoelectric absorption within lead is significant owing to its high atomic number (Z = 82). For this reason, many barriers (e.g., doors) in the diagnostic X-ray room incorporate a few millimetres of lead laminated with wood to give adequate radiation protection. Lead-glass windows are often fitted to such barriers to enable a visual contact to be maintained. The protection afforded by such a window must be at least the same amount as the protective barrier itself and there must be no gaps where the radiation is able to penetrate. The siting of such a barrier to protect staff must be such that the radiation must be scattered at least twice (greatly reducing its intensity) before reaching the opening in the barrier.

Wall thicknesses between X-ray rooms and adjacent areas must be such that any transmitted radiation will not produce a dose in excess of 1 mSv per year, which is the maximum dose for the general public. This figure must be calculated for all walls, floors, ceilings and windows of the X-ray rooms and is calculated by applying a use factor. The use factor is an estimation of the time when the radiation beam will be pointing towards that area. As a result of this calculation, the maximum dose received by a person sited on the far side of the barrier may be estimated and it must not exceed 1 mSv per year. In previous legislation, there was also an occupancy factor, which looked at the fraction of time a person was likely to spend in this area, but this factor has now been discontinued.

The materials used in the construction of the walls and floor of the X-ray room may contain lead sheeting or there may be sufficient thickness of other materials, such as concrete, to provide adequate absorption of the primary and scatter radiation produced in the room. The lead-equivalent of a concrete wall 15 cm thick is approximately 1.5 mm within the diagnostic energy range—this reflects the superior absorption of lead compared with concrete in this energy range. The lead-equivalent of such walls may be increased using barium sulphate plaster as a thin coating on the walls. This is because of the high atomic number of barium ($Z = 56$).

As the beam energy increases, the advantage of lead over concrete diminishes because there is a gradual shift from the predominance of photoelectric absorption to the predominance of Compton scattering. Thus the lead-equivalent of a barrier will increase with an increase in the photon energy—a greater thickness of lead will be required to give the same level of protection as the barrier. In the region of 1 MeV, the Compton scattering process predominates, and lead has no real advantage over concrete because all materials have similar mass attenuation coefficients owing to the Compton process. For this reason, many of the barriers used in radiotherapy departments are made of large thicknesses of concrete.

In conclusion, the design of a room, its wall thickness and the barriers must be such that the radiation doses received by patients, staff and members of the public are kept to a minimum in accordance with the ALARA principle. Further details of the design of diagnostic and therapy rooms can be found in specialised publications on this topic.

21.11　THE ROLE OF THE PRACTITIONER

The role of the practitioner is the justification of the request for the procedure. Practitioners are usually medically qualified individuals, although this role can be delegated to other radiographic professionals for some procedures, with the employer's approval.

Before justification can commence, the practitioner must check that the referrer has supplied sufficient data for the procedure requested. This includes the following:

- The patient's identification (and, depending of the area of study, if a female of childbearing age then the date of the patient's last menstrual period).
- Sufficient relevant clinical information to permit the practitioner to decide if there is sufficient net benefit to the patient to allow justification of the procedure and, if the patient is to undergo a procedure where radionuclides are administered, if the patient is breastfeeding an infant.

The logical suggestion is that no unnecessary radiation dose should be received by any person, but where there is a net benefit for the patient the request would be justified.

For instance, the mammography screening programme has increased the early detection rate of breast cancer, and this in turn increased the survival rate from this condi-

tion. In the case of other cancers, the risk of death to the patient is considerably higher if a course of radiotherapy treatment is not given. An undetected aneurysm may burst causing the patient's death or other serious medical complications.

Another possibility is that the same information about the patient's condition can be gained without using ionising radiation (e.g., ultrasound or magnetic resonance imaging) and, in these cases, the practitioner should suggest this change of imaging modality to the referrer.

If the patient is a female of reproductive capacity (i.e., between the ages of 12 and 55), the practitioner must consider the possibility that the patient is or may be pregnant. The operator is also responsible for checking this at the time of examination.

21.11.1　Radiological examinations of women of reproductive capacity

The current rules concerning radiological examinations of women of reproductive capacity are as follow:

- Any woman who has an overdue or missed period should be treated as though she were pregnant.
- If the woman cannot answer 'no' to the question 'are you, or might you be, pregnant?' then she should be treated as though she were pregnant.
- If the clinical indications are that an exposure should be made where the primary beam irradiates the fetus, then great care must be taken to minimise the number of views and the absorbed dose per view, but without jeopardising the diagnostic value of the investigation.
- Provided good collimation is used, and equipment is properly shielded, X-ray projections of areas remote from the fetus (e.g., chest, skull, hand) may be undertaken safely at any time during the pregnancy.

These recommendations do not reduce the care that should be taken in limiting the potential radiation dose to the fetus. The change in emphasis of the recommendations is that special precautions need be taken only if the woman is, or may be, pregnant—where 'pregnant' is defined as beginning when a menstrual period is overdue.

Other than this, there is no need for special limitations of exposures during a menstrual cycle, except for the normal requirements to keep all absorbed radiation doses as low as reasonably practicable. Good radiographic techniques should thus be used at all times to minimise radiation doses for all exposures.

A flow chart showing the progress of a woman of reproductive capacity presenting for a radiographic examination is given in Fig. 21.10.

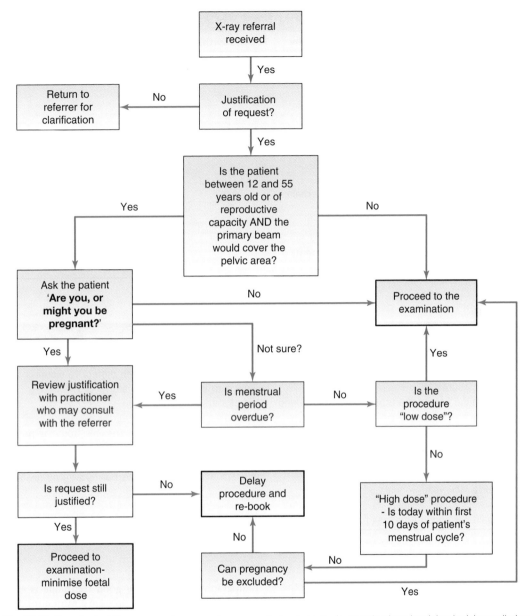

Fig. 21.10 Flowchart of the process for managing suspected pregnancy in examinations involving ionising radiation.

21.12 THE ROLE OF THE OPERATOR

The regulations define the operator as the individual (radiologist, radiographer or radiographic assistant) who is responsible for physically directing the X-ray exposure. They are the final link in the chain of radiation protection as they have a dual responsibility:

1. To keep the radiation dose to the patient, themselves and other staff and as low as reasonably practicable but consistent with the clinical requirements of the examination. This responsibility includes:
   - checking the patient's identity and that the practitioner has justified the procedure

TABLE 21.5 Methods of dose reduction to the patient

Factors within the operator's control in radiography	Factors within the operator's control in fluoroscopy
Selection of exposure factors, preferably using an anatomically programmed timer, so that the exposure is within the diagnostic reference level produced by the employer for the examination	Use of pulsed fluoroscopy and image storage systems
Use of the highest practicable kVp	Use of digital fluoroscopy
Making use of secondary radiation grids to reduce the scatter reaching the image receptor	
Use of tissue displacement techniques with obese patients	
Use of immobilization with patients who cannot remain in position or keep still during the exposure	
Limitation of the field size by collimation	
Utilizing gonad shields	
Use of the fastest image receptor system, consistent with the requirements of the examination	

TABLE 21.6 Methods of dose reduction to staff

Factors within the operator's control in radiography	Factors within the operator's control in fluoroscopy
Only those whose presence is required should be in the room during exposures	All staff must wear adequate protective clothing, as specified in the written systems of work
All staff should stand behind the protective barrier during exposure	Use of automatic collimation
The X-ray tube must have adequate shielding	Staff should stand as far as possible from the primary beam
Operators should not exposure themselves to the primary beam	Protective shielding should be incorporated into the system to reduce the dose from scattered radiation
Restless patients, where appropriate, should be supported by immobilization devices	
Operators should not support restless patients	

- if the procedure has not been justified, referring the request back to the practitioner
- if the patient is a female of reproductive age, assessing the risk of pregnancy. If a risk of pregnancy is present, referring the request back to the practitioner for approval to proceed.

2. Once these checks have been completed, the procedure can commence. The operator should bear the points listed in Table 21.5 and Table 21.6 in mind while carrying out the procedure.

Note: Many of the methods that reduce dose to the patient will also produce a reduction of dose to staff. Fluoroscopy results in higher radiation doses than conventional radiography and therefore good technique is even more essential to keep radiation doses to a minimum. The use of a modern flat-panel fluoroscopic unit with pulsed fluoroscopy, image storage, automatic collimation and digitisation of the image will result in a reduction of the radiation doses to patients and staff.

21.12.1 Reporting overexposure of patients

In the case of a known or suspected overexposure to a patient, the operator must inform the RPS/RPA. They will then report this to the CQC, who will conduct an investigation into the incident and make recommendations to prevent the reoccurrence of similar incidents.

SUMMARY

In this chapter, you should have learnt the following:

- The definition of exposure and the relationship between exposure and absorbed dose (Section 21.3).
- The definition of and the relationship between absorbed dose and kerma (Section 21.2).
- The effects of different media on the absorbed dose (Section 21.3.3).
- The meaning of the terms quality factor and dose equivalent and how their values vary for different types of radiation (Section 21.4).
- Measurement of radiation exposure and absorbed dose by the free-air ionisation chamber (Section 21.5.2).
- Measurement of radiation exposure and absorbed dose by chemical dosimeters (Section 21.5).
- Measurement of radiation exposure and absorbed dose by the thimble ionisation chamber (Section 21.6.1).
- Detection of the presence of radiation by the Geiger–Müller counter (Section 21.6.2).
- Measurement of radiation exposure and absorbed dose by scintillation detectors (Section 21.6.3).
- Measurement of radiation exposure and absorbed dose by TLD (Section 21.6.4).
- The use of photographic film in dosimetry (Section 21.6.5).
- Measurement of radiation exposure and absorbed dose by semiconductor detectors (Section 21.6.6).
- The purpose and scope of radiation protection (Section 21.7).
- An outline of the regulations affecting radiation protection (Section 21.8).
- The organisation of radiation safety in a hospital trust (Section 21.8.1).
- The responsibilities of the manufacturer (Section 21.8.2).
- Dose-equivalent limits in radiation protection (Section 21.9).
- The requirements for the designation of radiation workers (Section 21.9.1).
- Methods of personnel monitoring (Section 21.9.2).
- Procedure followed if an employee has been overexposed to radiation (Section 21.9.3).
- Local rules (Section 21.10).
- Designation of work areas in radiation protection (Section 21.10.1).
- The design of designated areas in radiography and radiotherapy (Section 21.10.1.1).
- The role of the practitioner (Section 21.11).
- Special precautions in the radiological examination of women of reproductive capacity (Section 21.11.1).
- The role of the operator and practical methods of radiation protection (Section 21.12).
- Reporting of overexposure to a patient (Section 21.12.1).

FURTHER READING

Allisy-Roberts, P. 2002. *Medical and Dental Guidance Notes – A Good Practice Guide on All Aspects of Ionising Radiation Protection in the Clinical Environment*. York: Institute of Physics and Engineering in Medicine.

Ball, J.L., Moore, A.D., & Turner, S. 2008. *Ball and Moore's Essential Physics for Radiographers*. 4th edn. London: Blackwell Scientific. (Chapter 21.)

Bushong, S.C. 2004. *Radiologic Science for Technologists: Physics, Biology and Protection*. New York: Mosby. (Chapters 33–40.)

HMSO. 2017. *2017/1075 The Ionising Radiation Regulations*. London: HMSO.

HMSO. 2017. *Statutory Instrument 2017/1322. The Ionising Radiation (Medical Exposure) Regulations*. London: HMSO.

HSE. 2000. *Working with Ionising Radiation – Ionising Radiation Regulations 1999. Approved Code of Practice and Guidance*. Sudbury: HSE Books.

Webb, S. (Ed.). 2002. *The Physics of Medical Imaging*. 2nd edn. Bristol: Institute of Physics. (Chapter 2.)

The gamma camera

22.1 AIM

The aim of this chapter is to introduce the reader to the basics of the gamma camera and how a diagnostic image is produced using radionuclides. The information available on a nuclear medicine scan will be compared with the information available on other forms of medical imaging.

22.2 BASIC CONCEPT OF RADIONUCLIDE IMAGING

The basic concept of radionuclide imaging involves a three-stage process:
1. A suitable pharmaceutical incorporating a radionuclide, referred to as a radiopharmaceutical, is introduced into the patient—the radionuclide is usually artificially produced.
2. The distribution of the radiopharmaceutical in specific organs or physiological systems within the body is compared with the normal distribution of the radiopharmaceutical.
3. The organ is scanned using an appropriate scanner (e.g., a gamma camera).

22.3 THE GAMMA CAMERA

The instrument used to detect the radiation from the radionuclide within the patient is called a gamma camera.

The gamma camera was first developed by Anger in 1958 and the camera and its associated technology have shown considerable progress since then. The gamma camera consists of a large detector; many modern gamma cameras are dual headed with two detectors so that scanning information in two planes can be collected simultaneously (see Fig. 22.1). The structure of

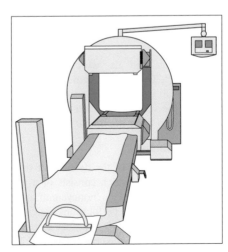

Fig. 22.1 A dual-headed gamma camera arrangement, which can be used for planar and SPECT radionuclide imaging studies.

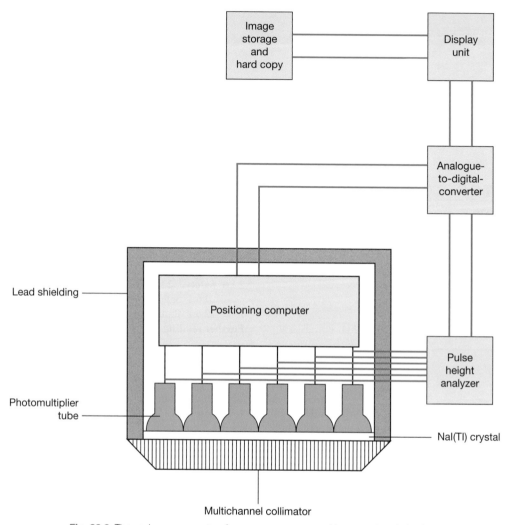

Fig. 22.2 The main components of a gamma camera and its associated circuitry.

the gamma camera and its associated circuitry are shown in Fig. 22.2. The gamma camera is a specialised type of scintillation counter where the position as well as the count of the scintillations are acquired. This information is used to form the image.

22.3.1   The collimator

The outermost component of the detector of the gamma camera is the collimator, which consists of a perforated lead plate giving the collimator a 'honeycomb' appearance. The walls of the honeycomb perforations are called septa. The function of the collimator is to absorb scattered radiation before it interacts with the crystal (see Fig. 22.3). The collimator is sensitive to physical shock and should be stored in a dedicated cart when not in use. A collision de-

tector is present above the collimator to stop the movement of the detector if pressure is exerted on it.

Collimators are very heavy, and most gamma camera systems have automatic or semiautomatic collimator changers to remove and attach collimators when required. The detector should never be left without a collimator and collimators are only removed when changed or when quality assurance acquisitions are being undertaken. The collimator has an outside wipeable cover which protects the crystal from moisture.

23.3.1.1   Types of collimator

Parallel hole collimators are the most commonly used collimators. The long axis of the holes is perpendicular to the detector crystal. The lead septa between the holes absorb

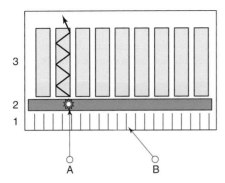

Fig. 22.3 Photon interactions in a gamma camera. Gamma ray photon (A), entering perpendicular to the gamma camera, passes between the septa of the collimator (1), causes light emission in the NaI(Tl) scintillation crystal (2) and electron multiplication in the photomultiplier tube (3), contributing usefully to the image. Gamma ray photon (B), entering the collimator at an oblique angle, is absorbed in the septa and gives no image data.

any gamma radiation not perpendicular to the crystal. Technitium-99m (^{99m}Tc) is the most commonly used radionuclide in radionuclide imaging, so standard low-energy high-resolution (LEHR) collimators are designed to absorb scatter from 140 KeV. For higher energy radionuclides such as iodine-131 (^{131}I) high-energy collimators with thicker septa are used so images are not degraded.

A general purpose low-energy all-purpose (LEAP) collimator can be used when a high count-rate of gamma events is required such as dynamic imaging or where little scatter is produced, such as imaging young children. General purpose collimators have larger holes than high-resolution standard collimators and therefore allow more radiation and scatter to reach the crystal.

Specialist collimators called pinhole collimators, working in the same manner as pinhole cameras, can be used to image thyroids. They produce very high-resolution inverted images, but they are hard to change and store in automatic collimator changers. The pinhole collimator has a restricted field of view.

22.3.2 The crystal

The detector is a crystal which absorbs energy from ionising radiation and emits visible light. This process is called scintillation and this is the basis of image formation in radionuclide imaging. Emission of visible light is because of excitation of electrons, which then drop back down to a lower energy level with the emission of light photons. The intensity of light is proportional to total energy absorbed within the scintillator. A crystal of sodium iodide with a thallium activator NaI(Tl) is one of the most efficient scintillators developed. The thallium impurities act as lumines-

cent centres, and about 10% to 15% of the energy deposited in the crystal is converted to light energy. The maximum light emission is in the blue part of the spectrum with a wavelength of 420 nm. The sodium iodide crystals are mounted in containers called cans to prevent them absorbing moisture from the atmosphere and becoming cloudy. One face of the crystal is attached to a transparent glass window and all other surfaces are in contact with a white reflective powder (magnesium oxide) so that as much light as possible is directed at the back of the crystal.

The crystal is very fragile and is sensitive to:
- rapid temperature change—air conditioning to regulate the temperature in the room is very important.
- humidity rise—after about 10 years crystals are no longer efficient because of the water absorbed.
- moisture—the crystal must be protected by the collimator to avoid fluid spills.
- external light—this can cause degradation to the crystal.
- physical damage—the gamma camera head houses one crystal and if this cracks, the camera will be unusable.

The crystal in the detector head on modern gamma cameras is normally 9.525 mm (3/8th inch) thick, which is the optimal thickness for ^{99m}Tc. Thicker or thinner crystals are less efficient because if the crystal is too thin, the gamma rays will pass through without interacting and scintillation will not occur. If the crystal is too thick, secondary scintillations will occur within the crystal which do not contribute to the image and even with a crystal of optimal thickness, 99% of the photons emitted from the patient are not recorded by the final processing computer.

The detector head contains one crystal; a dual energy system will have a crystal in each of its heads.

22.3.3 The photomultiplier tubes

Photomultiplier tubes (PMTs) are connected to the NaI(Tl) crystal by a light guide, which is clear, so light is not attenuated. A geometrical arrangement of PMTs allows the position and the intensity of the scintillation produced in the crystal to be measured. This allows us to display a picture of certain physiological processes within the body. This ability to image a dynamic physiological process makes the gamma camera a very powerful tool in the detection of pathologies where the physiology of the structure is disrupted.

The back of the crystal is in optical contact with a PMT, as shown in Fig. 22.5. If a gamma ray is absorbed by the crystal (at point *P* on the diagram), this results in the emission of light in all directions. A fairly high percentage of this light reaches the photocathode of the PMT. The photocathode consists of a thin coating of a mixture of alkaline salts deposited on the inner wall of the face of the PMT. About 10% to 25% of the light photons reaching the photocathode cause it to emit electrons by the photoelectric effect

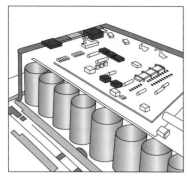

Fig. 22.4 A cutaway view showing the inside of a gamma camera, including the rows of photomultiplier tubes and electronic circuitry.

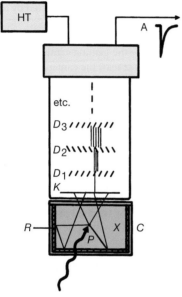

Fig. 22.5 A scintillation detector using sodium iodide. D_1, D_2, etc., dynodes; C, crystal can; K, photocathode; R, powdered reflector; X, Na(Tl) crystal. P, gamma ray photon absorption, HT, high tension voltage supply, A, signal pulse analyser.

(see Section 19.3), and these electrons are accelerated through the tube to a series of positively charged plates called dynodes (see Fig. 22.5). The surface of these dynodes is coated with a layer of a secondary electron emitter so that each dynode produces approximately six times as many electrons as fall on it. As a result of this process, one electron released at the photocathode may result in one million electrons being collected by the anode of the photomultiplier. The collection of this charge occurs at a very short time interval after the initial electron is released by the photocathode (normally $<10^{-6}$ s) and so a pulse of electricity is produced, the magnitude of the pulse being proportional to the

energy of the absorbed gamma-ray photon. Gamma cameras with higher numbers of PMTs have greater resolution because they are able to determine the intensity and location of the scintillation event more accurately.

> ### INSIGHT
>
> If the photomultiplier tube (PMT) contains n dynodes, each of which releases six electrons for one incident electron, then the electron gain in the PMT is 6^n. Thus for a 10-dynode tube, the gain would be 6^{10} which is just over 60,000,000 electrons and represents a charge at the anode of about 10 picocoulombs.

A spectrum of these pulses will not produce the discrete gamma energies emitted by the radioactive source because of the statistical nature of the light production in the crystal and the electron multiplication in the photomultiplier. This is shown in Fig. 22.6, where the numbers of pulses of a given height are plotted. The true spectrum would be a line at the centre of the photopeak, as this corresponds to the energy of the gamma rays absorbed by photoelectric absorption. In addition to the gamma rays being absorbed by photoelectric absorption, some of the gamma rays undergo Compton scattering (see Chapter 13) within the crystal and then escape from the crystal with no further interactions. Such scattering interactions result in energy being deposited in the crystal which is less than the energy of the gamma rays and so smaller pulses are produced in the photomultiplier. These pulses produce a 'photopeak' as shown in Fig. 22.6.

Some very-low-energy pulses are produced by the release of electrons from the photocathode by thermionic emission. There are also some positively charged ions produced at the dynodes which may strike the photocathode and cause it to release electrons. The electrons produced by both of the

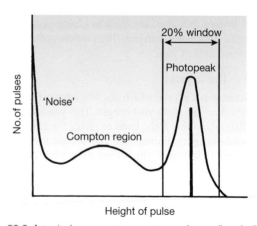

Fig. 22.6 A typical gamma-ray spectrum using sodium iodide.

above mechanisms produce no useful signal and are referred to as 'noise pulses' (Fig. 22.6). The intensity signal (Z) passes through the pulse-height analyser (PHA), which can discriminate between the photopeak, Compton scatter and noise sections of the signal from the PMTs. A window is set around the photopeak so only incident gamma photons from the photopeak area are accepted. For ^{99m}Tc, which has a peak energy of 140 KeV, a 10% window on either side of the peak is set (126–154 KeV).

There are fans present in the detector head to prevent overheating owing to the number of electronics in the detector head.

22.3.4   Shielding

The detector head is encased in lead shielding to prevent any radiation interference occurring during scanning.

22.3.5   The production of the image

The operator will have access to a number of preset protocols on the computer console and will select the appropriate one before acquisition of the image. A two-dimensional image is

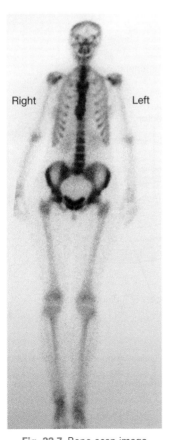

Fig. 22.7 Bone scan image.

produced by the processing computer on a planner gamma camera. The data received by the computer are position (X,Y) and intensity (Z). Gamma rays leaving the patient are at various angles; the collimator attenuates any gamma rays which are not perpendicular to the crystal. Scatter, noise and background radiation are still able to reach the crystal so the PHA discriminates via the set window to prevent scatter, noise and background radiation forming part of the image. A bone scan image is seen in Fig. 22.7.

22.4   PRODUCTION OF ARTIFICIALLY PRODUCED RADIONUCLIDES

Most radionuclides used in diagnostic imaging are produced artificially. These are produced:
1. using a generator
2. using a medical cyclotron.

22.4.1   The technetium generator (see Fig. 22.8)

Technetium is the most commonly used radionuclide in radionuclide imaging. A technetium generator is used in a hospital radiopharmacy to make technetium products for local use and for neighbouring hospitals. Technetium has a half-life of 6 hours so technetium products can be transported short distances.

The technetium generator consists of the radionuclide molybdenum-99 (^{99}Mo). ^{98}Mo can be made to absorb a neutron to produce the radionuclide ^{99}Mo in a nuclear reactor. The reaction may be shown using Eq. 22.1:

$$^{98}_{42}\text{Mo} + n \rightarrow {}^{99}_{42}\text{Mo} + \gamma \qquad \textbf{Equation 22.1}$$

The capture of a neutron raises the energy of the resulting ^{99}Mo nuclei and each loses this energy by the prompt emission of a gamma ray.

A ^{99}Mo/alumina column is in the centre of the generator, as shown in Fig. 22.8. The ^{99}Mo has a half-life of 67 hours and decays to form ^{99m}Tc by β⁻-particle emission, as shown by Equation 22.2:

$$^{99}_{42}\text{Mo} \rightarrow {}^{99}_{43}\text{Tc}^{\text{m}} + \beta^- + \nu^- \qquad \textbf{Equation 22.2}$$

The $^{99}_{43}\text{Tc}^{\text{m}}$ is eluted (or flushed) from the generator at regular intervals as sodium pertechnetate. This radionuclide, which is in liquid form, may be used for a number of radionuclide imaging situations. The $^{99}_{43}\text{Tc}^{\text{m}}$ decays to $^{99}_{43}\text{Tc}$ by the emission of a gamma ray of energy 140 keV. The metastable radionuclide has a half-life of 6 hours. Clearly, after a period of time, the activity of the ^{99}Mo, and hence its ability to produce ^{99m}Tc, will be reduced and the technetium generator must have its ^{99}Mo/alumina column replaced.

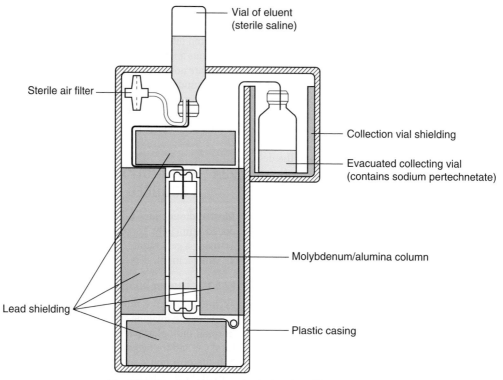

Fig. 22.8 Principle features of a technetium-99m generator.

The liquid is added to freeze-dried pharmaceuticals in a sterile environment in a clean room. Each pharmaceutical will demonstrate a specific system in the body when administered to the patient. Most radiopharmaceuticals for radionuclide imaging are produced in this way.

22.4.2 Production of radionuclides using a cyclotron

The type of cyclotron used in nuclear medicine to produce artificial radionuclides by the bombardment of stable substances will briefly be described. A simple diagram of such a device is shown (see Fig. 22.9). The cyclotron consists of an evacuated cylinder which has an ion source placed at its centre. Ions from this source are influenced by strong axial and radial magnetic fields. Two D-shaped electrodes, called "Dees", cause electromagnetic acceleration of the ions in circular paths of increasing radius. This causes acceleration of the ions in circular paths of increasing radius. This ion beam achieves significant velocity and can be made to interact with materials placed at the exit port of the cyclotron. This interaction causes nuclear changes in these materials and this can produce neutron-deficient nuclei (see Section 10.5.2.) which are capable of positron emission. Some radionuclides used for imaging on a gamma camera, such as thallium-201 (^{201}Tl), are produced in this way.

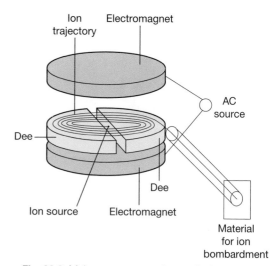

Fig. 22.9 Main components of a medical cyclotron.

Radiopharmaceuticals used in positron emission tomography (PET) scanning are produced in a cyclotron, but these radiopharmaceuticals cannot be imaged on a gamma camera.

Fig. 22.10 shows a photograph of such a medical cyclotron.

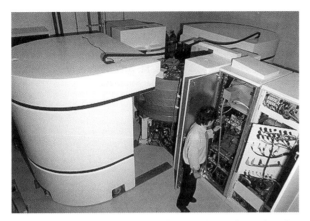

Fig. 22.10 A medical cyclotron. This cyclotron is undergoing maintenance. The position of the dees is clearly visible. (From the Department of Nuclear Medicine, Aberdeen Royal Infirmary.)

22.5 CLINICALLY USEFUL RADIONUCLIDES

Radionuclides are used to diagnose and treat certain conditions. When they are used for diagnosis, they may be labelled (chemically linked) to a certain pharmaceutical forming a radiopharmaceutical, thus encouraging their uptake by specific body parts. The labelled radionuclide may then be administered intravenously to or ingested by the patient. Such diagnostic techniques in nuclear medicine have three main uses:

- Static scans such as bone scans and static renal scans, dimercaptosuccinic acid (DMSA) scans.
- Dynamic renal scans, renograms showing renal function.
- Imaging patients who have received therapy doses such as ^{131}I.

Radionuclide imaging shows the physiology of the system or organ.

A list of the radioisotopes which are commonly used is given in Table 22.1.

For the diagnostic purposes of imaging or charting organ physiology, only gamma-ray emission or positron emission is useful. This is because particles (α or β) emitted are absorbed very efficiently by the patient's tissues. If the particles are absorbed by the patient and do not reach the imaging or counting device, they contribute a radiation dose to the patient but give no diagnostic information. α or β particles can be used for radionuclide therapy. ^{131}I emits both gamma rays and β particles, which means a patient can be treated with the ^{131}I and then imaged using a gamma camera to show the areas in the body being treated. In the case of positron emission, the positron itself is rapidly annihilated by collision with an electron (see Section 10.5.3) but the annihilation radiation is detected by suitable detectors in a PET scanner (see Chapter 23).

The ideal radionuclide for imaging should:

- have a short half-life—approximately twice the length of time from injection into the patient to completion of the scan
- emit gamma rays of relatively low energy, so that these are easily detected and do not pose a major hazard to others because of their penetrating power
- emit no particles as part of its decay pattern as these add significantly to the patient dose
- be readily labelled to allow its uptake by specific organs
- be readily excreted by the patient
- be easily generated in the radio pharmacy
- be produced economically.

In many ways $^{99}_{43}\text{Tc}^\text{m}$ is the almost ideal radionuclide for scanning purposes.

22.6 SAFETY

22.6.1 Safety of the gamma camera

The area around the gamma camera must be kept clear of objects to avoid collisions. The interlocks should be checked every day and every time a collimator is changed.

TABLE 22.1 Commonly used isotopes in radionuclide imaging

Isotope	Production	Half-life	Gamma emissions
Gallium-67	Cyclotron	78 hrs	93, 185, 296 keV
Krypton-81m	Generator	13 secs	190 keV
Technetium-99m	Generator	6 hrs	140 keV
Indium-111	Cyclotron	67 hrs	172, 247 keV
Iodine-123	Cyclotron	13 hrs	159 keV
Iodine-131 (used for therapy)	Nuclear reactors	8 days	364 keV
Xenon-133	Nuclear reactors	5 days	30, 80 keV
Thallium-201	Cyclotron	73 hrs	167 keV

22.6.2   Radiation safety

Radiopharmaceuticals are unsealed sources and should be handled carefully and safely to avoid contamination. During preparation of radiopharmaceuticals, the operator can be shielded using lead and tungsten shielding, and other personal protective equipment such as gloves and tongs should be used. A spill kit should be available, and staff should be adequately trained. The operator keeps a distance from the patient and applies the inverse square law for maximum protection from the radiation emitted from the patient.

SUMMARY

In this chapter you should have learnt the following:
- The basic concept of radionuclide imaging.
- The general operation of a gamma camera.
- The production of radionuclides.
- An overview of clinically useful radionuclides.

FURTHER READING

Chandra, R., & Rahmin, A. 2018. *Nuclear medicine physics: The basics*. 8th edn. Philadelphia: Wolters Kluwer Health.

Cherry, S., Sorensen, J., & Phelps, M. 2012. *Physics in nuclear medicine*. 4rd edn. Philadelphia: Saunders.

Positron emission tomography and single photon emission computed tomography

CHAPTER CONTENTS

23.1 AIM

The aim of this chapter is to introduce the reader to the principle of positron emission tomography (PET) and single photon emission computed tomography (SPECT) scanning as practised in diagnostic imaging. The assumption is made that the reader is familiar with the mechanisms of positron production from a radionuclide as described in Chapter 10 (Section 10.5.2).

23.2 POSITRON EMISSION TOMOGRAPHY

23.2.1 Revision of positron physics

As discussed in Chapter 10, if a nucleus has too few neutrons for stability, it is possible for the nucleus to achieve a more stable configuration by the emission of a positron. Positrons are the antiparticles of electrons and the positron and the electron will interact (within a very short distance in tissue), annihilating each other and producing two photons of annihilation radiation. These photons each have an energy of 0.51 MeV (511 keV) and detection of these photons forms the basis of PET. Each photon is produced at an angle close to 90 degrees to the direction of travel of the positron (see Fig. 10.7).

23.2.2 Detection of positrons

The first prototype PET computed tomography (CT) scanner was produced in 1998 from a proposal made 7 years earlier by Townsend, Nutt and coworkers.

If a positron-emitting radionuclide is introduced into the patient, it can be labelled in such a way that it concentrates in specific structures. The number of positrons emitted by these structures can be related to the activity of the cells within the structure. If we surround the patient with a ring of positron detectors (see Fig. 23.1), then each annihilation

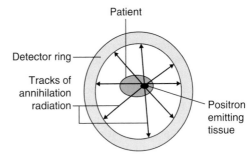

Fig. 23.1 Detection of annihilation radiation from a positron-emitting source within the patient.

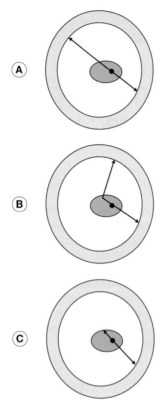

Fig. 23.2 Types of coincidence. (A) is a true coincidence. In (B), one of the photons is scattered and in (C), one of the photons is absorbed. This makes (B) and (C) false coincidences.

radiation from the positron–electron interaction can be registered, and the intersections of these points can be 'back-projected' to indicate the positron-emitting tissue in the patient.

23.2.3   Types of coincidence

For the annihilation radiation from the positron–electron interactions to give useful information, the two photons must travel in straight lines from the source of the radiation to the detectors. The photons in Fig. 23.2A are of this type.

Because the photons all travel with the velocity of electromagnetic radiation, they will each be detected by a detector almost at the same time—within less than 10×10^{-9} s of each other. These photons are said to be coincident. It is possible for one of the photons to be scattered (see Fig. 23.2B). If the position of these two photons were back-projected, it would be an incorrect position for the origin of the annihilation radiation. Because the scattered photon travels along a slightly longer route, the two photons will not be detected within 10×10^{-9} s of each other and so they are not said

to be coincident and the imaging computer can be programmed to ignore them. Similarly, in Fig. 23.2C, one of the photons has been absorbed. Because there is no matching coincident photon, the imaging computer will again ignore this event.

23.2.4   Positron emission tomography scanning system

23.2.4.1   Detector materials

Solid scintillation detectors are used to detect the 511 keV photons. This occurs by the absorption of the gamma ray in the scintillation crystal, which results in visible light being emitted.

In the gamma camera (see Chapter 22), the radiation is detected using a sodium iodide crystal. The radiation from technetium-99m has an energy of 140 keV. The energy of the annihilation radiation from the positron–electron interaction is 511 keV. The greater energy of this radiation requires a material of higher density and/or higher atomic number. Bismuth germinate (BGO) or lutetium oxyorthosilicate (LSO) are commonly used detector materials. When choosing a detector material the following characteristics should be considered:

- Stopping power of the detector for 511keV photons
- Scintillation decay time
- Light output per keV of photon energy
- Energy resolution of the detector.

The mean distance the photon travels until it stops after it completely deposits its energy is determined by the density and effective atomic number (Zeff) of the material. Materials with high density and high Zeff have high stopping power. The scintillation decay time is the time taken after the gamma ray interacts with an atom in the detector until visible light is emitted; during this time the atom is excited to a higher energy level and then decays to the ground state. Materials with shorter decay times are more efficient at higher count rates. A high light output per keV produces a well-defined pulse resulting in better energy resolution. PET detectors have relatively low energy resolution to the order of a few hundred nanoseconds to exclude random coincidences (see Section 23.2.3).

23.2.4.2   Detector mechanisms

The basic components of the detector mechanism are scintillation detectors over which photomultiplier tubes or photodiodes are positioned as shown in Fig. 23.3. These arrangements are known as *blocks*. Each photomultiplier tube detects the light emission as the result of the radiation photons interacting with the crystal. Groups of blocks (see Fig. 23.4) arranged with shared electronics form detector

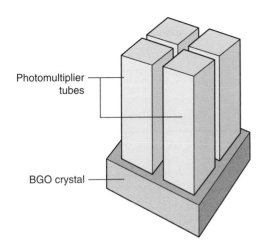

Fig. 23.3 Arrangement of bismuth germinate *(BGO)* crystal and photomultiplier tubes to make an imaging block.

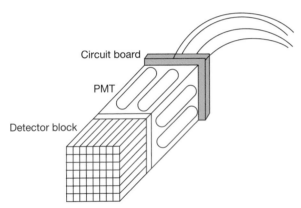

Fig. 23.4 A crystal block. *PMT,* Photomultiplier tubes.

cassettes, and a number of these detector cassettes form a detector ring around the patient.

Normally there is more than one ring so that information from a number of slices can be detected simultaneously. Photomultiplier tubes detect visible light at the photocathode and the interaction produces electrons. A high voltage is applied between the photocathode and the anode which accelerates the electrons between dynodes amplifying the signal. The amplified electrons are collected on the anode and the signal is delivered to the preamplifier which amplifies the signal to a detectable pulse and then to the pulse height analyser. The pulse height analyser accepts all signals from the centre (511 keV) to an acceptable window on each side rejecting scatter. An X,Y (position) and Z (intensity) signal is then fed to the computer.

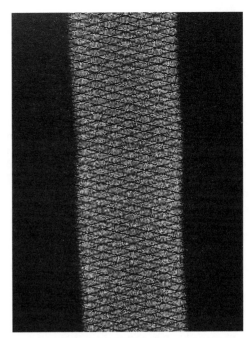

Fig. 23.5 PET sonogram.

23.2.4.3 Line of response

The two 511 keV photons from the annihilation event are detected simultaneously along a straight line connecting the two detectors; this is called the line of response (LOR). This provides accurate positioning of the event and contributes towards forming an accurate image. Each LOR is plotted to form a sinogram, a two-dimensional histogram (Fig. 23.5). The system has a coincidence time window which detects the two photons striking two detectors at the same time.

23.2.4.4 Random coincidences

Random coincidences occur when two photons not arising from the same annihilation event are incident on the detectors within the coincidence time window of the system. This contributes to the scatter within the system if the pulse height analyser does not filter out the photons because of their energy levels.

23.2.4.5 Bed movements

Whole body imaging is achieved by moving a computer-controlled bed through the aperture of the gantry. The axial plane is fixed and the patient moves through the axial plane of detectors. The scan time depends on the patient length, field of view (FOV) of the detector ring and the protocol. Overlap of FOV is required, because sensitivity decreases towards the periphery of the FOV. The resultant images are converted into a maximum intensity projection (MIP) giving a three-dimensional appearance as well as images in axial, sagittal and coronal planes.

23.2.5   Time of flight profiles

If we consider the method of producing images of the positron annihilation discussed so far, the radiation is detected by two detectors thus establishing the line in which the positron emission has taken place. The image of this event is then produced by 'back projection' of the information along the whole of this line. In time of flight (TOF) scanners, the precise time taken for each of the photons to reach its detector is measured. As can be seen in Fig. 23.6, the distance D_1 is greater than the distance D_2 so this first photon will take slightly longer to reach the detector than the second photon will. If we know the velocity of electromagnetic radiation (3×10^8 m.s^{-1}) then we can get a more accurate calculation of the distance travelled by each photon. Thus, in the back projection of the image, instead of simply saying the photons were emitted somewhere along this line, we can say more precisely the position of the emitted radiation on the line. This is illustrated in Fig. 23.7.

No timer is 100% accurate so there is always some degree of positional uncertainty. The fact that we can more accurately calculate the positions of the emitted radiation photons means that we get improved resolution

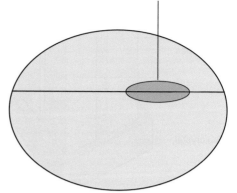

Fig. 23.7 Back-projected image showing the probable position of the area of increased activity from the TOF calculations.

in the image. Fig. 23.8 shows an attenuated corrected PET image.

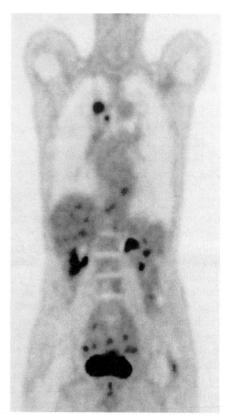

Fig. 23.8 Attenuated corrected positron emission tomography image.

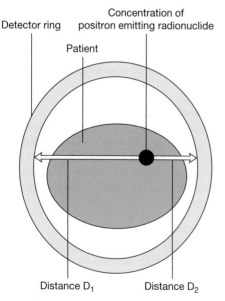

Fig. 23.6 Line diagram to explain TOF technology. The distances D_1 and D_2 from the source of activity to the detectors are shown by the *open arrows*.

TABLE 23.1   Positron emitters

Nuclide	Physical half-life (T1/2)	Mode of decay (%)	Energy (keV)	Mode of production
$^{11}_{6}C$	20.4 minutes	Beta + 100%	511	Cyclotron
$^{18}_{9}F$	110 minutes	Beta + 97%	511	Cyclotron
$^{68}_{31}Ga$	68 minutes	Beta + 89% EC 11%	511	Generator
$^{82}_{37}Rb$	75 seconds	Beta + 95% EC 5%	511 777	Generator

TABLE 23.2   Commonly used tracers

Radionuclide	Chemical form	Abbreviation	Route of administration
^{18}F	Fluoro-2-deoxy-D-glucose	^{18}F-FDG	IV
^{18}F	Choline	^{18}F-FCH	IV
^{18}F	Sodium fluoride	^{18}F NaF	IV
^{68}Ga	Prostate-specific membrane antigen	^{68}Ga PMSA	IV
^{68}Ga	Dotatate	^{68}Ga dotatate	IV
^{82}Rb	Chloride	^{82}RbCl	IV

IV, Intravenous.

23.2.6   Radionuclides used in positron emission tomography scanning

Tables 23.1 and 23.2 give details of positron emitters and some of the commonly used radionuclide tracers in PET scanning.

23.2.6.1   Positron emission tomography radiopharmaceuticals

PET radiopharmaceuticals are positron emitters with short physical half-lives. In the clinical environment they are administered intravenously. The image can only be obtained if the PET tracer is administered correctly because the image is formed from the photons interacting with a scintillator to produce visible light. The PET tracer is a noninvasive quantitative assessment showing the functional and biochemical processes within the body.

23.2.6.2 ^{18}F-Fluoro-2-deoxy-D-glucose

^{18}F-Fluoro-2-deoxy-D-glucose (^{18}F-FDG) is the most commonly used tracer at present. It is mainly used for oncology indications but can also be used for inflammation, infection and brain function. ^{18}F-FDG is an ^{18}F-labelled glucose analogue made when a synthetic sugar is bombarded with ^{18}F radionuclide in a cyclotron. FDG accumulation in tissue is proportional to the amount of glucose utilisation. In metabolism within the human body, ^{18}F-FDG is phosphorylated by hexokinase which is not metabolised any further. Most cancers have an increased consumption of glucose which is partly related to overexpression of the glucose transporter (GLUT) proteins and increased hexokinase activity. It is a sensitive imaging modality for detection, staging and therapy response in oncology.

^{18}F-FDG needs to be produced shortly before use because ^{18}F has a 110-minute half-life; the half-life is long enough for it to be transported from the cyclotron to hospitals.

23.2.6.3 ^{18}F-choline

^{18}F-FDG is not a sensitive radiotracer for prostate cancer because it has a low sensitivity and specificity. Phosphatidylcholine is an essential component of cell membranes, and malignant tumours have a high cellular membrane turnover rate because of their increased proliferation rate. ^{18}F-choline has a high sensitivity and specificity for prostate cancer.

23.2.6.4 ^{18}F-sodium fluoride

^{18}F sodium fluoride (NaF) is produced by irradiation of ^{18}O-water in a cyclotron, which can then be used in the synthesis of ^{18}F-FDG. ^{18}F NaF localises in bone by exchanging with PO_4 ion in the hydroxyapatite crystal. ^{18}F NaF is useful for bone scintigraphy, which would normally be performed with technetium-99m (^{99m}Tc) on a gamma camera. ^{18}F NaF has a higher patient dose than the conventional ^{99m}Tc bone scans, but has a higher target-to-background ratio creating higher resolution images.

23.2.6.5 ^{68}Ga prostate-specific membrane antigen

Prostate-specific membrane antigen (PSMA) is a trans-membrane protein primarily present in all prostatic tissues. Increased PSMA expression can be seen in a variety of malignancies, but most notably in prostate cancer, hence ^{68}Ga PSMA is used to image patients with prostate cancer. It is produced in a generator, and the 68-minute half-life of gallium-68 (^{68}G) makes it difficult to transport.

23.2.6.6 ^{68}Ga dotatate

^{68}Ga dotatate is used for information on the location of somatostatin receptor–expressing tumours; it is more sensitive and specific than ^{18}F-FDG.

23.2.6.7 ^{82}Rubidium choline

^{82}Rubidium choline (^{82}RbCl) is used for imaging the myocardium. It is made in a generator and delivered directly to the patient from the generator because it has a 75-second half-life. Strontium breakthrough needs to be measured before it can be administered to the patient. The heart is stressed chemically using a pharmaceutical before the ^{82}Rb is administered and another scan performed after the patient has rested. A high definition diagnostic CT scan is acquired at the same time, giving anatomical and functional information for the heart muscle and its blood supply simultaneously.

23.3 SINGLE PHOTON EMISSION COMPUTED TOMOGRAPHY

23.3.1 The single photon emission computed tomography scanning system

In the SPECT scanning system the gamma camera is mounted on a suitable gantry so that it can either rotate around the patient or move along the long axis of the patient. If the camera rotates around the patient, it produces a series of axial scans whereas the camera moving over the body produces a longitudinal scan called a planar scan. If we consider the production of an axial scan, the camera is made to rotate around the patient as a series of stepped rotations. Each step is an equal arc, for example, 1 degree, and information is collected at each step of the rotation. In the stepped rotation described, 360 different images would be collected in a complete rotation, and these are then reconstructed to produce an axial image. In practice most SPECT scanners have two gamma camera heads, which both acquire images at the same time so only 180 different images are acquired on each head. Only radiation emitted perpendicular to the gamma camera face will be detected. Typical movement in clinical practice is 3 degrees which would be 60 projections for a 180-degree orbit. Some information is lost owing to scatter. Light measured on each

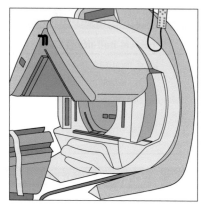

Fig. 23.9 A SPECT scanner set up for cardiac imaging, with the two gamma cameras positioned at 90 degrees to each other.

photomultiplier has a 3.5 to 4.5mm accuracy. The data area is created from a limited number of photons, which can result in image noise, so each event will look like a blurred dot instead of point source. SPECT scanning without the fused addition of CT data (as is obtained in hybrid imaging, see Chapter 26) has no anatomical data, no transmission scan and no attenuation correction maps. Fig. 23.9 shows a SPECT scanner set up for cardiac SPECT.

This technique has a number of uses in nuclear medicine, mainly in cardiac perfusion imaging, orthopaedic imaging and oncology (see Fig. 23.10 for cardiac SPECT images). In orthopaedic imaging and oncology a planar image is normally acquired before the SPECT scan.

23.3.2 The advantages of single photon emission computed tomography

The SPECT scan acquires images only of a specific system. It is a very sensitive type of scanning, giving better resolution and increased accuracy when compared with planar imaging. It shows function of a system in the body. Three-dimensional images in axial, coronal and sagittal planes can be created from reconstructions. It can be used with CT for SPECT/CT imaging—a type of hybrid imaging (see Chapter 26).

23.3.3 The disadvantages of single photon emission computed tomography

The gamma camera head needs to be moved very close to the body part being imaged; autocontouring is used to enable the camera head to be as close to the patient as possible. The typical effective radiation dose to the patient is higher than planar imaging because of the increased amount of radioactivity administered to the patient to produce a good quality image (see Table 23.3). The scan time is long, normally 30 to 60 minutes depending on the clinical protocol. Only one area can be scanned at a time, so the clinician would select the best FOV for the anatomical area.

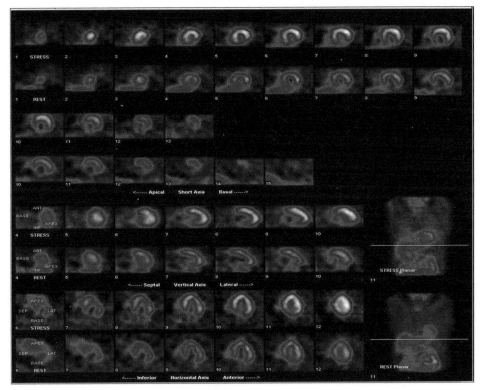

Fig. 23.10 Cardiac single photon emission computed tomography scan.

TABLE 23.3   Comparison of radiation exposure from SPECT and conventional chest X-ray procedures

	Typical effective dose (mSv)	Equivalent number of chest X-rays	Approximate equivalent period of natural background radiation[a]
Bone scan (99mTc)	3	200	1.4 years
Bone scan (SPECT) (99mTc)	4	267	1.9 years
Cardiac (SPECT) rest	7	460	3.2 years
Cardiac (SPECT) stress	6	400	2.7 years

[a]Assuming a typical natural background radiation dose of 2.2 mSv per year.

23.3.4 Typical effective doses in single photon emission computed tomography

The effective dose, measured in milliSievert (mSv), is an indication of "whole body" dose and may be used as an indicator of radiation induced cancer risk. It can be seen that effective doses from SPECT procedures are many times greater than those obtained from conventional chest X-ray procedures and are in fact more in line with those encountered during CT scanning. Thus caution should be advised when considering SPECT of patients who are vulnerable to ionizing radiation. As in any ionizing radiation procedure, doses should only be administered when the likely benefits of that procedure exceed the likely risks.

SUMMARY

In this chapter, you should have learnt the following:
- A basic revision of positron physics (Section 23.2.1).
- The process of acquiring a PET scan (Section 23.2.4).
- Some of the more common radionuclides used for PET scanning (Section 23.2.7).
- The process of acquiring a SPECT image (Section 23.3).

FURTHER READING

Chandra, R., & Rahmin, A. 2018. *Nuclear medicine physics: The basics.* 8th edn. Philadelphia: Wolters Kluwer Health.

Cherry, S., Sorensen, J., & Phelps, M. 2012. *Physics in nuclear medicine.* 4th edn. Philadelphia: Saunders.

Ultrasound imaging

CHAPTER CONTENTS

24.1 AIM

The aim of this chapter is to discuss the key properties of sound and explain how sound can be used to produce a diagnostic image. The Doppler principle, by which the velocity of moving tissues can be determined, is introduced. The clinical applications and advantages of ultrasound are described.

24.2 SOUND PROPERTIES

We tend to be more familiar with sound than with the other emissions used in radiography. From our own experience, we may have noticed that the light from a lightning bolt arrives more quickly than the following loud clap of thunder. This tells us something important about sound—it travels at about 340 metres per second in air, whereas light, like other electromagnetic radiations (including X-rays), travels at a staggering 300,000 kilometres per second in a vacuum. Sound, unlike electromagnetic radiations, needs a physical medium to travel through because it consists of a travelling series of vibrations passing through atoms and molecules. It cannot pass through the vacuum of space, and hence (perhaps fortunately!) we cannot hear the sun's activity, although we are bathed in its light and heat. Sound, unlike light and X-rays, cannot be considered as discrete packets or quanta of energy.

The speed and amplitude of sound is greatly affected by the medium through which it passes, much more so than are electromagnetic radiations such as light. In fact, the speeds of light and X-rays are generally regarded as constant. You may have noticed the very different pitches of

sound that you hear when your head is under water, compared with when your head comes back above the surface. Sound travels at slightly different speeds in different body tissues. The speed of sound is affected by the compressibility of the medium. It travels faster in more rigid materials which resist being compressed, and more slowly in materials such as fluids and gases which can be compressed easily. But conversely, sound loses a lot more of its intensity when travelling through a solid material than when travelling through fluid. You may have found that if you are swimming underwater you can hear other people quite far away, whereas it is rather hard to hear conversations through a door. Table 24.1 lists the speed of sound in air and biological tissues, and it can be seen that the more rigid substances allow sound to travel

TABLE 24.1 Approximate speeds of sound in different materials and tissues

Material or tissue	Speed in metres per second
Air at 20° C and normal atmospheric pressure	340
Lung	650
Fat	1460
Pure water	1500
Salt water	1530
Kidney	1560
Blood	1570
Muscle	1580
Bone	3000

faster. Reflection and refraction of sound can occur at boundaries between materials or tissues.

Reflection is a very important property of sound waves because it provides 'echoes' which are the returning signal, at tissue boundaries, and these are used to depict structures in diagnostic ultrasound. It also gives some information about the nature of tissues. A cyst, which mostly contains fluid, will return few or no ultrasound echoes (the signal is termed *hypoechoic* or *anechoic*) from within itself, as shown in Fig. 24.1, whereas a haemorrhage will return echoes from within itself (the signal is *echoic* or *hyperechoic*), as

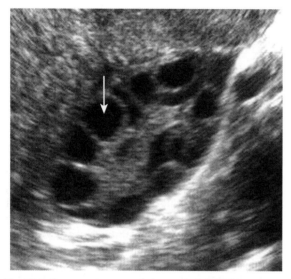

Fig. 24.1 The cysts (an example is arrowed) within this polycystic ovary contain watery fluid and appear anechoic (echo free).

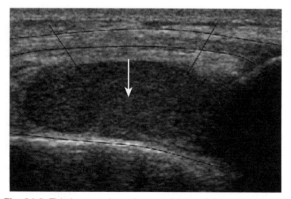

Fig. 24.2 This haemorrhage (arrowed) into a joint returns many small bright echoes from the substances within it, such as blood cells and proteins. It is echogenic (echo producing).

shown in Fig. 24.2. This is because a haemorrhage also contains blood cells and proteins (which return echoes) in addition to just fluid. The walls of a cyst may return strong echoes at the capsule–fluid boundary. Note that the technique of magnetic resonance imaging (see Chapter 25) also describes signals received from the human body as echoes, but these are very different from those found in ultrasound.

Whenever an ultrasound beam strikes a boundary between two materials with different acoustic impedances, some of the beam will be reflected, and the remainder transmitted. The acoustic impedance, symbol Z, refers to the amount of opposition that a medium presents to sound waves trying to pass through it and is affected by the compressibility and density of the medium. The greater the acoustic impedance between two tissues, the greater is the amount of sound reflection at the boundary between them.

- Soft tissue/air interface – large Z difference = large reflection.
- Soft tissue/bone interface – large Z difference = large reflection (about 100%).

The acoustic impedance values of body tissues can be seen in Table 24.2.

Large Z differences return good strong echoes but will prevent sound waves from penetrating beyond the boundary to show deeper structures. For this reason, it is almost (but not quite) technically impossible to see deep structures through the skull using diagnostic ultrasound in adults. The air-filled lungs and ribs also present barriers to ultrasound. Muscle/liver, muscle/fat and muscle/air boundaries reflect back about 2%, 10% and 99% of sound respectively. Good ultrasound images of deep structures result when there are moderate but not huge Z differences between tissues.

The process of reflection of sound at a boundary is illustrated in Fig. 24.3. Dense objects such as gallstones reflect

TABLE 24.2   Acoustic impedance (Z) values for air and body tissues

Material or tissue	Acoustic impedance (kg.m^{-2}.s^{-1})
Air	0.004×10^6
Fat	1.34×10^6
Water	1.48×10^6
Liver	1.65×10^6
Blood	1.65×10^6
Muscle	1.71×10^6
Bone	7.8×10^6

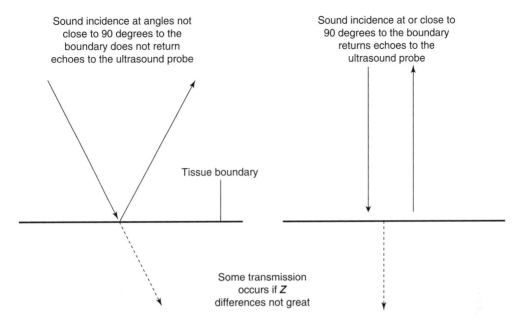

Sound incidence at angles not close to 90 degrees to the boundary does not return echoes to the ultrasound probe

Sound incidence at or close to 90 degrees to the boundary returns echoes to the ultrasound probe

Tissue boundary

Some transmission occurs if *Z* differences not great

Fig. 24.3 Possible ultrasound reflections at tissue boundaries.

back large amounts of sound, owing to the large acoustic impedance difference between themselves and surrounding substances. This may lead to the appearance of an acoustic shadow on an ultrasound scan. This takes the form of a dark echo-free band radiating out behind the stone, in a region where no sound has penetrated. An acoustic shadow can be seen in Fig. 24.4.

An alternative effect, refraction, although important for visible light, is not a major process in diagnostic ultrasound and so sound reflections are much stronger than sound refractions at tissue boundaries. In the process of refraction, a wave carries on from one material to another—it is not reflected back. Refraction is an alteration in propagation direction (direction of travel) which occurs at a boundary between two materials in which the speed of the wave differs. The wave is bent 'towards the normal' if the new speed is slower than the original, and 'away from the normal' if the new speed is faster. The process of refraction at a boundary is shown in Fig. 24.5. If refraction does occur, it can produce an artefact in ultrasound, by which the same body structure may appear in two positions.

An additional effect, scattering of sound, can occur when sound waves encounter small structures that are similar to or smaller than the sound wavelength. This pro-

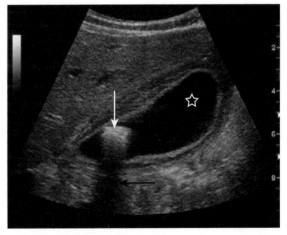

Fig. 24.4 A gallstone *(white arrow)* is returning many echoes and has a bright hyperechoic appearance on its leading face. Behind this there is an acoustic shadow *(black arrow)* where no sound has been transmitted. There are also bright echoes at the boundary between the wall of the gall bladder and its contained fluid, which appears dark and anechoic *(star)*.

duces a diffuse spread of weak signals within the image, deriving from sound scattering in all directions.

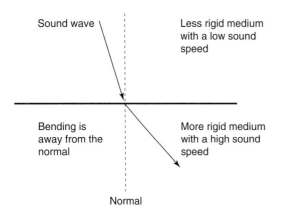

Sound wave

Less rigid medium
with a low sound
speed

Bending is
away from the
normal

More rigid medium
with a high sound
speed

Normal

Fig. 24.5 The process of refraction at a boundary between two media. In this case the sound is refracted away from the normal (the normal is at 90 degrees to the boundary).

INSIGHT

Although all electromagnetic radiations in a vacuum travel at the speed of light, c, which is about 299,792,000 metres per second (2.998×10^8 m.s^{-1}), visible light travels at slightly different speeds in different media. In water and glass, visible light travels at speeds of about 2.25×10^8 m.s^{-1} and 1.98×10^8 ms^{-1}, respectively. The alteration in speed of light (and sound) at boundaries is part of the process of refraction and, in the case of light, explains the production of a rainbow spectrum in a glass prism, with different light wavelengths being refracted to different extents. X-rays have a much higher frequency and energy than visible light. As a result, although X-rays do experience changes in speed in different media; this is to an infinitesimal degree of no practical significance. X-rays experience absorption and scattering in matter, rather than refraction and reflection, although diffraction effects can be seen in very low-energy X-rays whose wavelength is similar to the spacing between atoms in crystal structures.

Sound shares some properties with electromagnetic radiations, in that all can be considered as waves with a frequency, wavelength and amplitude. In all these cases, the velocity of the wave (in metres per second) is equal to the frequency (in Hertz) multiplied by the wavelength (in metres).

$$\text{velocity} = \text{frequency} \times \text{wavelength}$$

A key difference between sound and electromagnetic waves is that sound is regarded as a *longitudinal wave*. This

means that the oscillations of the wave (in this case, compressions and rarefactions in a medium) are in the direction of travel rather than at right angles to it. Fig. 24.6 shows the process of sound transmission through a medium.

Other examples of longitudinal waves include waves in slinky springs, ripples in a water tank, trucks shunting into each other on a rail track and a trick shot with a row of snooker balls!

The frequency of medical ultrasound is in the range of 2 to 20 MHz (megahertz). In medical ultrasound, low frequencies in this range penetrate deeper into the body but have a low resolution, whereas high sound frequencies can only penetrate a shallow depth in the body but have a high resolution. The term *ultrasound* means sound that is above the audible range of hearing for humans (the human range is roughly 20 Hz to 20 kHz). Dogs and younger people can hear slightly higher frequencies. It is interesting to know that there are also sound frequencies lower than the human audible range, termed *infrasound*, used by animals such as whales to communicate over very long distances and also emitted by natural sources such as earthquakes.

Table 24.3 summarises some key properties of sound, light and X-rays.

The 'intensity' of sound is measured in decibels (dB). We might describe it as 'loudness' although this is a rather loose term. It also relates to the amplitude and power of the sound. This decibel scale is a ratio measure and is also based on logarithms to the base 10. This means that sound of 80 dB is 10 times, or 10^1 times, more intense than that of 70 dB. Sound of 100 dB is 1000 times, or 10^3 times, more intense than sound of 70 dB. The decibel scale is useful in ultrasound for recording the attenuation (or loss of intensity) of sound as it passes through a medium such as human tissue because the relationship between incident and transmitted sound is a ratio measure. The ultrasound attenuation coefficients of different tissues are expressed in dB per cm of tissue, with dense tissue like bone attenuating sound much more strongly than soft tissue or water. The values are roughly 10, 1 and 0.002, respectively.

24.3   THE DOPPLER EFFECT

When an object which is emitting sound approaches an observer at speed, the waves become 'bunched-up' and the frequency (or pitch) of the sound increases. Similarly if an object which is emitting sound moves away from an observer at speed, the waves become 'drawn out' and the frequency (or pitch) of the sound decreases. This effect is shown in Fig. 24.7.

This principle has important clinical applications in diagnostic ultrasound because the altered sound frequency or 'frequency shift' of moving tissues, such as heart valves and flowing blood, can be used to determine their speed of

Compression waves passing through molecules

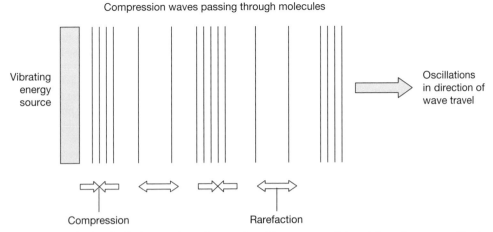

Fig. 24.6 Passage of a longitudinal wave through a medium. The waves radiate out from the source, like ripples moving away from where a pebble has splashed in a pool.

TABLE 24.3   Similarities and differences among sound, light and X-rays

Sound	Visible light	X-rays
Velocity = $f\gamma$	Velocity = $f\gamma$	Velocity = $f\gamma$
Slow velocity	Velocity is light speed, c, in vacuum	Velocity is light speed, c, in vacuum
Velocity much affected by medium	Velocity slightly affected by medium	Velocity not affected by medium
Longitudinal waves	Transverse waves	Transverse waves
Vibrations in atoms and molecules	Photons (quanta)	Photons (quanta)
Mainly absorbed, reflected	Mainly absorbed, reflected, refracted	Mainly absorbed, scattered
Non-ionising	Non-ionising	Ionising

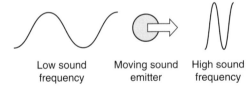

| Low sound frequency | Moving sound emitter | High sound frequency |

Fig. 24.7 A simple illustration of the Doppler principle.

movement relative to the ultrasound probe. In colour-coded Doppler imaging, motion towards the probe is traditionally depicted as red, whereas motion away from the probe is depicted as blue. The Doppler effect can be used to measure the speed of flowing blood, with the ultrasound probe held at about 45 to 60 degrees relative to the blood flow. If the probe was held at 90 degrees relative to the flow, there would be no measurable frequency shift in the direction of the probe. If the probe were held in the direction of the flow, then the frequency shift would be high, but the position would be impractical (the probe cannot be placed within the body). The flow speed can be calculated from the equation

$$v = cf_D/2f_T(\cos \theta)$$

where v is the speed of the flow, c is the average speed of sound in soft tissue, f_D is the Doppler frequency shift, f_T is the frequency of sound emitted from the flowing blood and $\cos \theta$ is the cosine of the probe angle θ.

INSIGHT

The Doppler effect can be observed when the speed of wave-emitting objects is significant relative to the speed of the waves. Doppler shift of light occurs in space when galaxies are moving away from us at tremendous speeds. At these high speeds, visible light becomes shifted towards the red end of the spectrum and this effect can be used to measure the expansion of the universe.

24.4   PRODUCTION AND APPLICATION OF ULTRASOUND

An ultrasound transducer (probe) typically consists of an array of individual elements. Each element contains a piezoelectric crystal, typically made of ceramic material combinations of lead titanate ($PbTiO_3$) and lead zirconate ($PbZrO_3$). An alternating voltage applied across the crystal will cause it to flex and emit sound vibrations at an adjustable frequency. Also, the crystal will generate an alternating voltage across itself in response to a returning sound wave, resulting in a signal. The crystal can be thought of as acting as both a sound speaker and a sound recorder. The elements of the transducer array can be focused to receive signal from shallow or deeper structures in the body. Transducers are usually either linear, producing a rectangular field of view, or curvilinear, producing a fan-shaped field of view that is wider at depth.

The various modes of ultrasound scanning available include the following:

- A mode—amplitude modulated. Produces a graph plot whose height on the *y*-axis shows the strength of the echoes received from the reflective boundary and whose position on the *x*-axis shows the depth of the boundary. Can be used to show motion in structures such as heart valves, if the data are converted to an *m mode* (motion) trace where the position of a reflective boundary is plotted against time.
- B mode—brightness modulated. Produces a two-dimensional anatomical slice through the body with a greyscale brightness based on the amplitude and frequency of reflected sound. This is the most common type of ultrasound scan and the easiest to interpret visually. The depth of the reflective structure (as with A mode scanning) is determined from the time it takes for the echo to return to the transducer.
- Doppler ultrasound—change in sound frequency indicates speed of tissue motion and may be plotted as a colour display plot. A spectral plot may be included, to indicate motion on the *y*-axis over time on the *x*-axis. Pulsed wave Doppler enables the operator to adjust the depth of tissue being visualised, by only accepting returning echoes with time lags in a particular range.
- Duplex scanning combines a Doppler scan with a B mode display which is used for localisation purposes.
- Endoscopic ultrasound uses small intracavity transducers which can show the insides of structures like the oesophagus and blood vessels.
- Three-dimensional transducer arrays provide a three-dimensional depiction of structures and are most popularly used to depict the fetus in utero.

Ultrasound imaging of tissue structures produces harmonic frequencies, which are multiples of the fundamental (or basic) returning sound frequency. For example, the second harmonic is twice the frequency of the fundamental. Harmonics are of great importance to the tones of sound we hear in music. In ultrasound, filters can be used to separate out the second harmonic, which, being of higher frequency, also provides greater resolution. Microbubble contrast agents in ultrasound include bubbles of gas just a few microns in size and are more compressible than surrounding substances. Thus, they return echoes and can be used to improve the visualisation of blood vessels and tissues such as the liver. The microbubbles resonate and produce harmonic frequencies in response to ultrasound waves and this further improves depiction.

Some of the clinical strengths and weaknesses of ultrasound are summarised in Table 24.4.

The biological effects of ultrasound are mainly heating and cavitation. Cavitation occurs in oscillating gas bubbles that may be produced and then collapse in tissues. To reduce these effects on the developing fetus in utero, there are recommended restrictions on the power output, scan time and duty cycle (pulse length and repetition frequency) during pregnancy. Thermal indices (TIs) are associated with heating effects, whereas mechanical indices

TABLE 24.4 Features of clinical ultrasound	
Strengths	**Weaknesses**
Inexpensive	Operator dependent
Quick	Images may be hard to interpret
Mobile	Suffers from image artefacts
Noninvasive	May be prone to giving 'false positives'
Can depict free fluid and aneurysms, e.g., in acute emergencies	Not good for deep structures
Can differentiate between solid and fluid structures	Cannot penetrate through bone or air
Can depict flow and motion	
Good for shallow structures	

(MIs) are associated with the pressure exerted by the ultrasound beam, which may cause cavitation effects. Both these indices are displayed on ultrasound screens. Although some researchers have proposed that dyslexia, left-handedness and reduced birth weight can result from ultrasound use in pregnancy, these studies have not been verified and there is no proven long-term harm resulting from ultrasound.

SUMMARY

In this chapter, you should have learnt the following:
- Medical ultrasound employs high-frequency sound waves which show boundaries between tissues by being reflected at them (Section 24.2).
- Sound waves are unlike the other radiations used in radiography and require a medium for transmission (Section 24.2).
- Reflections are strongest when there are sound transmission differences between tissues, but large differences may be unhelpful by preventing sound transmission to deeper structures (Section 24.2).
- Doppler ultrasound provides information on the speed of moving tissues (Section 24.3).

FURTHER READING

Allisy-Roberts, P.J., & Williams, J. 2007. *Farr's Physics for Medical Imaging*. 2nd edn. Edinburgh: WB Saunders.

Hoskins, P.R., Martin, K., & Thrush, A. 2010. *Diagnostic Ultrasound Physics and Equipment*. 2nd edn. London: Cambridge University Press.

Magnetic resonance imaging

CHAPTER CONTENTS

25.1 AIM

The aim of this chapter is to describe the technique of magnetic resonance imaging (MRI), which is a powerful imaging tool, uniquely able to provide both anatomical and functional information on living tissues. Although computed tomography (CT) imaging (see Chapter 20) is essentially based on the X-ray attenuation properties of tissues, magnetic resonance (MR) is able to examine a much greater range of tissue characteristics, such as proton (hydrogen density), fat and water content, magnetic susceptibility (iron content), water diffusion rate, chemical composition and blood oxygenation. This provides MR with power but also complexity, and the technique has acquired a language of its own, which is sometimes hard to decipher. Some operator-controlled MRI parameters, such as time to repetition (TR) and time to echo (TE), are introduced in this chapter and the appearances of standard MR image sequences are presented to allow their recognition in clinical practice. Available scanner technologies and MRI safety issues are summarised.

25.2 KEY PRINCIPLES OF MAGNETIC RESONANCE IMAGING

From the middle of the twentieth century, the technique of nuclear magnetic resonance (NMR) was widely used in laboratories to identify the nature and concentrations of chemicals by examining the frequencies and heights of their radio wave spectral peaks. Bloch and Purcell, working inde-pendently, had noted in 1946 that chemical samples placed in a strong magnetic field, when subjected to radiofrequency (RF) waves at specific resonant frequencies, returned detectable and characteristic RF signals. Radio waves are applied at a precise resonant frequency, at which energy may be transferred to the molecules. Following this, the molecules 'relax' and return radio waves in the form of a signal or 'echo', which are also at the resonant frequency. This is the basis of NMR and MRI. Atomic nuclei (hence the term 'nuclear' in NMR) have an angular momentum or spin, which means that they rotate on their axes, rather like tiny planets. This produces a rotating magnetic field, which 'precesses' like a playground roundabout, at a set frequency when placed in a magnetic field. This frequency is quite high and is measured in megahertz (MHz). If radio waves are applied at this exact precessional frequency, energy is transferred, and resonance is said to occur. This principle applies not just during NMR procedures, which produce graphical spectra, but also during MRI scans, which obtain two-dimensional or even three-dimensional images. NMR has evolved for clinical use into the technique of magnetic resonance spectroscopy (MRS) which provides chemical signatures of body tissue composition via spectra, using nuclei with useful magnetic properties, such as hydrogen-1 and phosphorus-31. But in MRI it is always hydrogen-1 which is used as the source of signal, and the brightness of individual pixels in the image matrix is based on the magnetic relaxation times of hydrogen nuclei found in different tissue environments, such as water and fat. It is fortunate that hydrogen-1 (the usual isotope of hydrogen, with a nucleus consisting of a single proton) not only has strong magnetic properties but is found in most body tissues at high concentrations. This concentration is termed the 'proton density'.

Hydrogen nuclei, used in MRI, have individual 'magnetic dipole moments'. This refers to the magnetic field orientation of each nucleus. Note that a 'moment' in this context means a vector quantity with magnitude and direction, not a brief moment of time! MRI has a language all of its own and the term 'spin' is commonly used to refer to the rotating magnetic field orientation of an individual atomic nucleus.

Normally the magnetic dipole moments of individual atomic nuclei, whether in a chemical sample or in a human body, are aligned randomly in all directions. There is no overall magnetisation in any particular direction. But if a powerful magnetic field is applied, the individual magnetic dipole moments tend to align:

- either with the external magnetic field (which is referred to in MRI as parallel or 'spin-up'). This is a low-energy state.
- or against the external magnetic field (which is referred to in MRI as antiparallel or 'spin-down'). This is a high-energy state.

There is normally a slight excess of magnetic dipole moments in the low-energy 'spin-down' state, an excess which increases as the external magnetic field strength increases. These states are illustrated in Fig. 25.1. The rotational or precessional frequency of the magnetic dipole moments is directly proportional to the external magnetic field strength. The Larmor equation describes this relationship:

$$\omega = \gamma B_0 \qquad \textbf{Equation 25.1}$$

where ω is the precessional frequency in Hertz, B_0 is the magnetic flux density of the external magnetic field in tesla and γ is a constant known as the *gyromagnetic ratio*. This dependence of precessional frequency on local magnetic field strength (because γ is constant) is a very important principle in MRI and has a lot of applications.

The gyromagnetic ratio is a constant for the particular atomic nucleus used in NMR or MRI to generate signal. The gyromagnetic ratio of hydrogen-1 is 42.6 MHz (million

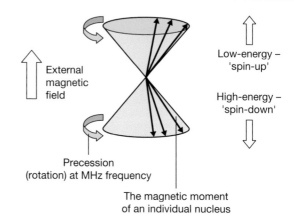

Fig. 25.1 The precession of individual magnetic dipole moments placed in a strong external magnetic field.

cycles per second) per tesla. Thus, hydrogen-1 nuclei precess at 42.6 MHz at a magnetic flux density of 1 T. Hydrogen is very abundant in water and biological molecules like fats, proteins and carbohydrates. This coupled with the fact that its most common (^{1}H) nucleus has a strong magnetic signal enables us to visualise many body tissues effectively.

Table 25.1 lists the gyromagnetic ratios of some nuclei used in MRI and MRS. MRI provides images of human anatomy, whereas MRS is an adaptation of NMR used to measure the strength of chemical signatures in living tissues, by providing spectra. Only hydrogen-1 has sufficient abundance and signal in the body to provide images.

The frequency of the returning radio wave signals received from nuclei in chemical samples or living tissues is influenced by the local chemical environment. This is largely attributed to the presence of electrons in chemical bonds, which slightly 'shield' nuclei to varying extents from the external magnetic field. Thus hydrogen nuclei (for

TABLE 25.1   Some atomic nuclei used in magnetic resonance imaging and magnetic resonance spectroscopy

Nucleus (mass number)	Gyromagnetic ratio (MHz per tesla)	Relative signal strength	Notes
Hydrogen-1	42.6	100	The main nucleus used in magnetic resonance imaging (MRI) and magnetic resonance spectroscopy (MRS) because it is very common in the human body and has a good magnetic signal. Consists of just a single proton.
Carbon-13	10.7	1.45	Only 1% of carbon occurs as the magnetically useful ^{13}C isotope. Used in MRS only. ^{12}C has no useful magnetic properties.
Fluorine-19	40.1	83	Not naturally present in the human body but can be used to label drugs and other molecules. Used in MRS only.
Phosphorus-31	17.2	6.6	Very useful for studying metabolic processes in molecules like adenosine triphosphate (ATP) and adenosine diphosphate (ADP). Used in MRS only.

example) in different chemical molecules (such as water, lactate, fat) precess at very slightly different speeds, according to the Larmor equation. This creates frequency shifts, known as *chemical shifts,* in the radio wave signals received within a spectrum. This effect is the basis of NMR and MRS. In MRI, the chemical shift effect can result in artefacts. Fig. 25.2 shows a hydrogen-1 spectrum obtained in an MRS procedure.

MRS is a powerful tool for providing chemical information on lesions such as tumours, but requires large voxels, high magnetic field strength, a very homogeneous magnetic field and cannot provide two-dimensional or three-dimensional images of human anatomy.

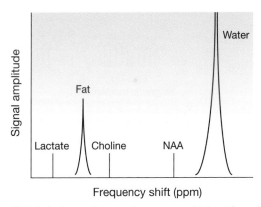

Fig. 25.2 A hydrogen-1 (proton) spectrum obtained from MR spectroscopy. Note that, to avoid confusion, frequency is plotted from low (*left*) to high (*right*) on the X-axis, although in practice this would be plotted in reverse order. Units of frequency are typically parts per million (ppm) frequency shift. The shift between fat and water is 3.5 ppm. The peaks for water and fat are very large (larger than shown) relative to other chemicals. Lactate levels increase in anaerobic conditions, for example, in tumours. Choline is a substrate for cell synthesis and reflects cell proliferation. N-acetyl aspartate (*NAA*) is a marker for neurons.

INSIGHT

A high magnetic field strength in the order of 1.5 tesla (T) or greater is needed in MRS to increase the frequency shift (chemical shift) between chemicals so that they show up more clearly as distinct spectral peaks. For example, although the shift between water and fat is always 3.5 parts per million, the actual frequency difference is three times greater at a field strength of 3 T (where hydrogen-1 precessional frequency is $42.6 \times 3 = 127.8$ MHz) than at 1 T (where hydrogen-1 precessional frequency is 42.6 MHz).

In 1971, Raymond Damadian provided an impetus to the development of clinical MRI by suggesting that the radio wave signal relaxation times of different tissues might be indicative of the degree of tumour malignancy.

Paul Lauterbur provided the first two-dimensional MR image of a chemical sample in 1973 and suggested the term *zeugmatography* for the technique. Developments in clinical MRI continued in the United States and in the United Kingdom, led by Peter Mansfield and colleagues in the latter, with the first clinical scanners appearing in about 1980.

Clinical MRI almost always uses hydrogen-1 nuclei as the 'MR-active' signal source in the human body. When RF radiations are applied to a patient's body, placed in a powerful magnetic field, at precisely the Larmor or precessional frequency of the hydrogen nuclei, then resonance occurs and energy is transferred to the nuclei. Subsequently, two types of tissue 'relaxations' or releases of radio energy from the patient (resulting in signals) occur simultaneously.

1. The longitudinal relaxation process occurs relatively slowly over a time period typically up to several hundred milliseconds. In this process the overall tissue magnetisation, which has been briefly 'flipped' by a flip angle α towards 90 degrees from the external magnetic field direction by the RF energy input, subsequently returns to a position of 0 degrees, parallel to the magnetic field. This is the basis of the T1 signal component in MRI.
2. The transverse relaxation process occurs relatively quickly over a time period typically up to several tens of milliseconds. In this process the rotating magnetic moments of individual nuclei, which have been brought briefly into line (or in phase) by the RF energy input, subsequently fan out (or dephase). This is the basis of the T2 signal component in MRI.

These relaxation processes are illustrated in Figs. 25.3 and 25.4.

INSIGHT

The two processes of (1) 'flipping' the overall magnetisation towards 90 degrees relative to the external magnetic field, and (2) putting the magnetic moments in phase, induces a strong electrical signal in a receiver coil placed at 90 degrees to the main magnetic field. The frequency of this signal matches the precessional frequency of the magnetic moments of the nuclei. When they are all in phase, a powerful alternating current is induced in the receiver coil. For an analogy, we could think of the way a bright rotating lighthouse beam sweeps periodically towards an observer. Imagine if the light fanned out and went diffuse—the beam would be less effective. As the magnetic moments of the nuclei dephase in magnetic resonance imaging, the signal in the receiver coil similarly fades out. This is called a *free induction decay*.

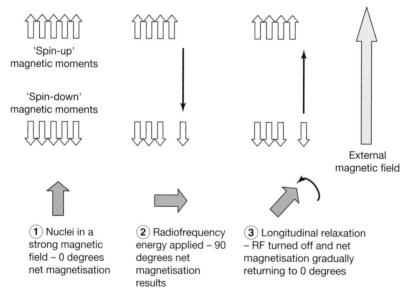

Fig. 25.3 The *longitudinal relaxation process* for the magnetic moments of hydrogen nuclei in a strong magnetic field. Before radiofrequency (*RF*) energy is applied, there is a small excess of low-energy 'spin-up' magnetic moments, giving an overall magnetisation of 0 degrees (*up in the diagram*) parallel to the magnetic field. On the application of RF at the resonance frequency, some spins are promoted to the higher-energy 'spin-down' state and net magnetisation is towards 90 degrees. Removal of the RF energy causes gradual 'recovery' of overall net magnetisation to 0 degrees, with some spins returning to the low-energy state.

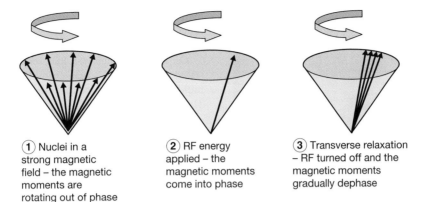

① Nuclei in a strong magnetic field – the magnetic moments are rotating out of phase

② RF energy applied – the magnetic moments come into phase

③ Transverse relaxation – RF turned off and the magnetic moments gradually dephase

Fig. 25.4 The transverse relaxation process for the magnetic moments of hydrogen nuclei in a strong magnetic field. Before radiofrequency (*RF*) energy is applied, the magnetic moments of individual nuclei are all precessing at the Larmor frequency and 'out of step' (out of phase) with each other. Think of them rotating at points occupying every minute of a clock face. When RF energy is applied, the magnetic moments all come briefly 'into step' (in phase), as if they were all rotating together in the 12 o'clock position on a clock face. When the RF energy is turned off, the magnetic moments all dephase.

TABLE 25.2 Relaxation of the radiofrequency signal in magnetic resonance imaging

Longitudinal relaxation	Transverse relaxation
Occurs slowly overall	Occurs quickly overall
Fat relaxes relatively quickly and water slowly	Fat relaxes relatively quickly and water slowly
Is the basis of T1 weighted imaging	Is the basis of T2 weighted imaging
Using T1 image weighting, fat appears bright and water appears dark	Using T2 image weighting, fat appears grey and water appears bright
Good for depicting anatomy	Good for depicting pathology (fluid filled)
Tissues which enhance with gadolinium contrast agent appear bright with T1 weighting	Tissues which enhance with iron oxide contrast agent appear dark with T2 weighting

The longitudinal relaxation process is also termed longitudinal recovery, or spin-lattice relaxation. It occurs relative to the longitudinal plane (0 degrees) and involves transfer of energy to the atomic lattice of the material. Note that although RF energy causes heating of human tissues, this is via electromagnetic induction and not flipping of the magnetic moments of nuclei.

The transverse relaxation process is also called spin–spin relaxation, because the process of dephasing occurs within the transverse plane and occurs between magnetic moments (spins).

Some important practical features of the longitudinal and transverse recovery processes are summarised in Table 25.2.

25.3 IMAGE WEIGHTINGS, SEQUENCES AND APPEARANCES

Leaving the physics aside for a moment, it is very important to be able to interpret the appearance of MRI images. In this section, we will first consider the appearances of T1, T2, proton density and fat or fluid 'saturated' images.

Remember that on a T1 weighted image, in terms of the longitudinal recovery process, fat relaxes quickly and appears bright. Fluid relaxes slowly and appears dark.

Look at Fig. 25.5, a T1 weighted image. The subcutaneous fat appears bright. Cerebrospinal fluid in the lateral ventricle appears dark. White matter in the corpus callosum of the brain appears relatively bright, because it

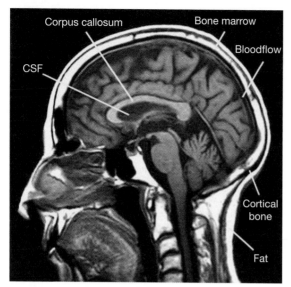

Fig. 25.5 A T1 weighted sagittal spin echo image of the head and neck. *CSF,* Cerebrospinal fluid.

contains axons with fatty myelin sheaths. Cortical bone appears dark, because its hydrogen-1 atoms are tightly bound within a crystalline lattice and transverse relaxation between spins occurs so quickly that no signal can be sampled. But bone marrow appears bright, because it contains fat. Flowing blood in the sagittal venous sinus appears dark, because in spin echo imaging the flowing

hydrogen atoms pass through an imaging slice before they can return a signal. This is known as the *time of flight effect.*

On an MRI image, you may see the terms TR and TE stated. The TR is the time in milliseconds between one radio wave excitation of the atomic nuclei and the next. The TE is the time in milliseconds between a radio wave excitation and the received signal (which is called an *echo*). This is not to be confused with echoes in ultrasound! T1 weighted images use a short TR and short TE and this contributes to making a T1 image relatively quick to acquire. It is often relatively free from motion blur. Fig. 25.6 illustrates the terms TR and TE.

Now let's look at Fig. 25.7, a T2 weighted image. On a T2 weighted image, fluid appears bright. Fluid relaxes more slowly than fat in terms of the transverse recovery process. The bright signal from cerebrospinal fluid in the lateral ventricles and oedema surrounding a brain tumour can be seen. Notice that fat and cortical bone appear grey or dark (the latter for the reason considered earlier) and are not well seen here. Grey matter, which contains many fluid-containing cell bodies, appears relatively bright, whereas the fatty myelinated axons of white matter appear grey. Once again flowing blood, seen here in two end-on blood vessels, does not give a signal as this is a spin echo image. T2 weighted images use a long TR and long TE, and this contributes to making a T2 image relatively slow to acquire. It is more often affected by motion blur than a T1 image.

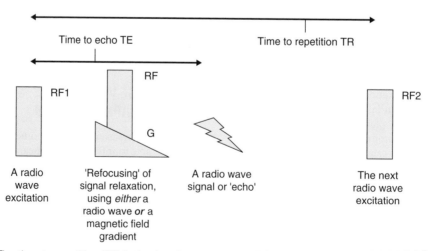

Fig. 25.6 The time to repetition (*TR*) is the time between two radiofrequency (*RF*) excitation pulses. The time to echo (*TE*) is the time between an RF excitation pulse and a signal. Adjustment of the TR and TE affects the image weighting in magnetic resonance imaging. *G,* Applied magnetic field gradient.

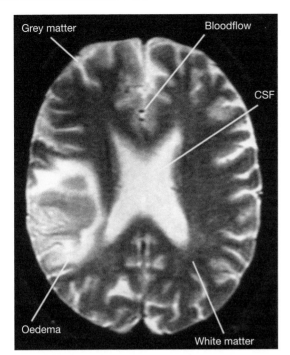

Grey matter

Bloodflow

CSF

Oedema

White matter

Fig. 25.7 A T2 weighted axial spin echo image of the brain. *CSF*, Cerebrospinal fluid.

INSIGHT

In magnetic resonance imaging (MRI), a gradient is a linear and regular variation in magnetic flux density, from low to high. There are many uses of gradients in MRI. In gradient echo imaging, a magnetic field gradient is used to refocus a signal, giving a gradient echo. Gradient echo MRI sequences are fast and have the characteristic that flowing blood appears bright. (Spin echo sequences, which use an RF pulse to refocus the signal and give a spin echo are relatively slow, high contrast and give no signal from flowing blood.) Gradients are also used in MRI to obtain slices in the sagittal, coronal and axial planes. Changing a gradient in a regular way across a patient alters the local precessional frequencies and phases of the rotating magnetic moments of hydrogen-1 nuclei. This enables a unique 'address' of the nuclei to be obtained. Direct multiplanar imaging is a major strength of MRI.

You may also encounter proton density weighted images in MRI. Such images tend to appear rather low in contrast compared with T1 or T2 images and are simply based on the number of 'protons' (in fact the numbers of hydrogen-1 nuclei) present within the image. Tissues with a high 'proton density' such as fluid and fat appear relatively bright. To achieve a proton density image, the contribution of T1 and T2 weighting must be minimised, and so a long TR (to reduce T1 weighting) and a short TE (to minimise T2 weighting) are used.

There are a number of imaging techniques commonly used in MRI, as summarised in Table 25.3.

25.4 MAGNETIC RESONANCE IMAGING EQUIPMENT—SCANNERS AND COILS

There are three main types of MRI magnet systems in clinical use, with most systems being superconducting because these offer the greatest field strength and image quality. High-field magnets, which typically operate at magnetic flux densities of 1.5 to 3 T, offer the advantages of high signal-to-noise ratios (which permit good image resolution and fast scanning) and suitability for a range of applications including MRS, diffusion imaging and functional imaging.

1. Superconducting magnets typically operate at magnetic flux densities up to 3 T for clinical use. They are powerful electromagnets whose coils of wire (typically niobium–tin or niobium–titanium alloy) show the phenomenon of zero electrical resistance at temperatures of around 4 Kelvin (−269° C) when cooled by liquid helium. The magnetic field is typically parallel to the floor, along the long axis of a patient, and is homogeneous over a wide volume. Signal-to-noise ratio is excellent. Drawbacks include large purchase and running costs, a *large fringe magnetic field* (which increases hazards and interference) and claustrophobia. Once 'ramped-up', such magnets cannot be switched off, except via a costly boil-off or 'quench' of liquid helium.

2. Resistive magnets are powerful electromagnets which rely on a large current density to create a strong magnetic field and operate at room temperature. Combination with permanent magnet materials can permit magnetic flux densities up to about 1 T. Such magnets often have a magnetic field vertical to the floor and provide the advantages of reduced claustrophobia (being 'open' designs) and reduced fringe field (which reduces hazards). They can also be switched off. However they tend to suffer from poor field homogeneity and low signal-to-noise ratio.

3. Permanent magnet designs are based around large ferromagnetic iron or alloy cores and may be quite bulky if even a moderate field strength is to be achieved. Relatively little used in clinical practice, they provide advantages of low fringe field and running costs but suffer from poor signal-to-noise ratio and field homogeneity.

TABLE 25.3   Common imaging techniques used in magnetic resonance imaging

Technique	Explanation
Spin echo (SE)	A standard magnetic resonance imaging (MRI) technique which uses a signal-refocusing radiofrequency (RF) pulse to generate a SE.
Short time inversion recovery (STIR)	A SE sequence based on RF pulses which reduces fat signal and increases the conspicuity of fluid-containing pathologies.
Fluid attenuated inversion recovery (FLAIR)	A SE sequence based on RF pulses which reduces fluid signal and increases the conspicuity of pathologies which could otherwise be masked by fluid.
Fat saturation or 'fat sat'	An alternative means of reducing fat signal which works by targeting RF pulses at the precessional frequency of fat.
Inversion recovery (IR)	A SE sequence which enables contrast between different tissues to be amplified and finely controlled.
Dual echo	A SE sequence which contains two refocusing RF pulses and simultaneously provides proton density and T2 image information.
Fast spin echo (FSE), also called turbo spin echo (TSE)	A rapid SE sequence which includes several signal-refocusing RF pulses rather than just one.
Rapid acquisition with relaxation enhancement (RARE) or single-shot FSE	A very fast SE sequence which uses a very long train of refocusing RF pulses and obtains all information from an imaging slice in a 'single shot'.
Gradient echo (GE)	A standard and fast MRI technique which uses a signal-refocusing gradient to generate a GE. Magnetic susceptibility effects are strong. Flowing blood appears bright
Echo planar imaging (EPI)	A very fast GE sequence which uses a very long train of refocusing gradients and obtains all information from an imaging slice in a 'single shot' or 'multi-shot'.
Magnetic resonance angiography (MRA)	A GE technique in which flowing blood signal is amplified and stationary tissue signal is suppressed. Includes time of flight (TOF) and phase contrast (PC) techniques that do not use gadolinium contrast media and contrast enhanced (CE) techniques that do.

Coils found in MRI are tuned to radio wave frequencies in the megahertz range employed. Transmit coils, as the name indicates, transmit RF waves into the patient at a finely controlled range of frequencies which affect slice thickness and image quality. They tend to be of 'volume coil' or bird cage designs which surround an area of patient anatomy. They may also have transmit–receive qualities. Receiver coils are designed to permit a good signal-to-noise ratio and should be positioned parallel to the external magnetic field and as close as possible to the anatomy of interest. Like transmit coils, they utilise Faraday's laws of electromagnetic induction. Small coils tend to provide good signal-to-noise ratios but poor volume coverage. This can be addressed by phased arrays of individual coils.

Whole-body imaging can be provided by extended arrays of coils. Parallel imaging is a very useful development in MRI, using receiver coils to perform part of the image reconstruction process, thereby reducing scan times.

25.5   MAGNETIC RESONANCE IMAGE CONSTRUCTION

Data from the MRI scan process must be organised as pixels or voxels, within the three orthogonal directions, which are z (head to toe), y (anterior to posterior) and x (left to right), assuming that the patient is lying supine within the scanner. We need to know precisely which pixel or voxel the RF signal is coming from, in three dimensions. This is achieved by superimposing magnetic field gradients on the main magnetic field in the x, y and z planes. A gradient is an applied subsidiary magnetic field which varies linearly in size over distance, adding to or subtracting from overall magnetic field strength, either side of the magnetic field isocentre. Essentially it provides a regular 'slope' of overall magnetic field strength. So if we consider hydrogen nuclei along the z direction, we will find that their processional frequency will vary in a predictable way, related to the local magnetic field strength, as stated by the Larmor equation. Using this relationship, we will find that the position of a voxel along the z axis (head to toe) can be identified by the returning RF frequency. Also, we can obtain an imaging slice by applying a particular range of frequencies (the transmit waveband) to the patient in an RF pulse. Voxel position within one direction in the plane of an axial slice (x or y) can also be determined using the RF frequencies in the returning signal. This employs either the x or y gradient as the 'frequency encoding gradient'. To obtain voxel position in the second direction within the axial slice, we use another property of the returning RF signal, known as 'phase'. To understand this, think of two cars driving around a circular track. The faster car will be passing around the circuit more often in a given time period, with a greater frequency. If we were to take a photograph of the two cars at a given point in time, their positions on the circuit are likely to be different. One car a quarter way round could be described as having a phase angle of 90 degrees, whereas one halfway round has a phase angle of 180 degrees. This extra property, the phase, can be detected in the RF signal and is determined by the second gradient in the xy plane, which we term the 'phase encoding gradient'. The functions of the x, y and z gradients, either slice select, frequency encoding or phase encoding, can be varied by the operator to obtain MRI slices in the axial, coronal and sagittal planes.

Once signal information has been obtained from each pixel or voxel, this is assigned to an area of temporary computer storage that is termed 'k-space'. Information related to image contrast and signal is stored in the central portion of k-space, whereas information related to resolution and detail is stored in the periphery. K-space sounds like a rather abstract concept but it is very important to the way in which MRI works, because all fast scanning techniques, such as fast spin echo and echo planar imaging, are based on putting data into k-space more quickly. Each 'echo' fills a line of k-space. Some fast scan techniques, such as 'keyhole imaging' and partial averaging, are speedy because they fill only a portion of k-space, with some loss of image quality as a result.

25.6   MAGNETIC RESONANCE IMAGING BIOEFFECTS AND SAFETY

Although MRI does not generate ionising radiation and is not thought to induce cancers, there are a large number of biological effects of MRI scanning, some of which can be fatal. This is a surprise to many people. Thus MRI must be operated within strict guidelines, although most effects are transient and reversible. Sources of hazard in MRI arise from:

- the static (constant) external magnetic field which operates at magnetic flux densities of several tesla
- time-varying magnetic fields produced by magnetic field gradients
- radiofrequency electromagnetic fields used to excite the nuclear spins.

The projectile effect is the most dramatic demonstration of the influence of the static magnetic field. This exerts a rotational torque and translational force on ferromagnetic objects, tending to align them with the field and draw them towards greater magnetic flux densities. An exclusion zone of 5 gauss surrounds an MRI scanner, designed to prevent objects like scissors and oxygen cylinders from becoming projectiles and also to prevent damage to magnetically sensitive devices like pacemakers. The static field also affects the T-wave amplitude in the cardiac cycle.

Time-varying (gradient) fields can induce electrical currents and cause resistive heating effects in patients, particularly if 'loops' are created in wires or even by a patient clasping their hands or legs together. Current and heating are greatest in conductors. Induced currents can cause tingling or spasm but are not sufficient to cause fibrillation of the heart. Flexing of the gradient coils as a result of changing current flow creates the loud banging sounds which may reach 120 decibels and require patients to use ear protection (recommended >85 decibels).

RF waves can cause heating of body tissues, especially shallow tissues, by electromagnetic induction. The specific absorption rate (SAR) is controlled in MRI to prevent temperature rises above 1° C. The power, repetition rate and wavelength of the RF pulses, as well as the size of the patient, are factors which influence heating.

The trend towards higher field MR magnets, with 3 T now much more common in clinical practice, has improved scan capabilities but also resulted in an increase in potential hazards. RF frequency increases in accordance with field strength and this can result in increased tissue heating. In addition, a greater amplitude and/or duration of RF is required to achieve a given flip angle at high field strength. Gradient performance, as expressed by amplitude and slew rate, also tends to be greater in high-field scanners and this can increase induced electrical currents as well as sound levels. Finally, 'projectile effects' on ferromagnetic objects within the scan room will be greater at high field, and items regarded as 'MR safe' at 1 T may not be safe at 3 T.

Note that MRI is not recommended for use in the first trimester of pregnancy. Although no studies of pregnant radiographers or patients have indicated increased adverse effects, some animal studies have suggested caution, albeit at exposure durations greater than those likely to be encountered in MRI practice.

25.7 ADVANCED MAGNETIC RESONANCE TECHNIQUES

There are a number of exciting advanced MR techniques available.

- Functional MRI (fMRI) examines areas of neuronal activation in the brain in response to motor activity and sensory stimuli. This is because there are subtle changes in the amount of oxygenation in the blood supply, which are revealed as differences in magnetisation. The technique is referred to as blood oxygen level-dependent contrast (BOLD).
- Diffusion weighted imaging (DWI) examines changes in the diffusion rate of water molecules, which can occur in conditions such as stroke and tumour. Generally 'restricted diffusion' occurs in these conditions and shows up as areas of increased signal intensity (brightness) on a basic diffusion image and reduced intensity on an apparent diffusion coefficient (ADC) map.
- Susceptibility weighted imaging (SWI) can show subtle haemorrhages as areas of signal loss, caused by the magnetic properties of iron in haemoglobin.
- MRS, as previously mentioned, is based on a spectral display rather than an image. It allows the chemical composition of tissues to be assessed without needing a biopsy and is particularly useful for investigating the grade of tumours.

SUMMARY

In this chapter, you should have learnt the following:
- MRI developed from an earlier nonimaging technique called NMR which is still used today in MRS (Section 25.2).
- MRI makes use of the relaxation properties of hydrogen nuclei placed in a powerful magnetic field and subjected to RF energies. These relaxation properties provide characteristic signals from different body tissues (Section 25.2).
- T1 and T2 weighted images are the standard visualisation method in MRI (Section 25.3).
- There are many available techniques in MRI, which enable visualisation of stationary tissues and flowing blood (Section 25.3).
- Most magnets use superconductivity (Section 25.4).
- MRI has many hazards and biological effects (Section 25.6).

FURTHER READING

Hashemi, R.H., Lisanti, C.J., & Bradley, W.G. 2017. *MRI – The Basics.* 4th edn. Baltimore: Lippincott Williams & Wilkins.

McRobbie, D.W., Moore, E.A., Graves, M.J., & Prince, M.R. 2017. *MRI from Picture to Proton.* 3rd edn. Cambridge: Cambridge University Press.

Westbrook, C., & Talbot, J. 2018. *MRI in Practice.* 5th edn. Oxford: Wiley–Blackwell.

Hybrid scanners

CHAPTER CONTENTS

26.1 AIM

The aim of this chapter is to introduce the reader to the basic principles and development of hybrid scanners.

26.2 BACKGROUND

In medical imaging, we wish to produce images which will enable us to diagnose, treat (if possible) and monitor a disease process. Some images will produce good anatomical images (e.g., computed tomography [CT] and magnetic resonance imaging [MRI]) of pathology but will give little information about the physiological process occurring around the pathology. Other imaging devices will produce good images of the physiological processes involved in pathology (e.g., radionuclide imaging [RNI] and positron emission tomography [PET]) but give little information about associated changes in the anatomy around the pathology. Hybrid scanners attempt to collect both anatomical and physiological data and to merge this information to give a composite image, and for this reason they are sometimes referred to as *multimodal imaging* (MMI). Such has been the success of hybrid scanners that no manufacturer now produces a 'stand-alone' PET scanner.

26.3 HISTORICAL DEVELOPMENT

Historically there have been two approaches to producing the composite images. These will now be discussed.

26.3.1 The software approach

The software approach took images produced by two different scanners and then merged these images using appropriate software. To achieve effective fusion of the images, accurate spatial and temporal alignment is crucial. This is difficult to achieve when the images have been produced on two separate scanners, and so this approach is susceptible to differences in patient position and noise artefacts because of the patient being in different phases of the respiratory cycle. In recent years, this has been superseded by the hardware approach.

26.3.2 The hardware approach

The hardware approach utilises a hybrid system where two (or more) scanners are housed in a single device. The principal advantage of this system is that the imaging modalities collect data sequentially while the patient is in the same position on the couch, thus limiting noise artefacts caused by inaccurate alignment. Careful patient positioning with maximum patient comfort is required because if patients

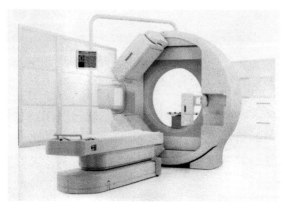

Fig. 26.1 An example of a single photon emission computed tomography/computed tomography hybrid scanner. (Image courtesy of Phillips Healthcare.)

move between the two sequences even in a hybrid system a true fused image will not be produced. These systems will now be discussed in more detail.

26.4   THE SINGLE PHOTON EMISSION COMPUTED TOMOGRAPHY/COMPUTED TOMOGRAPHY HYBRID SCANNER

This system consists of a patient couch and two gamma cameras ring-mounted in front of an adapted CT scanner. The system has been around in various forms since 1999 but has seen significant improvement over the years. Fig. 26.1 shows the layout of such a scanner.

The gamma cameras can rotate around the patient and so can collect single photon emission computed tomography (SPECT) scan data. This produces an axial SPECT scan. The CT scanner part will produce an axial CT image of the same area. The two images can be displayed separately and a merged image can also be displayed. The ability to collect anatomical and physiological information simultaneously has great merit in oncology and also has potential in cardiac studies.

26.5   THE POSITRON EMISSION TOMOGRAPHY/COMPUTED TOMOGRAPHY HYBRID SCANNER

This is again an example of a hybrid scanner which will collect functional data (from the PET scan) and anatomical data (from the CT scan). The first of these entered clinical use in 2001. In the PET/CT gantry the CT element of the PET/CT scanner is in front of the PET element, so the patient is scanned initially in the CT component and then the PET component. Fig. 26.2 shows such a scanner.

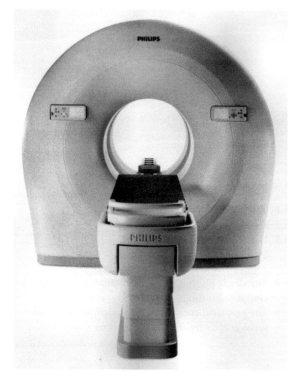

Fig. 26.2 An example of a positron emission tomography/computed tomography hybrid scanner. (Image courtesy of Phillips Healthcare.)

Data from both scanners can be displayed separately or merged to produce a composite image of the anatomy and physiological detail of a lesion. Clinical image reporters may use both merged and unmerged data when reporting the scans. The main use of this type of scanner is oncology and cardiac studies where it gives functional and anatomical data. The CT scan in a PET/CT scan for oncology is normally an attenuation scan, not a full diagnostic scan.

26.5.1   Attenuation computed tomography scan in positron emission tomography/computed tomography for oncology

Attenuation is when the detected photons are greatly reduced compared with the original source photons attributed to scatter out of the detector field of view or absorption within the patient. In PET most attenuation is caused from Compton scatter outside the detector ring. A CT transmission scan produces a low-noise, high-contrast image for attenuation correction in PET/CT. The attenuation CT scan in PET/CT is a low-dose CT scan which helps delineate the outline of the body and internal organs proving attenuation

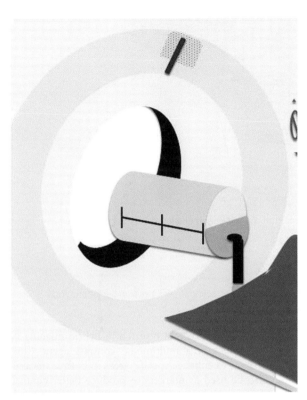

Fig. 26.3 Daily positron emission tomography quality assurance with phantom.

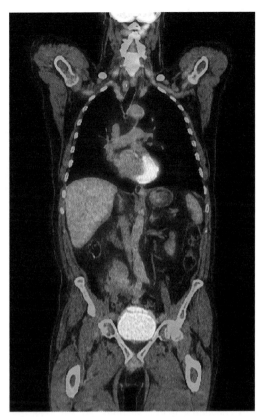

Fig. 26.4 Positron emission tomography/computed tomography scan.

correction. A fused PET-CT image can be created providing anatomical and functional information as long as the patient remains still throughout the whole scan. Images are acquired from base of orbits to mid-thigh for most oncology indications; if the arms are elevated, less beam-hardening artefact occurs in the trunk of the body. The patient is normally scanned 60 to 75 minutes postadministration of the tracer. Patients need to lie flat because the bore of the combined CT and PET scanners is longer than a standalone CT unit, the scanning couch has a long run and the couch cannot be as low in the bore as conventional CT scanners because of the table support mechanism. The patient breathes normally throughout the CT and PET elements of the scan, which takes approximately 30 minutes, although modern scanners can complete a scan in 6 minutes. Iterative reconstruction is used to reconstruct the images. Oral or intravenous contrast media is not used for a PET/CT scan.

Artefacts can occur in the area of the liver because of the difference in respiratory patterns in the CT and PET scans; patients are advised to breathe normally throughout both scans. Motion compensation can be used to avoid this

artefact. A wide-field CT image reconstruction, 70 cm instead of 50 cm, is required for the CT images or a truncation artefact can occur.

The CT element of the PET/CT scanner is a normal full-ring diagnostic CT scanner which can be used independently to the PET scanner. PET/CT cardiac studies require a diagnostic CT scan.

The complete system should be tested daily as part of the quality assurance programme, to check that the CT and PET elements are synchronised. Fig. 26.3 shows daily PET phantom testing.

Fig. 26.4 shows a PET/CT patient image.

26.6 THE POSITRON EMISSION TOMOGRAPHY/MAGNETIC RESONANCE IMAGING HYBRID SCANNER

Images from a PET/MRI hybrid scanner were first published in 2007. The logic of moving from a PET/CT hybrid to a PET/MRI hybrid is that MRI provides better contrast

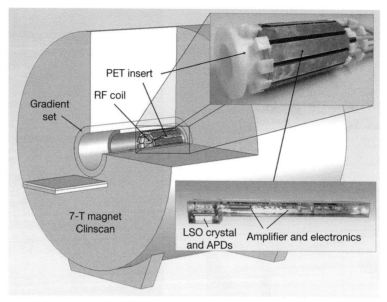

Fig. 26.5 Positron emission tomography (*PET*)/magnetic resonance imaging scanner. *APD,* avalanche photodiode detector; *LSO,* lutetium orthooxysilicate; *RF,* radio frequency.

in soft tissues than CT and therefore enhanced anatomical detail. MRI can also deliver specific information about molecular cell structure. One of the problems in designing such a hybrid scanner is that the photomultiplier tubes used in conventional PET scanners are very sensitive to magnetic fields. These photomultipliers are replaced in the hybrid scanner by solid-state scintillation detectors, silicon avalanche photodiode detectors. Heating is an issue in an MRI/PET, so scanners are water cooled to dissipate heat (see Fig. 26.5). Lutetium orthooxysilicate (LSO) PET crystals produce only small magnetic distortion. The unit consists of a PET scanner and an MRI scanner in the same housing, with the PET detector ring placed between the gradient and the radiofrequency body coil. PET attenuation correction based only on MRI data is challenging. The images from this type of scanner are still being evaluated but are producing encouraging results in neurological studies, where tumours are revealed earlier, and in more detail than with other scanners, and in oncology.

26.7 OTHER HYBRID SCANNER COMBINATIONS AND CURRENT RESEARCH

Efforts to develop an ultrasound/MRI hybrid are currently ongoing.

Hybrid interventional imaging with image intensifiers and cone-beam CT have been produced for operating theatres to aid surgeons during intervention ion procedures.

Another area of current research in hybrid imaging is the development of a multimodal contrast agent. This could be used to enhance specific areas in both scans and could also be used as markers to produce better control points for image alignment. At present only very limited clinical studies have been published.

SUMMARY

In this chapter, you should have learnt the following:
- The historical development of hybrid scanners (Section 26.3).
- The general operation of the SPECT/CT hybrid scanner (Section 26.4).
- The general operation of the PET/CT hybrid scanner (Section 26.5).
- The general operation of the PET/MRI scanner (Section 26.6).
- Areas of current research in the area of hybrid scanners (Section 26.7).

FURTHER READING

Most of the up-to-date material regarding hybrid scanners can be found on the Internet by searching for that particular mode of hybrid scanner. See also Chapter 19 in Cherry, S., Sorensen, J., & Phelps, M. (2012). Physics in nuclear medicine. 4th edn. Philadelphia: Saunders.

Medical informatics and radiology

CHAPTER CONTENTS

27.1 AIM

The aim of this chapter is to consider the principles of medical informatics within the radiology and medical imaging environment. Information technology (IT) systems have been deeply embedded in radiology practice for many decades. It is important to understand the IT systems available and how they can contribute to a more efficient radiology service. Computer technology in healthcare is constantly being developed, and an appreciation of potential future developments for medical imaging informatics is also important.

27.2 INTRODUCTION

Radiology is under increased pressure to add more value to medical imaging examinations, essentially, to provide more educated, accurate, useful and efficient interpretations in the face of increasingly large and complex imaging studies and to communicate this information quickly and in the most useful manner. Ultimately, radiology needs to be better, faster and cheaper if it is to continue to grow and survive.

In previous chapters we have seen the variety of imaging examinations available and that all medical imaging examinations are capable of producing significant quantities of data. These include both textual (i.e., reports/episode data) and image data that must be managed effectively. Medical informatics (MI), when applied to radiology, includes many of the processes needed to help achieve these goals. Medical imaging informatics is the develop-

ment, application and assessment of IT for radiological imaging. It includes the interfaces between IT and people. Within radiology departments MI is already deeply embedded in the requesting of examinations and in the reporting and disseminating of imaging findings. Picture archiving and communication systems (PACS) and radiology information systems (RIS) are readily available in almost all imaging departments and healthcare institutions. Despite the heavy reliance on MI systems, there can be significant variation in productivity between departments. To achieve the maximum possible benefits from MI, these systems must be fully understood by all users and carefully integrated into departmental workflows and practices.

27.3 HOSPITAL INFORMATION SYSTEMS

A hospital information system (HIS) is essentially an information management system used in hospitals and healthcare facilities. The HIS will generate a wealth of data around the clock, 365 days a year, all of which needs to be well managed to ensure efficient functionality. An HIS will include basic patient demographic data (name, address, age and gender) together with information on hospital admissions and visits to outpatient facilities and the emergency department. Such systems often include data on the patient's primary care physician and next of kin details. Such systems must be accurate, modifiable (for example, able to change a surname) and capable of communicating with a variety of associated systems, for example, laboratory management systems. Within private practice such systems will often have integrated commercial modules which can be used to track payments and help facilitate accounting. The key requirements of a modern HIS are described in Table 27.1.

Depending on the developer, cost and age of the HIS, a variety of add-on modules can be procured. Some examples of such additional 'add-on' modules are described in Table 27.2.

TABLE 27.1 Requirements of a modern health information system

Ability to use a unique patient identifier (unique reference number) or hospital reference number.
Facilitation of quick registration in times of emergency.
Facilitation of regulatory compliant data security, patient confidentiality and privacy.
Use of sound processes for access (passwords, smartcards and biometrics).
Ability to facilitate appropriate financial systems for reimbursement.
Ability to integrate with other systems (RIS, PACS, ORMIS).
Ability to review records securely, both on and off site.
Ability to track and request written (paper-based) hospital case notes.

ORMIS, operating room management information system; *PACS*, picture archiving and communications systems; *RIS*, radiology information system.

TABLE 27.2 Add-on modules for a hospital information system

Module	Description
Patient administration system (PAS)	Allows the management of preadmissions, waiting lists and bed management.
Master patient index	Allows the management of patient-related information (patient searches, merges and demergers) and the allocation of unique reference numbers.
Appointment scheduling	Manages the scheduling of patient events including admissions, investigations and procedures, and resources (human, equipment and facilities).
Patient billing	Important from a hospital's business perspective. Details chargeable items, waivers and discounts.
Financial accounting	Manages accounts payable, accounts received, cash management, purchase ordering, general ledger and budgetary control.
Equipment management system	Management of instruments (clinical and nonclinical) which require regular maintenance and occasional replacement.
Human resource management	Provides functionality for resource scheduling, payroll management, resource engagement and separation management.
Nursing management system	Provides functionality for general nursing information, bed management, order tracking, medication administration, patient assessment and classification.
Order management	Module for managing patient-related orders (radiology, laboratory, pharmacy, etc.).
Medication therapy evaluation	Module for the management of medications and usually reserved for inpatients. Prescribed medications are listed according to their recommended doses, route and schedule.
Operating theatre management	Specialist appointment system for operating theatres.
Laboratory information system	This module can be subdivided into pathology, microbiology, biochemistry, haematology, serology, etc. This allows the management of sample collection, specimen registration, work scheduling, results management, verification and reporting.
Blood bank	Manages orders for blood transfusion products.
Radiology information system (RIS)	Manages patient administration, examinations, reporting and system administration in relation to radiology processes. Supports workflows between imaging modalities and related information technology systems, i.e., PACS.
Picture archiving and communication system (PACS)	Medical imaging technology to securely store and digitally transmit images and clinically relevant reports.

27.4   RADIOLOGY INFORMATION SYSTEMS

RISs provide opportunities for recording when patients are scheduled for imaging examinations, when they arrive, when their examinations are ready for interpretation, when reports are finalised and information on all of the intermediate steps. Report turnaround time (RTT) is a commonly cited metric for quality and typically measures the time from examination completion to the finalised report.

27.5   PICTURE ARCHIVING AND COMMUNICATIONS SYSTEMS

A PACS is the whole system managing medical images and related data in a digital imaging and communications in medicine (DICOM)-compliant manner. In the medical imaging community, there are a number of different interpretations as to which components fall within the definition of a PACS. The following are normally considered components of a PACS:
- The acquisition modalities, for example, computed tomography (CT) and magnetic resonance imaging (MRI) scanners, ultrasound systems and digital radiography units.
- The imaging archive, known as the *PACS server.*

- Diagnostic workstations, which can be primary or secondary depending on the task.
- The network connecting the above components.

The principal components of a PACS are illustrated in Fig. 27.1.

27.6   DIGITAL IMAGING AND COMMUNICATIONS IN MEDICINE AND RADIOLOGY

DICOM is an international standard related to the exchange, storage and communication of digital medical images and other related media. DICOM seeks to achieve a number of goals including making medical imaging information interoperable and allowing the integration of image-acquisition devices, PACS, workstations, vendor neutral archives and printers. The freely available DICOM standard benefits from being actively developed and maintained to meet the demands of evolving technologies and requirements from the medical imaging community. The DICOM standard facilitates the interoperability of medical imaging equipment by specifying:
- For network communications, a set of protocols to be followed by connected devices.

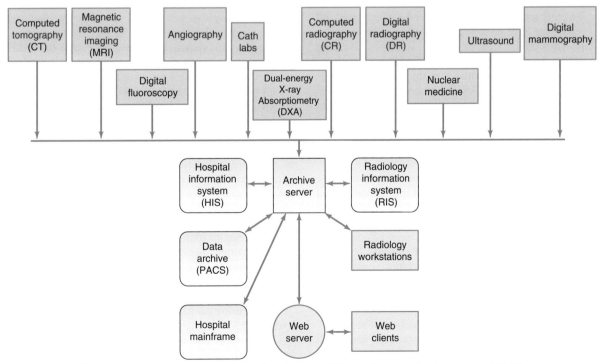

Fig. 27.1 Principal components of a typical picture archiving and communications system (*PACS*).

TABLE 27.3 Description of the main <u>d</u>igital imaging and <u>c</u>ommunications in <u>m</u>edicine (DICOM) services

DICOM service	Description
Verification	This is used to verify the connectivity between two DICOM devices. This is similar to the 'ping' command on a standard PC when checking that there is network connectivity.
Storage	Used to transfer DICOM images and other related digital data from one DICOM node to another. This allows the exchange of data among multiple devices over the DICOM network.
Storage Commitment	This is an advanced DICOM service allowing a DICOM application to request a commitment to a server for safekeeping of certain DICOM images and related data. This is a useful service when planning the deletion of patient data from an individual imaging modality. Before undertaking this task the modality sends a Storage Commitment request to the PACS server to check that the images have previously been stored on the archive and it is safe to locally delete the images.
Query/Retrieve	This service is used to query a DICOM archive in relation to its content. As its name implies this service is made up of two components. The query phase is technically a search of the PACS server. The retrieve phase is when the PACS server is requested to transfer the images to another DICOM node, e.g., an imaging workstation.

- The syntax and semantics of commands and associated information that can be exchanged using these protocols.
- For media communication, a set of media storage services to be followed as well as a file format and medical directory structure to facilitate access to the images and related information stored on interchangeable media.
- Information that must be supplied when implementing equipment meeting the DICOM standard.

Having computer standards within radiology is not new. Back in the early 1980s, the American College of Radiology (ACR) and the National Electrical Manufacturers Association (NEMA) formed a joint committee to develop communication of digital information and to facilitate the development and expansion of PACS and the interface with related systems.

The DICOM standard covers the formats that should be used for the storage of digital medical images and related digital data, and the protocols that need to be adopted to implement communication services which are useful in the medical imaging workflow.

The main objective of the DICOM standard is to ultimately allow cross-vendor interoperability amongst devices and information systems dealing with medical images. If all medical imaging vendors adhere to the DICOM standard, it should be possible for images to be sent from a CT scanner of vendor 'A' to a digital archive of vendor 'B' and be displayed on a diagnostic workstation of vendor 'C'. Within the standard there are four key DICOM services, which are detailed in Table 27.3.

27.7 ELECTRONIC PATIENT RECORD

In many healthcare institutions, new hospital-based clinical information systems are being implemented which are being commonly referred to as the *electronic patient record* (EPR). The EPR comprises a series of software applications which bring together key clinical and administrative data into one place. There are numerous benefits from implementing an EPR system; the main advantage is the ability of clinicians to view a patient's medical record when and where they need it. This removes the need for having to wait for paper-based hospital notes to be located and distributed. Further benefits include greater legibility of clinical information and increased accuracy of data. For example, the EPR systems have features for promoting the safer identification of patients at the bedside and confidentiality is also safeguarded through the strongest security measures for handling data. Access to EPR information is typically only available to users with a smartcard (similar to a chip and pin bank card) and a clinical relationship with the patient. Each time a patient's information is accessed, an electronic record of this is logged in the system. There are some limitations because while institutions develop their EPRs there will be a period of transition in which both electronic and paper-based records will be in operation and greater resources will be required.

When using an EPR system clinicians can be guided and supported through the process by:
- The development and use of decision-support systems, which can be built into EPR systems.

- Multidisciplinary electronic integrated care pathways.
- Protocols (local, national or international) embedded within the EPR system.

EPR systems can support quality and risk-management strategies, including clinical governance. Quality data for audit purposes can be extracted from them, providing access to up-to-date evidence and information about best practice at the point of clinical decision making. For example, the OptimiseRx tool developed by First Data Bank provides the option for integrating pharmaceutical-prescribing protocols within the EPR. With such a system any deviation from acceptable protocols, in terms of prescribing, would alert the clinician to the local guidance/evidence. Such systems are likely to be integrated into EPR systems for radiology referrals and again can look at imaging histories and local protocols before allowing the referrer to request examinations. An example of this would be whether a patient has had skeletal radiography before a referral for MRI.

27.8   DOSE MANAGEMENT SOFTWARE

Within medical imaging there are a growing number of radiation dose management software technologies (see Table 27.4) that can automatically gather and analyse information on a patient's exposure to medical ionising radiation. These technologies are designed to support the facilitation of the best diagnostic image quality while minimising the radiation exposure to the patient. In such systems, dose information can be collected from DICOM-compliant devices including:

- directly from the imaging device, for example, a specific CT scanner within a healthcare institution.
- by using PACS.
- from RIS records.

The most common methods used in dose management software for recording and analysing dose data are:

1. Through the Radiation Dose Structured Report (RDSR). This is contained within the DICOM dataset and has various dose-related parameters, for example, for CT scans the dose-length-product (DLP) and the volumetric CT dose index ($CTDI_{vol}$).
2. Modality-performed procedure steps (MPPS). This is a report generated by the imaging modality and contains information about the examination, including the number of images, scan length and the radiation dose delivered.
3. By using the image file header, which again is part of the DICOM dataset, and contains the general imaging acquisition parameters.

In the dose management software, the main functions are to collect, store and monitor radiation dose data across different imaging modalities, departments and hospitals. The dose data evaluated will typically be from CT scanners, interventional suites, cardiology catheter labs and other medical imaging equipment (typically focused around high-dose examinations).

Analyses from the captured data can include:
- Trends in the number of different examinations performed each year.
- Radiation doses for individual examinations and all examinations performed.
- Comparisons between patient-level data and population-based information on radiation dose.
- Set protocol-specific diagnostic reference levels.

From the analysis, reports can be generated, for example, on the range of doses given for each type of study to identify examinations with the highest dose.

TABLE 27.4   A description of the common dose management software solutions currently available

Software name (company)	Installation	Access	Modalities
DOSE (Qaelum)	Local	Web	CT, XA, DR, MG, RF, NM, PET
DoseM (Infinitt)	Local	Web	CT, XA, DR, MG, RF, NM, DXA
DoseMonitor (PACS Health)	Local	Web	CT, XA, DR, MG, RF, NM, DXA
DoseTRack (Sectra)	Cloud	Web	CT, CA, DR, MG, RF, PET
DoseWatch (GE Healthcare)	Local	Web	CT, XA, DR, MG, PET
DoseWise (Philips)	Local	App	CT, XA, DR, MG
OpenREM (OpenREM)	Local	Web	CT, CA, RG, DR, MG
Teamplay (Siemens Healthcare)	Local and cloud	Web	CT, XA, DR, MG, RF, NM, PET

CT, Computed tomography; DR, digital radiography; DXA, dual-energy X-ray absorptiometry; MG, mammography; NM, nuclear medicine; PET, positron emission tomography; RF, radiation fluoroscopy; XA, fluoroscopy.

27.9 ADVANCED INFORMATICS IN RADIOLOGY

Advances in technology have led to developments in image quality, review and analytical tools. These, together with image digitisation and mobile solutions, have changed the way we work within imaging departments. Such developments have provided new opportunities in how we view images and ultimately how we diagnose illness. The rationale for such developments has been focused not solely around clinical outputs but also on value. With this brings expectations for faster diagnosis and the greater availability of imaging data in an institution. Working with technologies has brought greater emphasis on efficiency in imaging workflows.

Modern radiology informatics allows the combined handling of CT, MRI, radiography, ultrasound, fluoroscopy and nuclear medicine data, even from multiple vendors, in a single multimodality viewing environment. This provides the opportunity for a fully immersive review of a patient from a single seat anywhere within the healthcare system. Such systems can provide the opportunity for complex three-dimensional modelling, image fusion, CT virtual colonoscopy, CT liver and lung analysis, diffusion and perfusion analysis and multimodality tumour tracking, to name but a few. Such applications play vital clinical roles in cardiovascular medicine, neurology and oncology.

Radiology report writing has also evolved with developments in technology, and reports are now almost exclusively dictated and electronically transcribed using voice recognition software. This brings the possibility of standardised reporting, and data mining to identify and respond to trends. Historically, reports were dictated on a tape recorder, transcribed by a medical secretary and then verified by the reporter (radiologist or radiographer), and this was a time-consuming process. Now, with electronic dictation (voice recognition), reports can be typed and verified almost immediately, speeding up patient throughput and time to diagnosis.

27.10 FUTURE OF RADIOLOGY INFORMATICS

The rapid growth in the amount of radiology data being recorded electronically brings opportunities for big data technologies, machine learning and artificial intelligence (AI).

Big data is a term that can be applied to an extremely large amount of data available to imaging departments. There is a future possibility that big data will allow smart

and intelligent RIS systems to be developed, providing assistance to reporters in terms of decision support, virtual quality assurance and forensic radiology. For example, patients presenting with acute right upper quadrant pain will be automatically triaged and scheduled for urgent ultrasound. Patients scheduled for hysterosalpingography appointments, after the date of the last menstrual period is entered, will have the best dates for conducting the examination automatically identified. Moving further forward, tagged areas on imaging examinations (for example, nodules on CT) can be intelligently compared on future scans for changes in volume. For certain pathologies (e.g., intracerebral bleeds), the system can be automatically set up to mention the size, shape and presence of midline shift.

With regards to machine learning there are a growing number of prominent applications within radiology. These include medical image segmentation, registration, computer-aided detection and diagnosis; brain function or activity analysis and neurological disease diagnosis from fMRI images; content-based image retrieval systems for CT and MRI images; and text analysis of radiology reports using natural language processing (NPL) and natural language understanding (NLU). Machine learning can identify complex patterns automatically and can help the reporter make intelligent decisions based on radiology data.

The principal focus of AI in radiology has been on improving diagnosis. Encouraging reports on this are frequently being published in the literature, and two AI systems have been reported as having human-level performance. Beyond improving diagnosis accuracy, AI systems can work in a number of additional areas. These could include assisting in the optimisation of worklists to prioritise key cases; preanalysis of high volume cases where observer fatigue may be a factor; extracting information from the image which is not apparent to the human eye; and improving the quality of reconstructed images. The final role of AI in radiology and its ultimate impact on reporters is not fully apparent. AI does provide a promising set of new tools for evaluating imaging data, and these should be explored to optimise patient care in future.

FURTHER READING

Dreyer, K.J., Hirschorn, D.S., Thrall, J.H., & Mehta, A. 2005. *PACS: A guide to the Digital Revolution.* New York: Springer.
Huang, H.K. 2010. *PACS and Imaging Informatics: Basic Principles and Applications.* Hoboken, NJ: John Wiley & Sons Inc.

Safety and protection for non-ionising radiations

CHAPTER CONTENTS

28.1   AIM

The aim of this chapter is to discuss the safety issues connected with those 'radiations' used in medical imaging which can be described as non-ionising. These are emanations which lack the ability to eject electrons from the shells of atoms and hence this chapter will not consider the effects of X-rays or gamma rays. The possible effects of the non-ionising radiations found in magnetic resonance imaging (MRI) and ultrasound may not seem so worrying for patients attending for examination or treatment but are nevertheless real and varied. These procedures are not thought to be cancer inducing, but MRI if undertaken carelessly can cause immediate fatality. Computed tomography (CT), by comparison, may present stochastic risks of cancer after a long latent period (see Section 21.7) but should not cause severe harm on the day of attendance. What do we mean by the term 'non-ionising radiations?' These include wave-like electromagnetic radiations such as radio waves, microwaves, ultraviolet, infrared and visible light. A further category includes static (constant) and time-varying (changing) electric or magnetic fields. Ultrasound is categorised as a form of non-ionising radiation within most medical imaging textbooks, although its properties are distinct from those of electromagnetic radiations (see Chapter 24). In general, the effects of MRI and ultrasound on the human body are mild and transient. However, their effects do increase with the magnitude of exposure (MRI field strength, ultrasound power output) and these effects may exhibit

threshold exposure levels below which no harm will occur. These dose-effect relationships are rather analogous to those of the deterministic (nonstochastic) effects observed during high dose X-ray exposures (see Chapter 21), although the term 'deterministic' effect is not typically applied to MRI or ultrasound. It is important to minimise risk by reducing the magnitude and likelihood of harm. This is achieved via published safety guidelines for MRI and ultrasound which set out recommended exposure limits and practices. Although these documents are not necessarily legal regulations, there is an expectation that they should be adhered to within the overall framework of health and safety in clinical practice. Failure to abide by published safety guidelines could be regarded as negligence in a court of law, in an instance where harm resulted to patients or staff.

28.2   MAGNETIC RESONANCE IMAGING SAFETY

Healthcare workers are often surprised to learn that injury or even death can occur as an immediate result of an MRI scan, although there is thought to be no risk of cancer. A patient is immersed in a powerful static (or unvarying) magnetic field which may be 60,000 times the magnitude of the earth's field in a 'high field' 3 tesla (T) scanner. He or she is also subjected to time-varying magnetic fields (which may create induced electrical currents) and bombarded with pulsed radiofrequency electromagnetic waves in the megahertz (MHz)

TABLE 28.1 The possible biological effects of magnetic resonance imaging	
Source of effect	**Effect**
Static (unvarying) magnetic field	Force exerted on ferromagnetic objects—resulting in motion
	Alteration of cardiac pacemaker function
	Altered cardiac electrocardiogram (ECG) waveform
	Nausea and vertigo at high field
	Magnetophosphenes ('flashing lights') affecting vision at high field
	Possible effects on concentration and memory ('mag lag')—but unproven
	Potential effects on the embryo in utero—but evidence from animal studies only
Changing (time-varying) magnetic fields	Induced electric fields and currents—nerve and muscle stimulation, associated heating owing to electrical resistance in conductive materials
Radiofrequency electro-magnetic waves	Tissue heating, especially at the skin surface and in conductive materials such as iron-containing tattoos

frequency range (which may induce heating). He or she may be startled by loud sounds which may reach over 100-decibels level, attributed to the action of the time-varying magnetic field gradients. There may also be feelings of claustrophobia and doses of gadolinium contrast media. There are in fact a wider range of biological effects to be found in MRI than in any other medical imaging procedure. Although this makes interesting physics, it can result in discomfort or even harm to the patient. Table 28.1 summarises the sources of the main non-ionising radiation effects in MRI.

28.2.1   Static magnetic fields

The effects of the main or constant magnetic field (termed B_0) of an MRI scanner increase directly with field strength. 'High field' magnets of 3 T are increasingly common in clinical MRI, and even more powerful magnets exist for research studies involving volunteers. Effects such as feelings of nausea and vertigo, as well as visual disturbances (called magnetophosphenes—'flashing lights' before the eyes) are more common in high field strength scanners but are typically absent in low field scanners. These changes may cause slight discomfort but are temporary and will disappear when the patient leaves the scanner. Reports of slight headaches are inconsistent. Nausea and visual disturbances are most pronounced when the patient moves within the field. A few published articles have reported a phenomenon known as 'mag lag', this being a loss of memory and concentration, affecting both patients and staff. However, this mag lag effect is unproven and has even been noted in a wooden 'mock-up' of an MRI scanner. It is a good precaution to prepare patients for the previously mentioned minor possible effects. Much more serious is the so-called 'projectile effect' which causes ferromagnetic materials (such as iron, cobalt and nickel) to line up parallel to the magnetic field (experiencing a 'torque' or twisting force) and to be attracted to its strongest point of the field. This can cause objects such as scissors or even oxygen cylinders to be propelled at up to 40 miles per hour (65 kilometres per hour) as they fly across the scanner room towards the magnet isocentre, with occasional fatal consequences. Within the patient's body, ferromagnetic shrapnel, surgical aneurysm clips or intraocular foreign particles can move and cause injury. It is for this reason that metal surgical implants inserted since the 1980s have been of nonferromagnetic titanium alloy. The static magnetic field may also affect the function of cardiac pacemakers at a field strength of a little over 5 gauss (0.5 mT), causing several reported fatalities. Although the projectile effect is well known, fewer people are aware that the static magnetic field can also produce changes in the cardiac electrocardiogram (ECG) waveform and in blood pressure. The waveform becomes much more 'spikey' and irregular and in particular the T-wave amplitude is raised. This is caused in part by the 'magnetohydrodynamic' effect, which affects induced electrical potentials in flowing blood, but subsides when the patient is removed from the scanner.

MRI is not recommended in the first trimester of pregnancy. This is because some animal experiments have suggested possible reductions in birth weight or length following exposure to strong or time-varying magnetic fields. The evidence is inconclusive and might not be applicable to humans; however, there are possible theoretical mechanisms by which cells and ions in a developing embryo might be affected by powerful magnetic fields. It is reassuring to note that no published study of pregnant MRI staff or patients has yet indicated any significant detriment from MRI scanning of the child in utero. It should also be remembered that in the case of a clinical emergency, MRI would be regarded as a safer option than CT during the first trimester of pregnancy because pelvic CT involves deterministic effects at embryonic doses greater than 100 mGy. The International Commission on Non-Ionizing Radiation Protection

(ICNIRP) has set normal, controlled and research limits for static magnetic field exposure to patients and volunteers of 4 T, 8 T and above 8 T respectively. Little is known about the effects of fields above 4 T on infants or fetuses. Most clinical MRI scanners do not exceed 3 T.

It should be noted that the field strength of each MRI scanner has a set value in practice, determined by its design features; this field cannot be varied to suit individual patients. It is recommended that effects such as vertigo are reduced by restricting the speed at which patients are brought into or out of an MRI scanner. In view of the previously mentioned effects of static magnetic fields on pacemakers and ferromagnetic implants, all regulatory agencies recommend that strict screening and control of patient and public access to an MRI scanner area must be applied. It must be remembered that most MRI scanners are of a 'superconducting' category and are 'on' 24 hours a day, 7 days a week. In fact they cannot be turned off without a costly 'quenching' away of liquid helium. A controlled area exists around the scanner, set at the 0.5 mT (5 gauss) magnetic field strength contour, and no patient, member of the public or staff member can enter this unless they have been magnetic resonance (MR) safety screened by a trained operator using a questionnaire. This field strength limit is chosen to avoid effects on pacemakers or other implanted medical devices. Additionally, access to the controlled area is by lockable doors or other physical restrictions. The United Kingdom Medicines and Healthcare Products Regulatory Agency (MHRA) also defines a 3 mT (30 gauss) inner controlled area, into which no ferromagnetic object may be brought, to avoid the 'projectile effect'.

INSIGHT

Metal items that may be brought into the controlled area of a magnetic resonance imaging (MRI) scan room are generally classified as magnetic resonance (MR) safe, MR conditional (safe provided precautions are applied) or MR unsafe. This situation is complicated by the fact that items which may be tested as MR safe in a 1 tesla (T) scanner may be unsafe at 3 T. Also, there may be composition differences within batches of items such as metallic aneurysm clips, even from the same manufacturer. Implants such as hip pins are unlikely to move within the MR magnet, provided that they are adequately fixed at surgery. Recent improvements in pacemaker design have made most modern pacemaker devices MR conditional, meaning that they may be safe to scan under certain conditions, whereas older designs are MR unsafe. These issues present challenges for safe working practice within the MRI community. It is important that people with pacemakers and other insertions are not denied the facility of MRI diagnosis, while also avoiding MR-related injury.

28.2.2 Time-varying magnetic fields

Magnetic fields of time-varying and distance-varying amplitude are applied across a patient during the course of an MRI scan, by gradient coils which perform functions such as slice and pixel localisation and gradient echo (signal) formation. These gradients induce electric fields and currents in body tissues, which are proportional to the frequency and rate of change of the applied time-varying magnetic fields. The electrical permittivity and conductivity of tissue also influence the magnitude of the induced currents. Larger currents can be expected in highly conductive tissues, tattoos (which may contain metal particles) or metal implants. As MRI technology has developed, the amplitude and rate of change of the time-varying magnetic fields have increased and patients are more commonly experiencing tingling, twitching or spasm during scan procedures. This indicates that induced electrical conduction is occurring in nerves and muscles. However these currents are an order of magnitude lower than those that would be needed to cause heart muscle fibrillation. There are ICNIRP and International Electrotechnical Commission (IEC) limits for patient and volunteer exposures to time-varying magnetic fields. In terms of the IEC definitions, the normal limit (no physiological stress risk) is set at 80% of the value for peripheral nerve stimulation. The 'first level controlled operating mode' (at which there may be physiological stress) is set at 100% of the value for peripheral nerve stimulation, whereas a 'second level controlled mode' (at which there may be significant risk) exceeds it. Nerve and muscle stimulation appears to be unaffected by body age, size and fat content. The induced currents in metal pigment-containing tattoos and surgical implants might contribute to heating—in fact burns have been reported to patients' tattooed skin. The strength of induced currents in tissues is increased if conductive 'loops' are created, for example, if the patient's legs are touching or the hands are clasped together. This has even been known to cause skin burns. Incidentally, the time-varying magnetic fields cause the gradient coils to flex and bang during MRI, creating a lot of sound and requiring patients to wear ear protection at levels above 85 decibels.

INSIGHT

Magnetic gradient performance, expressed by amplitude, rise time and slew rate (rate of change of magnetic field), is a less well-known scanner specification than field strength but is a very important factor to consider when defining overall scanner performance. High specification gradients have the advantages of permitting small fields of view and thin slices (improving image resolution) and also permitting rapid scanning. Many of the imaging sequences used in magnetic resonance (MR) functional imaging are fast gradient echo techniques, sometimes acquiring each image in a 'single shot', as in echo planar imaging. This is all good news for scan capability but may expose patients to greater induced currents. Gradient and radiofrequency-induced burns are usually the largest category of MR safety incident.

28.2.3   Radiofrequency electromagnetic radiation

Radio waves of about 21 to 127 MHz frequency (at 0.5- to 3-T magnetic field) are directed into a patient during an MRI scan. As the radio waves pass through the patient, electrical resistivity effects cause tissue heating. The energy transfer to the patient's body is expressed in watts per kilogram and is termed the specific absorption rate (SAR). The heating effect increases with the radio wave frequency, which in turn is proportional to magnetic field strength, because the frequency needed for magnetic resonance increases with it, according to the Larmor equation (see Chapter 25). Heating also depends on the number and amplitude of radio wave 'pulses' applied within a given time, as well as on the patient's size and weight. Particular care is needed when scanning infants and other patients with a reduced thermoregulatory capacity, and SAR limits are set automatically by MRI scanners to ensure that core body temperature cannot rise by more than 1° C. Superficial tissues such as the eye and testes may be especially vulnerable to temperature rises. Although human data are limited, animal experiments have indicated that deep tissue temperature rises might reach 4° C in some circumstances. The ICNIRP and IEC have set limits for whole body temperature rises in MRI. The ICNIRP levels are illustrated by Table 28.2. Temperature rises are controlled by restriction of SAR levels in scanners, especially by restricting the magnitude and number of RF pulses.

> **INSIGHT**
>
> Fast spin echo pulse sequences and additional pulses (for example, fat saturation pulses) place more radiofrequency (RF) energy into the patient's body. This situation provides another potential 'trade-off' between scan quality and safety. Tissue heating does not result from the 'relaxation' of hydrogen nuclei after an RF pulse is applied (see Chapter 25). In fact the oscillating RF causes charged ions in body tissues to move, generating tiny electrical currents, which in turn cause heating. Thus the heating can be termed a resistive effect. This heating effect will tend to be more pronounced at high field strength because the RF frequency will be increased, according to the Larmor equation, and the electromagnetic field oscillation rate will be greater. Cooling can be achieved by blood flow, which may differ between patients. It is interesting to note that induced currents and consequent heating should be greater in tissues with a high iron content, such as the liver.

28.2.4   Magnetic resonance contrast media

MR contrast media most commonly contain gadolinium ions (Gd^{3+}) which are paramagnetic (weakly reinforce the magnetic field) and shorten tissue longitudinal relaxation times at T1 imaging, causing brightening. This is valuable for demonstrating lesions such as tumours and abscesses. These media are rather safer overall than the iodine-containing media used in CT, owing to reduced overall osmotic load and reduced incidence of anaphylactic reactions. However, the MR community was affected by a scare in 2007, when it became clear that so-called linear chelates such as Omniscan could release free (and highly toxic) gadolinium ions into body tissues in patients with very poor renal function. This effect appeared to be related to altered pH (acidity) and resulted in a very damaging condition termed nephrogenic systemic fibrosis (NSF). Linear chelates have now been replaced by cyclic chelates such as gadovist and dotarem. Equally concerning is the fact that linear chelates may release gadolinium into the human

TABLE 28.2   International Commission on Non-Ionizing Radiation Protection limits for whole body temperature rise in magnetic resonance imaging

Operating mode	Temperature rise limit
Normal mode—patients and volunteers	0.5° C
Controlled mode with monitoring—patients and volunteers	1° C
Research/experimental mode—volunteers	>1° C

brain, as revealed by scans of patients who have received numerous previous MR contrast procedures.

28.2.5 Claustrophobia

Most superconducting magnet designs offer a very enclosed environment and scan times are long in MRI compared with CT. As a result, many patients experience claustrophobia, which is severe enough to cause the scan procedure to be abandoned in about 5% of examinations. This can be alleviated by thorough explanations and reassurance, personal contact and 'feet first' patient positioning. Some scanner designs are more 'open' at each end of the scanner bore, reducing claustrophobic effects but also limiting the length of the 'homogeneous' magnetic field. Field homogeneity is important for maintaining resonant conditions between the applied RF field and the precessing nuclear spins, thereby achieving a high signal-to-noise ratio.

28.3 ULTRASOUND SAFETY

Although a wide range of adverse effects have been claimed for medical ultrasound at various times in published studies, these have not been proven conclusively. Ultrasound is a very safe method of examination when undertaken in accordance with published safety guidelines. Sound waves are not electromagnetic radiations or fields; they consist of vibrations that pass through matter and cause the substance of that matter to compress and rarefy. Ultrasound refers to sound waves with a frequency greater than 20 kHz, and sound frequencies in the 1 MHz to 20 MHz range may be used in diagnostic imaging. The body presents 'opposition', partly in the form of acoustic impedance, to the passage of sound waves and as a result energy is transferred from the sound waves to the body,

via heating and cavitation. Rigid tissues such as bone provide more opposition than soft tissues and thus they will experience a greater temperature rise. Also, tissues adjacent to bone, or to the ultrasound probe, will experience heating attributed to heat conduction. We saw in Section 28.2 that many effects of MRI involve the whole of the patient's body within the scanner, but in ultrasound the effects are localised to those body parts directly within the ultrasound beam. The intensity of the beam decreases as energy is transferred to tissues during passage through the body and thus body parts closer to the ultrasound probe or transducer will tend to receive more energy than those which lie deeper.

The physical mechanisms are complex but ultrasound energy transfer to body tissues will be increased by:
- High transducer (probe) power output
- Use of a wide ultrasound beam
- Use of a stationary transducer (e.g., in Doppler studies)
- Long scan time
- High sound frequency
- Tissue proximity to the transducer
- High tissue density or rigidity (e.g., bone)
- The presence of microbubbles in fluids (e.g., because of the use of bubble-producing contrast media).

28.3.1 Heating effects

As mentioned previously, the passage of ultrasound through the human body creates a heating effect. Tissues which have a low thermal conductivity and poor blood perfusion can be expected to heat up more. The developing embryo or fetus in the womb is especially vulnerable to temperature rises, both because tissues are developing and because the unborn child has a poor capacity to dissipate heat. Tissues at risk from heating in fetuses, infants and adults include bone (and tissue adjacent to it), brain and the eye. The 'thermal index' (TI) is an indication of the magnitude of the acoustic power being applied compared with that acoustic power which would cause a tissue temperature rise of 1° C. So $TI = W/W_{deg}$, where W is the applied power and W_{deg} is the power needed to cause a 1° C temperature rise. In adults, local temperatures of less than 43° C can normally be tolerated in tissues, but the developing embryo or fetus may be at risk of harm if the temperature reaches 41° C for about 5 minutes. The IEC publishes standards for reporting acoustic outputs but does not specify maximum permissible TI values. The IEC does specify that the temperature of the ultrasound probe should not exceed 43° C when in contact with body tissue. In reality it is hard to predict actual temperature values at depth in particular tissues or patients. As a result, the use of thermal indices (which are displayed by ultrasound scanners during operation) is designed to restrict likely temperature rises in patients to levels below those which could cause harm. It is the sonographer's responsibility to pay attention to TI values during scanning. Thermal indices for bone and soft tissue may be displayed separately by scanners. The average thermal indices for bone may be up to four times greater within pulsed Doppler ultrasound scans than in B-mode ultrasound. But the average thermal indices for soft tissue are only marginally greater within Doppler scans. The British Medical Ultrasound Society (BMUS) recommends that during obstetric ultrasound, thermal indices should not exceed 3.0 and scans need to be time-limited above a value of 0.7. It should be noted overall that the routine use of medical diagnostic ultrasound is unlikely to result in hazardous heating levels.

28.3.2   Cavitation effects

Sound waves exert an 'acoustic pressure' on tissues, which is the difference between atmospheric pressure and the local pressure caused by the ultrasound beam. This pressure can be positive (during compression) or negative (during rarefaction). Negative pressure is used within the definition of the mechanical index (MI), which is another measure displayed by ultrasound scanners during operation. As used in practice, MI is proportional to peak rarefaction and is a dimensionless quantity. MI values are smallest at higher ultrasound frequencies. The MI is important because large values increase the likelihood of 'cavitation'. What do we mean by cavitation? This term refers to processes by which high energy sound waves can cause bubbles to form, oscillate, expand and collapse. During the collapse of bubbles, there may be very high local temperatures and pressures (within a tiny volume), causing mechanical damage to cells and the formation of free radicals. Free radicals are very chemically reactive atoms, ions or atomic groups that have a lone unpaired electron. Cavitation effects are unlikely in most body tissues at diagnostic ultrasound energies, unless bubble-forming ultrasound contrast media are present. Bubble collapse could potentially damage cell membranes and capillary walls. Fortunately, cavitation is most likely to occur in extracellular fluid and thus any free radicals formed are unlikely to affect cellular DNA (free radical damage to DNA is a major cause of risk resulting from the intracellular absorption of X-rays). In addition, cavitation within a cell would likely result in cell death. Cells need to survive and suffer DNA mutation damage for cancer to be initiated and thus there is unlikely to be a cancer risk from

cavitation in ultrasound. The lungs are potentially an at-risk tissue for cavitation effects, because of the presence of air and fluid. The BMUS recommends that during obstetric ultrasound, MIs above 0.3 might risk minor damage to the fetal lungs and values above 0.7 carry a risk of cavitation when using ultrasound contrast media.

INSIGHT

Microbubble contrast agents can be used in ultrasound to improve the echogenicity (echo production) of the vasculature, providing more signal. The carrier particles often consist of albumin or phospholipids and the contained bubbles are typically perfluoropropane gas. The bubbles, whose diameter is measured in microns, oscillate in size in response to mechanical pressures created by the passage of ultrasound waves, and the effect is greatest when sound is applied at the resonant frequency of this oscillation. This can result in cavitation collapse of the bubbles which is of low risk in diagnostic studies but can be used therapeutically in association with high energy-focused ultrasound to ablate unwanted tissue.

28.3.3   Streaming

Acoustic streaming is thought to be a relatively minor factor as far as the biological effects of ultrasound are concerned. It arises in fluid attributed to differences in radiation pressure across an ultrasound beam, both with depth and width. This can result in a movement of fluid. In theory streaming might affect molecular transport but evidence for this is weak in vivo.

28.3.4   Developmental effects

Because ultrasound is routinely used in pregnancy, a number of research studies have examined the possible effects of ultrasound on fetal and child development. The potential mechanism for any such effects would be heating in utero. There is no conclusive evidence for any significant effect on birth weight, dyslexia, attention deficit, speech development, neurological development, hearing, sight, left-handedness or school performance. Research may be biased by the fact that complicated pregnancies (which might potentially result in subsequent effects) can often be accompanied by more ultrasound scanning. Some published studies have suffered from methodological weaknesses. Thus despite occasional alarms in the press and media concerning the use of ultrasound in pregnancy, firm evidence of detrimental effects is lacking.

SUMMARY

In this chapter, you should have learnt the following:

- Non-ionising radiations are encountered in MRI. They are not believed to cause cancers but do present a wide range of biological effects and hazards. Most effects are mild and transient. In general the effects are determined by the magnitude of exposure and occur above a threshold value.

- The biological effects of MRI include tissue heating and induced electrical currents. Ferromagnetic objects including patient implants may be subject to motion, termed the 'projectile effect' and this can be harmful in some circumstances. Occasional deaths have been reported in MRI, mostly because of the effects of the main magnetic field on pacemakers. Other effects of MRI include acoustic noise and claustrophobia.

- Diagnostic ultrasound may cause tissue heating, cavitation (microbubble formation and collapse) and streaming of fluid. These effects are not thought to be harmful so long as operators restrict the output of the ultrasound probe to safe levels.

FURTHER READING

Gibbs, V., Cole, D., & Sassano, A. 2009. *MRI – Ultrasound Physics and Technology: How, Why and When.* London: Churchill Livingstone.

Medicines and Healthcare Products Regulatory Agency. 2015. *Safety Guidelines for Magnetic Resonance Imaging Equipment in Clinical Use.* London: MHRA.

McRobbie, D. 2020. *Essentials of MRI Safety.* Chichester: John Wiley.

Wood, A., & Karipidis, K. 2017. *Non-ionizing Radiation Protection: Summary of Research and Policy Options.* Oxford: Wiley–Blackwell.

Putting it all together—showing tissues with science

29.1 AIM

Radiological physics is not a theoretical subject—its 'reason for being' is to display human body tissues by differentiating between their properties. The aim of this chapter is to apply the science coverage of the previous sections of this book, by considering the broad spectrum of ways in which medical imaging modalities can depict normal and pathological tissues. Visualisation is achieved by obtaining a signal difference between living substances, which we can term 'contrast' in a broad range of situations. Depiction can be anatomical, which is based on the physical and biochemical structure of tissues, or functional, obtained via imaging of properties such as metabolic rate, molecular concentration, blood flow and water diffusion. Imaging methods such as 'plain' or conventional X-ray and computed tomography (CT) are chiefly anatomical depiction approaches, although both can image tissue blood flow/perfusion via radiological contrast enhancement. Radionuclide imaging (RNI), including single photon emission tomography (SPECT) and positron emission tomography (PET), is principally a functional approach, although it can be fused with CT via hybrid imaging to provide an 'anatometabolic' imaging capability (see Chapter 26). Ultrasound and magnetic resonance imaging (MRI) have special properties because they are able to provide both anatomical and metabolic information, via a range of techniques.

29.2 ANATOMICAL DEPICTION USING SCIENCE

29.2.1 Depiction using X-rays

X-ray imaging, whether it be in 'plain' (or conventional) radiography or CT, is based on the attenuation of X-ray photons by body tissue (see Chapter 13). This in turn is related to the atomic number, density, thickness, and in the case of X-ray scatter, to the electron density, of that tissue.

The atomic numbers of atoms found in the body, or in contrast media introduced into the body, are especially important to X-ray attenuation at low kVp values because photoelectric absorption is a key factor at low kVp. Table 29.1 displays the atomic numbers of some elements that are commonly found in the body and/or in radiographic contrast media. Both in conventional radiography and in CT, use of a reduced kVp can help to emphasise atomic number differences between tissues, by increasing relative absorption differences. We saw in Chapter 18 that low-energy X-rays of about 20 keV are used in mammography to demonstrate microcalcifications in the breast. Table 29.1 indicates that fat can be expected to have a slightly lower 'average' atomic number than, for example, water or protein because it contains relatively more carbon. Haemorrhage, liver and spleen will have a higher average atomic number than most soft tissue, because they contain more iron and will therefore appear bright on CT (see Fig. 29.1).

TABLE 29.1 Atomic numbers of some important elements	
Element	**Where found**
Hydrogen Z = 1	In most tissues, including in fats, carbohydrates, proteins, water
Carbon Z = 6	In most tissues and especially in fats
Nitrogen Z = 7	In most tissues in small amounts and especially in proteins
Oxygen Z = 8	In most tissues and especially in water
Phosphorus Z = 15	Especially in bone
Calcium Z = 20	Especially in bone and calcified tissue
Iron Z = 26	Especially in haemorrhage, liver, spleen
Iodine Z = 53	In contrast media and the thyroid
Barium Z = 56	In contrast media

Body tissues consist of a mix of different elements and hence we need to think in terms of an 'average' atomic number for tissues such as fat or bone, which can be difficult to calculate owing to variations in tissue composition and atomic number measurement. However, Table 29.2 provides some indicative average atomic numbers and densities for different tissues. These values may vary a little depending on the technicalities involved in their estimation, but the following points emerge:

- There will be good X-ray contrast between air and body tissues attributed to a large density difference.
- There will be good X-ray contrast between bone and soft tissue, particularly at low kV, because of a large average atomic number difference (photoelectric absorption is proportional to Z^3).
- There will be X-ray contrast between fat and other soft tissues, especially in CT, because fat has a lower average atomic number and density (see Fig. 29.1).
- There will be poor X-ray contrast between most soft tissues because their average atomic numbers and densities are similar.

INSIGHT

People often talk about the speed and resolution of computed tomography, but its main advantage is that it amplifies the visible image contrast between body tissues. It does this in various ways. Firstly it reduces the effects of X-ray scatter, by the use of pre- and postpatient collimators, metal partitions between detector elements and 'tidying' of the image during mathematical postprocessing. Secondly it removes the obscuring superimposition of organs that occurs during 'plain' X-ray imaging, obtaining a sectional 'slice'. Thirdly it converts small X-ray attenuation coefficient differences between body tissues into a scale of relative signal intensities, termed the Hounsfield scale.

At high kVp, photoelectric absorption becomes less important in body tissues although it is still maintained in high atomic number elements such as iodine and barium. At high kVp, Compton scatter becomes the predominant X-ray attenuation mechanism in body tissues, and it is

TABLE 29.2 Some indicative 'average' atomic numbers and densities for body tissues and air		
Tissue	**'Average' atomic number**	**Density g/cm³**
Air	About 7	0.001
Fat	About 6	0.9
Water	About 7	1.0
Soft tissues	About 7	1.03–1.06
Cortical bone	About 14	1.8

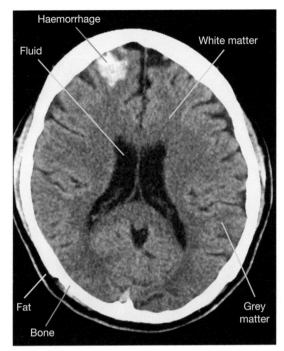

Fig. 29.1 A computed tomography (CT) scan of the head. This image demonstrates the X-ray attenuation differences among fat (Hounsfield units −100), fluid (Hounsfield units zero), haemorrhage (Hounsfield units +200) and bone (Hounsfield units +500 plus) in a CT head scan at 120 kVp. It is hard to discriminate attenuation differences between white and grey matter, although the former will attenuate X-rays a bit less, owing to the presence of fatty myelin.

proportional to the electron densities of those tissues. Table 29.3 shows the electron densities of some important tissues. This indicates that at high kV, image contrast will still exist among lung, fat, other soft tissues and bone, as is indeed the case in CT, which typically uses kVp values in the range of 120 to 140.

TABLE 29.3 Some electron densities for body tissues and air

Tissue	Electron density $\times 10^{23}$/cm^3
Air	0.004
Lung	2.3
Fat	3.1
Water, most soft tissues	3.3–3.4
Liver, thyroid, haemorrhage	3.5–3.6
Bone	5.5

INSIGHT

Within the Compton scatter process, X-rays can interact with any of the electrons orbiting an atom, in inner or outer electron shells. Compton scatter is proportional to electron density. It might be thought that electron density would rise directly in line with atomic number because the number of electrons found in neutral atoms equals the number of protons in the nucleus. But in fact the electron density of atoms (excluding hydrogen) does not vary much between elements because density relates to the number of electrons per unit volume and the volume of atoms rises overall in accordance with their electron number. In practice the electron density of tissues relates more closely to how densely the atoms are 'packed' together, than to the size of these atoms. Atoms are much less closely packed together in air or lung than in the crystalline matrix of bone.

X-ray imaging is mainly based on just a single tissue characteristic—X-ray attenuation. By comparison, magnetic resonance imaging makes use of a much wider range of tissue properties.

29.2.2 Depiction using magnetic resonance imaging

The simplest tissue property observable using MRI is termed 'proton density'. This is a bit misleading and could perhaps be better termed 'hydrogen density' because it refers to the numbers of hydrogen nuclei contained per unit volume of body tissue (see Fig. 29.2). Protons are found in the nuclei of all elements, but it is only hydrogen nuclei which are employed in MRI. Hydrogen is found in most body tissues, within water, fats, proteins, carbohydrates, cartilage and even in cortical bone. In practice, MRI can only obtain signal from 'free' or 'mobile' hydrogen nuclei which are not tightly bound in rigid molecular structures.

INSIGHT

Hydrogen nuclei within water and fat provide lots of signal in magnetic resonance imaging (MRI), whereas hydrogen nuclei in fibrocartilage and cortical bone do not, resulting in signal 'voids'. This is because the hydrogen atoms in fat and water are not bound too tightly in their respective molecules. Their nuclei are termed 'mobile protons' which have some freedom of movement and are hence able to transfer magnetisation between each other. This permits a 'decay' of magnetisation which provides signal in MRI after the radiofrequency excitation pulse is turned off (see Chapter 25). If hydrogen atoms are rigidly bound in crystalline structures such as bone, their nuclei are termed 'restricted' or 'bound' protons. These protons are held in such close proximity to each other that transfer of magnetisation occurs very rapidly between them. This results in a decay of magnetisation which occurs too quickly for signal to be received and sampled. It should be noted that the 'free' protons do not wander about—they are contained in hydrogen atoms which are covalently bound to carbon or oxygen atoms in fat and water molecules, respectively.

MRI does not just obtain signal from water molecules. In fact fat has a similar proton density (hydrogen density) to water, as shown by Table 29.4. The percentage composition of hydrogen by weight in both water and fat is about 11% and this similarity can be explained by thinking about their chemical structures. Fat molecules contain long chains of $-CH_2-$ groups, whereas water consists of H_2O. In both cases the amount of 'H' is similar. In clinical practice, proton density-weighted MRI is often used to show increases in water content within tissues, such as occur in brain tumours, 'strokes' and multiple sclerosis, especially if the competing high signal from fat is 'saturated' out (suppressed). It should also be mentioned that adipose tissue (fatty tissue) contains water in addition to fat. Lung tissue is not well seen using MRI, because its low proton (hydrogen) density provides very limited signal. Cortical bone does not provide signal, because its available hydrogen nuclei are restricted rather than mobile.

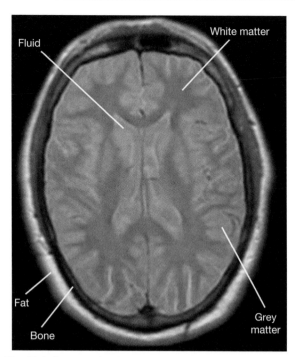

Fig. 29.2 A proton density magnetic resonance imaging (MRI) scan of the head. This image demonstrates that both fat and fluid have a high signal on proton density-weighted imaging in MRI, attributed to their high mobile hydrogen content. White matter has a lesser proton density than grey matter and hence appears less bright. Cortical bone provides a signal void because of the presence of tightly bound hydrogen.

MRI is very good at depicting the fat and water content of different tissues, via 'T1 weighting' which depicts fat as bright and 'T2 weighting' which depicts water as bright (see Chapter 25). But this is not achieved by comparing their proton densities. Separation is achieved based on their magnetic spin relaxation times, which are fast for fat and slow for water. Essentially the magnetisation in fat, which is achieved after the application of a RF pulse, disappears quickly, whereas that in water is retained for a longer period. The term 'relaxation' (or recovery) in MRI refers to a decay in the overall magnetisation of a tissue sample, both in the longitudinal and transverse planes.

TABLE 29.4   Relative mobile proton densities (hydrogen densities) of some body tissues

Tissue	Relative mobile proton density
Water	100
Fat	Similar to water
Brain tumour	85–90
Multiple sclerosis lesion	85
Grey matter of the brain	80
White matter of the brain	70
Lung	10
Cortical bone	<1

INSIGHT

The differences between the relaxation times for fat and water can be understood in terms of their structural properties. Hydrogen nuclei can be considered as magnetic dipoles, which may interact depending on their distance apart and their relative motion. A magnetic property, here termed a dipole, exists in association with a proton because there is a looped flow of charge as the proton rotates. In fat, the hydrogen nuclei (single protons) are held in close proximity, attached to long chains of carbon atoms, and hence the dipole–dipole interactions are strong. This gives rapid spin relaxation. In water, the hydrogen nuclei are in greater state of relative motion within the fluid and in lesser proximity. Thus their dipole–dipole interactions are weak and spin relaxation is slow.

TABLE 29.5 Relative values of ultrasound reflection at different tissue boundaries

Tissue boundary	Percentage of sound reflected
Liver/kidney	0.01%
Soft tissue/water	0.2%
Fat/muscle	1%
Bone/soft tissue	40%
Soft tissue/air	99%

Fat depiction in MRI is very useful for showing human anatomy because many organs and tissues are separated by fat. Water depiction in MRI is very powerful for outlining disease processes because pathologies such as tumour, cyst, oedema and inflammation tend to have an increased water content. MRI can also depict the fat and water content of tissues by making use of a property known as 'phase'. The spins associated with hydrogen nuclei in water rotate at a faster rate than those of hydrogen nuclei in fat. This precessional speed difference (not to be confused with relaxation times) is an example of a 'chemical shift' and is because electrons within an O–H chemical bond are held further away from the hydrogen nucleus than in a C–H chemical bond, thereby exposing the hydrogen to a slightly greater magnetic field in a magnetic resonance (MR) magnet. It was mentioned in Chapter 25 that the rotational speed of spins is proportional to the magnetic field strength, according to the Larmor equation. Imagine for a moment that the fat and water spins are like two cars travelling around a circular racetrack. Every so often the faster car (fat) will be alongside the slower car (water) and the two spins can be termed 'in phase'. At other times they will be at different points on the track and not side-by-side, a state that can be termed 'out of phase'. The consequence of this is that if fat and water are in phase within the same tissue voxel, there is bright signal, whereas if they are out of phase there is loss of signal. 'In phase–out of phase imaging' will show signal loss at some echo sampling times if fat and water exist in the same voxel (e.g., if there is some replacement of fat by tumour in an adrenal gland) but will give a constant signal if there is only fat.

29.2.3 Depiction using ultrasound

Ultrasound imaging depends upon sound reflections at boundaries between tissues of different density and hence upon their different acoustic impedance values (see Chapter 24). Table 29.5 shows the relative sizes of these reflections. Reflections do not occur within a homogeneous medium such as water. As mentioned earlier, fat has a lower X-ray attenuation than that of other soft tissues as a result of its reduced density. Similarly in ultrasound fat has a lower acoustic impedance than other soft tissues, again owing to its reduced density. Thus it is possible to obtain sound reflections at fat/muscle boundaries, as shown in Fig. 29.3. Strong echoes produced at dense structures such as stones in the body can be useful in revealing their presence, via acoustic shadows. Sound intensity falls off with increasing depth in body tissue, to a greater extent than does X-ray intensity in CT, with sound of low frequency having greater penetrative ability, but reduced anatomical resolution capability, than sound of high frequency. Anatomical depiction can be improved by the use

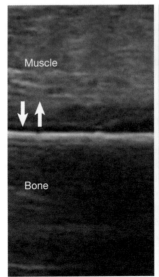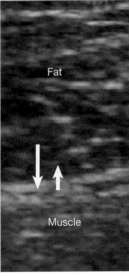

Fig. 29.3 Ultrasound reflections at tissue boundaries. The boundary between muscle and bone produces a lot of sound reflection (*arrows*), giving a bright layer on the image with not much sound received from beneath the bone barrier. By comparison, less sound is reflected at the boundary between fat and muscle, permitting deeper transmission of sound and enabling echoes to be received from within both tissues.

of microbubble-producing contrast agents, which generate a lot of extra reflections and can be useful in specialist applications such as ultrasound of the liver.

29.3   FUNCTIONAL DEPICTION USING SCIENCE

29.3.1   Tissue perfusion

Perfusion refers to the blood supply which all functioning organs and tissues receive via a network of small capillary vessels. Local tissue perfusion can be increased where there are conditions such as malignant cancer, abscess/infection and inflammation. Cancers may attract an increased blood supply to themselves via a process of new blood vessel formation, termed angiogenesis. Infections and inflammations trigger a migration of white blood cells and other substances to the affected site, requiring an increase in blood supply. In some cases it is the surrounding rim of a cancer or abscess which receives a particularly high perfusion, creating a 'ring' enhancement pattern with radiographic contrast agents. Some factors, such as vessel occlusions caused by thrombus, or haemorrhages from vessels, create a state of reduced perfusion resulting in tissue ischaemia (loss of blood supply) and infarction. Infarction, which is the death of a tissue attributed to obstruction of blood supply, may manifest itself as an initial state of 'misery perfusion' during which blood supply is reduced, followed by a state of 'luxury perfusion' during which large numbers of white blood cells arrive at the site to assimilate the dead tissue. All of these altered states of perfusion can be imaged using CT, MRI, RNI and ultrasound, generally in conjunction with contrast agents or radionuclides (the latter in RNI only). Perfusion differences result in altered signal using CT and MRI, 'hot spots' or 'cold spots' using RNI methods and changes in reflectivity using ultrasound. Cancers and abscesses will often manifest themselves via a signal brightening termed 'contrast enhancement' when increased perfusion is shown via uptake of iodinated contrast agents in CT or gadolinium agents in MRI. Infarcts will generally appear as 'perfusion deficits'.

Often a technique known as *dynamic contrast enhancement* is used in CT and MRI to differentiate malignant tissues from other tissues on the basis of their contrast enhancement properties. These are illustrated by Fig. 29.4. The signal intensity of a malignant tissue will often show:

- A steep 'rise to peak' because of a high blood perfusion rate
- A high peak, because of increased capillary permeability, which permits a lot of contrast agent to leak into the extracellular space
- A long plateau, because of the slow diffusion of contrast media through the tumour tissue, before 'wash out' into the venous circulation occurs.

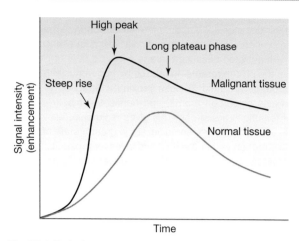

Fig. 29.4 Typical contrast agent enhancement curves for malignant and normal tissues.

INSIGHT

Computed tomography (CT) perfusion imaging is a special technique which employs X-rays beams of two energies (dual energy CT). This can be achieved by using two X-ray tubes, or a single X-ray tube with 'kVp switching' or two layers of X-ray detectors (each layer sensitive to a different X-ray energy range). The use of two X-ray beam energies permits very accurate measurements of voxel Hounsfield unit values to be obtained during tissue enhancement with iodinated contrast medium. This allows accurate maps of quantitative tissue perfusion to be obtained.

29.3.2   Tissue uptake of radionuclides

Tissue perfusion is a factor affecting the uptake of radionuclides in RNI and this can help to demonstrate 'hot spots' in cases such as tumour, infection and fracture healing. However, the functional depiction capabilities of RNI also depend on a host of additional factors. Radionuclides may be attached to pharmaceutical 'carrier' molecules, whose biodistribution will depend on their mode of administration (vascular, oral, inhaled), their uptake, binding and assimilation within target tissues, their metabolism, biochemical transformation and excretion route. It is even possible to provide radiolabelled antibodies and blood cells, which will enter complex physiological pathways. In all cases it is intended that radiopharmaceuticals should demonstrate 'specificity', concentrating only in intended pathological target tissues, not in normal tissues nor in tissues affected by unrelated changes. Radiopharmaceuticals have a 'biological half-life', which defines their excretion rate from the body, in addition to their radioactive half-life, which was discussed in Chapter 10. An ideal radioactive isotope for RNI should have a radioactive half-life sufficiently long to permit practical imaging, but also sufficiently short to avoid high radiation doses to patients if retained in the body for a prolonged period. It should also emit gamma rays of high energy, to enable good transmission through the body and hence into a detector. Attenuation of gamma rays in the body plays no part in forming an image in RNI. The image is based purely on emission of rays from areas of increased activity and thus RNI images need to be registered or 'fused' with CT to provide anatomical detail.

29.3.3 Tissue diffusion

Diffusion refers to the slow movement of water molecules, which may be random and equal in all directions (isotropic) as in a homogeneous fluid, or affected by direction (anisotropic). In the human body, anisotropy can occur when tissues have directional properties, such as nerve fibres and muscle fibres which have long axes along which water can move relatively freely, and cross-sectional axes which may offer more resistance to the flow of water. In addition, diffusion may be slowed or 'restricted' when there are pathological changes in tissue, such as in tumours, infarcts, trauma or toxicity. This is because of a restriction in the extracellular fluid space between cells as well as an increase in the 'debris' that results from cytotoxic effects on cells and cell death. These changes result in more opposition to the movement of water through the tissue. Diffusion weighted imaging (DWI) is an MRI technique and results in two major types of image. These are basic diffusion images, in which restricted diffusion appears bright, or apparent diffusion coefficient (ADC) maps, in which restricted diffusion appears dark. The ADC represents the mean diffusion in a voxel, taking account of directional differences and also other factors such as blood perfusion which may affect measurements. Typical water diffusion rates in different tissues are shown in Table 29.6.

INSIGHT

Why does diffusion of water cause signal loss on a basic diffusion image in magnetic resonance imaging (MRI)? In MRI, diffusion imaging is achieved by applying magnetic field gradients. These are magnetic fields additional to the main magnetic field, varying linearly in magnetic field 'strength' over distance. They are often drawn as 'slopes', with a 'high' end and a 'low' end. If a water molecule diffuses rapidly (i.e., a long distance along the gradient), its hydrogen nuclei will experience a considerable change in local magnetic field strength, leading to spin–spin dephasing and signal loss. The hydrogen nuclei in a slowly diffusing water molecule will not be so affected. The amplitude and timing of the applied gradients will affect the appearance of the diffusion image.

29.3.4 Metabolic rate

Tumours often have rapid cellular division rates and may therefore have high demands for energy, especially in the form of increased glucose utilisation. PET makes use of glucose labelled with fluorine-18 as fluorodeoxyglucose (FDG) to show 'hot spots' of increased metabolic activity (see Chapter 23). This makes use of what is essentially a natural molecule and is a very 'physiological' way of imaging body function. Areas of

TABLE 29.6 Typical apparent diffusion coefficient values in different tissues	
Tissue	**Mean ADC value ×10–3/mm² per s**
Lung—pleural fluid	3.6
Lung—consolidation	1.5
Lung—tumour	0.8
Prostate—normal peripheral zone	1.9
Prostate—normal transition zone	1.6
Prostate—cancer	1.0
Brain—normal white matter	0.8
Brain—normal grey matter	0.75
Brain—cerebrospinal fluid	3.4
Brain—oedema	1.7
Brain—infarct	0.3

ADC, apparent diffusion coefficient.

activity may be attributed to cancer but can also occur in normal brain (which consumes a lot of glucose), brown adipose tissue and in conditions such as inflammation, arthritis, fracture healing, infection and diabetes. PET is particularly useful at detecting 'hard to detect' tumours, monitoring cancer treatment and depicting cancer recurrence. It can also provide unique information in other conditions, such as Parkinson disease. Tumour response to therapy can be quantified using standardised uptake values (SUVs), which are measures of relative tissue or organ uptake and must take account of patient size, blood glucose level and administered radionuclide activity. Signal-to-noise resolution may be limited in PET, owing to detector spatial resolution and the number of effective gamma-ray counts. SUVs are generally greater in tumours than in normal tissue but can vary between institutions and do not provide a reliable absolute scale. Non imaging methods have shown that the basal metabolic rates of tissues such as the heart, brain and liver are much greater than the corresponding values for muscle and adipose tissue, when expressed in kcal/kg per day.

29.3.5 Magnetic susceptibility

In addition to its portrayal of tissue relaxation times (see Section 29.2.2), MRI has the ability to demonstrate the magnetic susceptibility of tissues. This refers to the amount to which substance becomes magnetised within a magnetic field. Most body tissues are diamagnetic, which means that they weakly oppose the field. However, some substances, such as melanin and methaemoglobin (the latter being a component of subacute haemorrhages) are paramagnetic, meaning that they weakly oppose the magnetic fields. In so doing, they shorten tissue longitudinal relaxation times and appear bright on T1 weighted images.

> **INSIGHT**
>
> Gadolinium-based contrast agents used in magnetic resonance imaging are paramagnetic. Hence, they brighten tissues that 'enhanced' during increased blood perfusion on T1 weighted images, by shortening longitudinal relaxation times. In fact, their effect is on hydrogen nuclei contained within a sphere of water molecules surrounding a gadolinium chelate. A chelate is an organic molecule which surrounds and stabilises the gadolinium ion. Exchange of water molecules between a binding site on the chelate complex and the surrounding water sphere has the effect of increasing dipole–dipole interactions and promoting spin relaxation.

Other substances, such as haemosiderin, which is found in haemorrhage, are superparamagnetic and show a magnetic susceptibility effect, due to containing small particles of iron oxide. This means that they are more strongly magnetised by the field. In practice this leads to a 'drop-off' of signal, resulting in a signal void. This can be utilised in susceptibility weighted imaging (SWI) which amplifies the signal loss using gradients and is a good way to demonstrate small bleeds. The magnetic properties of oxygenated and deoxygenated blood are used in an interesting way in MRI, within a technique known as *functional MRI* (fMRI), which employs blood oxygen level-dependent (BOLD) contrast. This can show blood oxygenation in tumours and also neuronal activation in the brain, in response to sensory stimuli or motor tasks.

> **INSIGHT**
>
> Oxyhaemoglobin is diamagnetic and deoxyhaemoglobin is paramagnetic. During neuronal activation affecting specific functional areas of the brain, an increased blood supply results in greater levels of oxyhaemoglobin in the draining blood capillaries. This results in a lengthening of transverse relaxation times (T2* times) and thus more signal, providing the basis of the blood oxygen level-dependent effect. On T2 weighted imaging, activation and nonactivation images, which show a signal difference, can be subtracted to provide a map of functional neuronal areas which are related to the sensory or motor task being performed.

29.3.6 Elasticity

In ultrasound, mechanical compressions and rarefactions resulting from the passage of sound through tissues can be used to show the elasticity of those tissues. Malignant masses tend to be 'stiffer' (less compressible) than benign masses or cysts. For example the elasticity of malignant breast masses is about 0.3 to 0.5 kilopascals (kPa), whereas the elasticity of benign masses is about 0.7 to 1.1 kPa. Static elastography uses physical compression of the ultrasound probe itself for shallow lesions, whereas dynamic elastography is based on the use of a high-powered ultrasound pulse to compress deeper tissues, via shear waves. As mentioned in Chapter 24, the speed of sound in tissue is proportional to tissue density, and thus a 'harder' lesion will permit sound to pass through it more rapidly. The hardness of lesions on physical palpitation has long been a feature of clinical examinations and now imaging science is able to quantify this process.

29.3.7 Blood flow

Blood flow may be affected by vessel stenosis or occlusion, as well as by altered circulation in the case of congenital variants or tumour. Ultrasound can quantify the velocity of blood flow via the Doppler effect, whereas MRI can use pulse 'tagging' of flowing blood to measure its speed.

SUMMARY

In this chapter, you should have learnt the following:

- The tissue depiction abilities of plain X-ray techniques and CT are based on tissue atomic number, density, electron density and thickness. CT provides improved tissue discrimination (tissue contrast) relative to plain X-ray.
- Dynamic contrast enhancement is available in CT and MRI and can demonstrate tissue blood perfusion, which is often increased in the case of malignancy or infection.
- MRI provides a wide range of tissue depiction capabilities, including proton density weighting, T1 and T2 weighting, water diffusion, magnetic susceptibility and BOLD contrast. More than any other modality, MRI combines anatomical and functional imaging approaches.
- RNI, including PET, has the ability to demonstrate functional uptake and metabolic rate.
- Ultrasound imaging is chiefly based on the reflective properties of tissue boundaries. It can also show tissue elasticity and blood flow.

FURTHER READING

Barrie Smith, N., & Webb, A. 2010. *Introduction to Medical Imaging: Physics, Engineering and Clinical Applications*. Cambridge: Cambridge University Press.

Carver, E., & Carver, B. 2012. *Medical Imaging: Techniques, Reflection and Evaluation*. 2nd edn. London: Churchill Livingstone.

Lisle, A. 2012. *Imaging for Students*. 4th edn. Boca Raton, Florida: CRC Press.

Rockall, A., Hatrick, A., Armstrong, P. & Wastie, M. 2013. *Diagnostic Imaging*. 7th edn. Hoboken, New Jersey: Wiley-Blackwell.

SECTION 3

Appendices and tables

291

Mathematics for radiography

APPENDIX CONTENTS

This appendix on the revision of mathematics is directed primarily at those whose mathematics is a little weak. However, many of the worked examples shown are chosen from topics in radiography.

For those studying for examinations, the following remarks may be of help. Examiners frequently complain of cramped, untidy mathematics which is difficult to follow. What they are hoping to see in the answer is a clear statement of the problem and an easy-to-follow development of the mathematics used to obtain the solution. This may be more important (and hence gain more marks) than simply obtaining the correct numerical answer. In fact, the correct answer simply recorded on its own with little or no supporting mathematical reasoning will not achieve many marks—remember that the examiner cannot know how you achieved the final answer unless you tell them. In practice, you should use phrases and sentences to tell the examiner how you have progressed from one step of the problem to the next as you move towards the eventual solution. This should also help you to think more clearly about what you are doing and also to check the integrity of your final answer; this is probably even more important with the widespread use of pocket calculators and computers. A study of the worked examples in this appendix should clarify these points.

A.1 ALGEBRAIC SYMBOLS

The letters of the English and Greek alphabet (see Table D following the appendices) are often used to represent the magnitude of an unknown quantity. For example, an electrical potential difference may be represented by V volts, an angle by θ (i.e., theta) degrees or radians and an energy by E joules. Such a practice enables the symbols to be used in place of the actual numerical values of the quantities, and is of great practical use in solving equations (see Appendix A.4).

A.1.1 Suffixes

Suffixes are used to denote a specific value of a particular quantity. If we use the symbol I to denote the intensity of radiation from a particular source, then I will depend upon the distance from the source at which the intensity is measured (see Chapter 14). We may call a particular distance x, say, and denote the intensity of this distance by Ix—*meaning the intensity at x*. For another distance y, the corresponding value of intensity is Iy.

Similarly, if a quantity, N, changes with time, t, the value of N at any given time may be denoted by Nt.

Suffixes are used, then, to avoid ambiguity and are used as such in many chapters of this book.

A.2 FRACTIONS AND PERCENTAGES

Although fractions are infrequently used in radiographic calculations because they have been largely replaced with decimals, a knowledge of how to manipulate fractions mathematically is useful in calculations involving Ohm's law (see Chapter 5) and capacitors (see Chapter 5). For this reason, a section on fractions and percentages is still included in this appendix.

A.2.1 Percentages

If a quantity increases in value by 50 per cent (%), then this means that it has become greater by one-half of its previous value. Thus, if the electric current passing through an X-ray tube is 200 mA, then an increase of 50% would bring this to 300 mA. Alternatively, it may be said that the new value is 150% of the original value.

In general terms, if a is the original value of a quantity and b is its new value, then:

$$\text{the percentage change} = 100 \times \frac{b-a}{a}$$

$$\frac{100b}{a} = \text{the percentage of } b \text{ compared to } a$$

$$\gamma\% \text{ of } a \text{ is just } \frac{\gamma}{100} \times a$$

EXAMPLES

a. Original value = 40; new value = 90

The percentage change is then $100 \times \dfrac{40}{90} = 44.4\%$

and the new value is $100 \times \dfrac{90}{40} = 225\%$ of the original.

---

b. A quantity has reduced by 30%. What is the new value if it was 700 originally?

$$30\% \text{ of } 700 \text{ is just } \frac{30}{100} \times 700 = 210$$

$$\text{so the new value is } 700 - 210 = 490$$

A percentage is a special case of a fraction, where one number is divided by another. The following sections describe how fractions may be added together and multiplied.

A.2.2 Addition of fractions

Suppose we have the fraction a/b, where a and b represent general numbers. Now the addition or subtraction of a/b to another fraction c/d rests on the fact that we can take any fraction and multiply top and bottom by the same factor (k, say) *without* altering its value:

$$\text{i.e., } \frac{a}{b} = \frac{ka}{kb} \text{ (because the } k\text{s cancel)}$$

It is the appropriate selection of k for each fraction which makes for the easy addition of fractions. For example, suppose we have:

$$\frac{2}{3} + \frac{5}{6}$$

If we multiply 2/3 by 2 (top and bottom), we shall have a fraction expressed in sixths, just like the second fraction:

$$\frac{2}{3} + \frac{5}{6} = \frac{2 \times 2}{2 \times 3} + \frac{5}{6} = \frac{4}{6} + \frac{5}{6} = \frac{9}{6} = 1\tfrac{1}{2}$$

Notice that we multiplied only the first fraction—we need not do the same thing to the second. This method is often very quick, particularly when only two or three simple fractions are involved, and is in fact entirely equivalent to the more general method of using the lowest common denominator (LCD), as illustrated in the following example:

$$\frac{2}{3} + \frac{3}{4} - \frac{5}{6} = \frac{4 \times 2 + 3 \times 3 - 2 \times 5}{12}$$

$$= \frac{(8 + 9 - 10)}{12} = \frac{7}{12}$$

Here, the LCD of the denominators 3, 4 and 6 is 12 and is therefore used as the overall denominator on the right-hand side. The individual denominators are then divided into 12, the result being multiplied by the respective numerator and summed (observing the correct signs) as shown in the example.

EXERCISE A.1 (Answers at the end of this appendix)

a. $\dfrac{11}{12} - \dfrac{5}{6}$

b. $\dfrac{7}{9} + \dfrac{2}{3}$

c. What is 20% of 50?

d. $\dfrac{2}{3} + \dfrac{1}{4} + \dfrac{3}{5}$

e. $\dfrac{7}{11} + \dfrac{2}{9} - \dfrac{2}{3}$

f. What is the percentage change if a quantity increases from 80 to 90?

A.3 MULTIPLYING AND DIVIDING

A.3.1 Positive and negative numbers

It is obvious that $1 \times 8 = 8$, but what are -1×8, -1×-8 and 8×-1?

To avoid having to work out such problems from first principles every time, a simple rule has been developed which we may call Rule 1.

Rule 1
When multiplying or dividing two numbers together:
   Two (+)s make a (+).
   Two (−)s make a (+).
   A (+) and a (−) make a (−).

That is, only when the signs are dissimilar is the result negative.

EXAMPLES

a. $-3 \times 4 = -12$
b. $14 \div -7 = -2$
c. $\dfrac{-40}{-4} = 10$
d. $-2 \times 4 \times -3 = 8 \times -3 = -24$

EXERCISE A.2

a. $28 \div 7$
b. $\dfrac{-36}{6}$

c. $\dfrac{144}{-4}$
d. -13×-3
e. $-7 \times \dfrac{-8}{-2}$

A.3.2 Fractions

The multiplication of two or more fractions is just a matter of simplification by cancellation (where possible) and then multiplying all the numerators together to form the new numerator, and all the denominators together to form the new denominator.

EXAMPLES

a. $\dfrac{2}{3} \times \dfrac{7}{5} = \dfrac{14}{15}$

b. $\dfrac{2}{3} \times \dfrac{9}{4} = \dfrac{\cancel{2}^{1}}{\cancel{3}_{1}} \times \dfrac{\cancel{9}^{3}}{\cancel{4}_{2}} = \dfrac{3}{2}$

The division of two fractions is straightforward provided that the following rule is obeyed.

Rule 2
When dividing by one or more fractions, turn those in the denominator upside down and multiply.

Let us say, by way of illustration, that we wish to divide 4 by ½:

$$\text{i.e., } \dfrac{4}{\dfrac{1}{2}}$$

Applying Rule 2, we turn ½ upside down and multiply:

$$\dfrac{4}{\dfrac{1}{2}} = 4 \times \dfrac{2}{1} = 8$$

Is this the answer we would expect intuitively? Well, the problem may be expressed as 'how many halves are there in 4?', and then it is obvious that the answer is 8. Here are some more examples to clarify the method:

a. $7 \div \dfrac{14}{9} = 7 \times \dfrac{9}{14} = \dfrac{9}{2}$

b. $\dfrac{\dfrac{3}{8}}{\dfrac{7}{11}} = \dfrac{3}{8} \times \dfrac{11}{7} = \dfrac{33}{56}$

c. $\dfrac{\dfrac{4}{9}}{\dfrac{-8}{27}} = \dfrac{4}{9} \times \dfrac{-27}{8} = \dfrac{-3}{2}$

d. $\dfrac{\dfrac{2}{3}}{\dfrac{4}{7} \times \dfrac{3}{5}} = \dfrac{2}{3} \times \dfrac{7}{4} \times \dfrac{5}{3} = \dfrac{35}{18}$

EXERCISE A.3

a. $\dfrac{\dfrac{-4}{11}}{\dfrac{7}{22}}$

b. $\dfrac{\dfrac{2}{9}}{\dfrac{7}{3} \times \dfrac{-2}{11}}$

c. $\dfrac{\dfrac{1}{3} \times \dfrac{2}{9}}{\dfrac{9}{1} \times \dfrac{1}{2}}$

A.3.3 Brackets

A bracket links two or more quantities together such that the bracket and its contents may be treated mathematically as a single quantity. If we wish to remove the brackets, then care over the plus and minus signs must be taken (Rule 1).

EXAMPLES

a. $2 \times (a - b) = 2 \times a \times b = 2a - 2b$

Thus, each term in the bracket is multiplied by the term outside the bracket, with due regard for the sign convention.

b. $-4(c - 2d) = -4c + 8d$

Note that the multiplication sign, present in Example a, has been omitted, as is usually the case.

c. $-3\left(\dfrac{-2a}{3} + b - \dfrac{1c}{7}\right) = 2a - 3b + \dfrac{3c}{7}$

Multiplying two or more brackets together can become quite involved. However, it is rare for problems in radiography to require even the multiplication of two brackets, but the method is outlined here for the sake of completeness.

Assume we wish to calculate:

$$(a + b)(c + d)$$

That is, $(a + b)$ multiplied by $(b + c)$

To perform this calculation, we take the first term of the first bracket, a, and multiply it by $(c + d)$. Then we add the result to the multiplication of the second term, b, by $(c + d)$:

i.e., $(a + b)(c + d) = a(c + d) + b(c + d)$
$$= ac + ad + bc + bd$$

Again, we must be careful of the sign convention (Rule 1), as the following two worked examples show.

EXAMPLES

a. $(7 + c)(d - 8) = 7(d - 8) + c(d - 8) = 7d - 56 + cd - 8c$

b. $(4 - a)(3 - b + 2c) = 4(3 - b + 2c) - a(3 - b + 2c)$
$$= 12 - 4b + 8c - 3a + ab - 2ac$$

EXERCISE A.4

a. $7a - 4(a - 2)$
b. $-6(-x + y - 3)$
c. $2(3a - 4) - 3(-a + 6)$

A.4 SOLVING EQUATIONS

Many of the types of equations encountered in problems associated with radiography are those in which a single 'unknown' (whose numerical value we wish to calculate) is 'mixed up' with several other numbers which may occur on both sides of the equation. (The solution of several equations involving several unknowns, i.e., simultaneous equations, is not normally required, and so will not be discussed here.) Our task, then, in the equations encountered, is to 'unscramble' the unknown so as to leave it on one side of the equation and all the numbers on the other side—the equation is then said to be 'solved'. This process is straightforward, provided that the following simple rule is obeyed:

Rule 3
Always perform the same operation to both sides of an equation.

This rule is intuitively obvious if it is imagined that the equals sign of the equation is the pivot of a pair of scales which is in exact balance. Whatever weight we now add to or subtract from one scale-pan must be added to or subtracted from the other or the scales will no longer be in balance. Similarly, if we double (say) the weight on one side we must do the same to the other; thus, provided we multiply by the same factor, balance is preserved and one side is equal to the other side. For example, consider the simple equation:

$$x - 2 = 3$$

If we add 2 to the left-hand side of this equation the -2 will be cancelled, leaving x only. However, in accordance with Rule 3 above, we must add 2 to the right-hand side to preserve equality:

$$\text{i.e., } x - 2 + 2 = 3 + 2 \text{ thus } x = 5$$

Putting $x = 5$ in the original equation, we have $5 - 2 = 3$, which is correct.

As another example, consider: $15 - y = 7$. Subtracting 15 from both sides so as to eliminate it from the left-hand side:

$$15 - y - 15 = 7 - 15, \text{ i.e., } y = -8$$

Multiplying both sides by -1 to make both terms positive (Rule 1), we have:

$$-1 \cdot -y = -1 \cdot -8, \text{ i.e., } y = 8$$

Note that the symbol '$\cdot$' is often used, as earlier, to denote multiplication.

Substituting our solution into the original equation to serve as a check, as in the previous example, we have:

$$15 - 8 = 7$$

thus, verifying our answer.

It is apparent from these examples that a convenient way of picturing this type of mathematical operation is that of transferring a quantity from one side to the other and changing its sign. Obviously, this only applies to the elimination of variables by addition or subtraction, not multiplication, which will be discussed in the next example.

EXAMPLE

$$2 = 7 - \frac{5x}{2}$$

Proceeding as before,

$$\frac{5x}{2} = 7 - 2 = 5$$

$$\text{i.e., } \frac{5x}{2} = 5$$

We cannot now add or subtract anything to leave x on its own—we have to multiply by 2/5:

$$\text{i.e., } \frac{2}{5} \cdot \frac{5x}{2} = \frac{2}{5} \cdot 5$$

This last step is known as *cross-multiplication* and may be pictured in the following manner:

 (cross-multiplication)

The double-ended arrows indicate that movement may be in either direction. Note that there is no change of sign.

One incorrect use of cross-multiplication occurs so frequently that it is worth a special mention here. Suppose we have the equation:

$$\frac{7x}{2} = \frac{3}{8} + \frac{x}{3}$$

if we cross-multiply in the following manner:

$$\frac{2}{7} \times \frac{7x}{2} = \frac{3}{7} \times \frac{3}{8} + \frac{x}{3} \text{ (incorrect)}$$

we obtain:

$$x = \frac{2 \cdot 3}{7 \cdot 8} + \frac{x}{3} \text{ (incorrect)}$$

The fault lies, of course, in the fact that Rule 3 has been disobeyed, that is, the term $x/3$ remains unaltered although we were intending, by our cross-multiplication, to multiply both sides by 2/7. Hence, if we wished to cross-multiply at this stage, we should have obtained:

$$x = \frac{2 \cdot 3}{7 \cdot 8} + \frac{2 \cdot x}{7 \cdot 3} \text{ (correct)}$$

which may be further simplified to solve for x.

EXERCISE A.5

a. $\dfrac{2}{3}x = 4$

b. $\dfrac{7}{9}y - 1 = 13$

c. $q + \dfrac{3}{10} = \dfrac{5}{12}q$

d. $3\frac{3}{5}z - 12\frac{4}{5} = 1\frac{2}{5}z - \frac{7}{10}$

A.5 POWERS (INDICES)

An index is written at the top right of a quantity (the base) and refers to the number of times the quantity is multiplied by itself. For example, 5^3 means $5 \times 5 \times 5$ (i.e., 125). It is a convenient mathematical 'shorthand' to write powers of a number in this way. In this example, the index is a positive integer (i.e., 3), but this need not be the case for it may be positive, negative, fractional or decimal, as described later.

A.5.1 Combining indices

Let us assume that we have two numbers, 2^3 and 2^2, which we wish to combine by addition, multiplication and division to elicit general rules for the handling of indices.

A.5.1.1 Addition

Using the definition of an index as described:

$$2^3 + 2^2 = 2 \cdot 2 \cdot 2 + 2 \cdot 2 = 8 + 4 = 12$$

Thus, when adding such numbers, each term is calculated separately before addition (or subtraction).

A.5.1.2 Multiplication

Again, from first principles, we have:

$$2^3 \cdot 2^2 = \left(2^3\right) \cdot \left(2^2\right) = 2^5 = 2^{(3+2)}$$

Hence, when multiplying two or more such numbers together, the rule is to add the indices.

A.5.1.3 Division

$$\frac{2^3}{2^2} = \frac{2 \cdot 2 \cdot 2}{2 \cdot 2} = 2 = 2^{(3-2)}$$

Thus, when dividing such numbers, the rule is to subtract the indices.

A.5.2 Negative indices

Suppose that we wish to divide 4^2 by 4^4. From first principles (Section A.5), we have:

$$\frac{4^2}{4^4} = \frac{(4 \cdot 4)}{4 \cdot 4 \cdot 4 \cdot 4} = \frac{1}{4^2} \qquad \textbf{Equation A.1}$$

Also, by the rule on division as described above, we may subtract indices:

$$\frac{4^2}{4^4} = 4^{(2-4)} = 4^{-2} \qquad \textbf{Equation A.2}$$

Because Equation A.1 and Equation A.2 are equal:

$$4^{-2} = \frac{1}{4^2}$$

In general, therefore:

$$x^{-n} = \frac{1}{x^n} \qquad \textbf{Equation A.3}$$

That is, to change a negative index to a positive index, just take the reciprocal, as shown in Eq. A.3.

EXAMPLES

a. $10^{-2} = \dfrac{1}{10^2} = \dfrac{1}{100}$

b. $\dfrac{1}{10^{-6}} = \dfrac{1}{\frac{1}{10^6}} = 1 \times \dfrac{10^6}{1} = 10^6$

c. $\dfrac{420 \times 10^2}{2 \times 10^4} = 210 \times 10^{-2} = \dfrac{210}{10^2} = \dfrac{210}{100} = 2.1$

A.5.3 Fractional indices

What is meant by, say, $x^{1/2}$?

Now,

$$x^{1/2} \cdot x^{1/2} = x^{1/2+1/2} = x^1 = x$$

Also,

$$\sqrt{x \cdot \sqrt{x}} = x$$

from the definition of a square root.

Thus from inspection of these two equations:

$$x^{1/2} = \sqrt{x}$$

That is, $x^{1/2}$ is just the square root of x. Similarly, $y^{1/2}$ is the cube root of y, etc.

EXAMPLES

a. $9^{1/2} = \sqrt{9} = \pm 3$

b. $3^{3/2} = \left(9^{1/2}\right)^3 = \left(\pm 3\right)^3 = \pm 27$

c. $64^{1/3} = \sqrt[3]{64} = 4$

A.5.4 The zero index—x^0

A general number x raised to a power m is x^m. If we divide x^m by itself, the answer will obviously be 1. But $x^m \div x^m$ is x^{m-m} by the rules discussed above. Thus $1 = x^{m-m} = x^0$. Because we took any general number, this result is also general (except for 0^0, which is indeterminate).

Thus any number raised to the power zero is *unity*.

A.5.5 Indices to different bases

A problem on the inverse square law (see Chapter 14) frequently involves calculation of the form:

$$\frac{a \cdot b^2}{c^2}$$

Here a, b and c represent numbers whose values are known, having been specified by the problem. We wish to determine the best way of obtaining the final result, because b and c are frequently large numbers, whose squares are therefore even larger. This means that the probability of making an arithmetical error can be quite high if a labourious method of calculation is undertaken. However, a great simplification is possible if we remember that:

$$\frac{b^2}{c^2} = \left(\frac{b}{c}\right)^2 \qquad \textbf{Equation A.4}$$

EXAMPLE

If $b = 90$ cm and $c = 60$ cm then b^2/c^2 the 'hard' way is:

$$\frac{b^2}{c^2} = \frac{90^2}{60^2} = \frac{8100}{3600} = \frac{81}{36}$$

which may be cancelled to give 2.25—this exercise being left to the reader. The 'easy' way is to use Equation A.4, that is,

$$\frac{b^2}{c^2} = \left(\frac{b}{c}\right)^2 = \left(\frac{90}{60}\right)^2 = \left(\frac{3}{2}\right)^2 = 1.5^2 = 2.25$$

Note that the answers are the same, as we should expect, but that the second method involves cancelling of smaller numbers so that there is less likelihood of an arithmetical error.

A.6 POWERS OF 10

When 10 is used as a base for indices, all the findings of the previous section apply. In addition, powers of 10 are very useful when measuring very large or very small quantities of a given unit, as shown in Table A.

It is advisable for the student to memorise most of these terms because they are in very common usage in radiography. The following exercise is included for this purpose.

EXERCISE A.6

a. An X-ray tube has a current of 0.4 amperes passing through it. How many milliamperes (mA) does this correspond to?

b. If the X-ray tube has a peak potential difference of 90,000 volts across it, what is the value in kilovolts (kVp)?

c. Express a capacitance of 0.000065 farads in microfarads (μF).

d. A photon of light has a wavelength of 550 nanometres (nm). What is this in metres?

A.7 PROPORTIONALITY

A.7.1 Direct proportion

If a car is travelling at constant speed such that the petrol consumption is a steady 60 km.L^{-1}, then:

0.5 litres has been used after 30 km
1.0 litres has been used after 60 km
1.5 litres has been used after 75 km, etc.

Thus the amount of petrol consumed is in direct proportion to the number of miles travelled, and we may write:

$$\text{litres} \propto \text{mileage}$$

where the sign '$\propto$' means *is proportional to*. Alternatively, we may write:

$$\text{litres} = \left(\frac{1}{60}\right) \times \text{mileage}$$

In general, therefore, if two quantities y and x are directly proportional to each other, then:

$$y \propto x \text{ or } y = kx$$

where k is called the *constant of proportionality*. Some examples of direct proportionality which are discussed in the main text include the following:

- The electric current (I) through a metallic conductor is proportional to the potential difference (V) across it, that is, $I \propto V$ (Ohm's law; Chapter 5).
- Intensity of an X-ray beam $\propto$ tube current (mA) (Chapter 14).
- Intensity of an X-ray beam $\propto$ kilovoltage squared, that is, intensity $\propto$ kV^2 (Chapter 14).

A.7.2 Inverse proportion

Suppose that we have many rectangles of equal area, k, but of differing heights (h) and widths (w). However, in each case the area is the same, so that:

$$h \times w = \text{constant} \, (k)$$

Then, because k is constant, we may write:

$$h = \frac{1}{w}$$

In this case, therefore, h and w are in *inverse* proportion because w is halved if h is doubled, and vice versa. This is opposite to direct proportion, of course, where doubling (say) one quantity also doubles the other.

Examples of inverse proportion discussed in the main text include:

- The capacity (C) of a parallel-plate capacitor is inversely proportional to the separation (d) between its plates, that is, $C \propto 1/d$ (Chapter 5).

- The intensity (I) from a point source of electromagnetic radiation is inversely proportional to the square of the distance (x) from the source, that is, $I \propto 1/x^2$ (Chapter 14).
- The electrical resistance (R) of a given length of wire varies inversely as the area of cross-section (A), that is, $R \propto 1/A$ (Chapter 5).

A.8 GRAPHS

A.8.1 Drawing and interpretation

A good understanding of the construction and interpretation of graphs is of great value in radiography, radiotherapy and nuclear medicine. The following simple but effective rules are offered in the drawing of good graphs:

- Each graph should take at least one-third of a page – use as large a scale as practicable so that you can make accurate readings.
- Each graph should have a clear, appropriate title.
- The axes, which should be drawn with a ruler, should be of approximately equal length.
- Both axes must be clearly labelled to show what is being measured and should contain units (cm, s, kg, etc.) where appropriate.
- The independent variable is normally on the x-axis, and the dependent variable on the y-axis, that is, the variable which is being measured is plotted on the y-axis whereas the variable causing the change in y is plotted on the x-axis. If we consider plotting the radioactivity from a sample over a period of time, then the independent variable is time (plotted on the x-axis) whereas the dependent variable is the radioactivity (plotted on the y-axis).

The following examples have been chosen to illustrate both the drawing and the interpretation of graphs.

EXAMPLE 1 – DIRECT PROPORTION

As described in the last section, two quantities, x and y, are directly proportional to each other if $y = kx$, where k is a constant. Fig. A.1 shows $y = kx$ in graphical form. The following points should be noted:

- The graph passes through the origin, because when $x = 0$, y is also equal to zero.
- The slope (or gradient) of the straight line produced is a measure of how steep it is and is defined as *the change in y divided by the corresponding change in x.* Because the graph passes through the origin, this is a convenient place from which to measure the changes. From this it can be seen that the slope is y/x. But from the equation $y = kx$ it can be seen that $y/x = k$. Thus the slope increases as k increases.

- The general equation for a straight line will be in the form $y = mx + c$ where m is the gradient of the line and c is the intersection of the line with the y-axis – the value of x when $y = 0$.

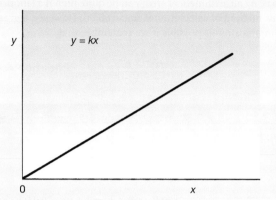

Fig. A.1 Graph of $y = kx$, illustrating a directly proportional relationship.

EXAMPLE 2 – INVERSE PROPORTION

Fig. A.2 shows a graph of the inverse relationship between the capacitance, C, of a parallel-plate capacitor and the distance of separation of its plates, d, where $C \propto 1/d$ or $C = k/d$ for a specific capacitor.

From the graph it can be seen that as the distance between the plates increases, so the capacitance of the capacitor decreases.

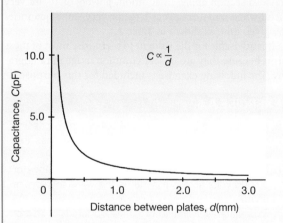

Fig. A.2 Graph of $C \propto 1/d$, illustrating an inverse proportional relationship.

EXAMPLE 3 – RATING GRAPHS

Rating charts are supplied by the manufacturers of X-ray tubes, and contain a lot of information in graphical form which is an essential guide to the radiographer in the selection of 'safe' exposure factors, that is, the combination of focal-spot size, kVp, mA and exposure time which will not cause damage to the X-ray tube.

An example of a rating chart is given by Fig. A.3, where a family of curves represent the maximum permissible exposure factors for different settings of kVp. The use of rating graphs is discussed in detail in Chapter 12 and we only need to make the point here that points below a particular curve for one kVp setting are 'safe', whereas points above it lead to tube damage by overheating the anode.

Note the nonlinear (logarithmic) scale on the x-axis. Logarithmic scales are discussed in Chapter 12.

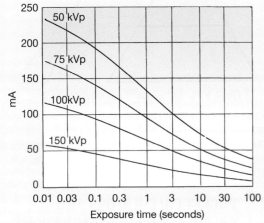

Fig. A.3 Rating graph for an X-ray tube. Note the nonlinear (logarithmic) scale on the x-axis.

A.8.2 Interpolation and extrapolation

It is often the case that a graph is drawn using a relatively small number of points, and that these points are joined together with a curve or straight line passing through them. The smooth curve or line makes it possible to 'read off' values from the graph, even when such values lie between the original points used to construct the graph. This procedure is known as *interpolation* and is one of the advantages of the graphical method.

If it is desired to determine the value of one of the plotted variables when it lies outside the range of the points used to plot the graph, the curve may be extended, or extrapolated, to reach this region. However, such an extrapolation can lead to large inaccuracies because several different curves may seem equally suitable and there may be no way of knowing which one is correct!

EXERCISE A.7

a. Draw a graph of $y = 0.2x$, choosing values of x from 1 to 10 in steps of 1. Hence read from the graph in Fig. A.4 the value of y when x is (i) 1.5, (ii) 9.5, (iii) 12, (iv) 0.5. Verify your answers by substitution into the original equation.

b. Repeat the same procedure for the equation $y = 0.2x^2$. (Note the increased uncertainty in obtaining the extrapolated value of y when $x = 12$.)

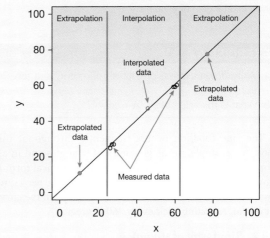

Fig. A.4 An example of interpolating and extrapolating data from a graph.

A.9 THE GEOMETRY OF TRIANGLES

A.9.1 The right-angled triangle

Consider the right-angled triangle shown in Fig. A.5. The trigonometric functions of sine, cosine and tangent are defined as:

$$\sin A = \frac{\text{opposite}}{\text{hypotenuse}} = \frac{a}{b}$$

$$\cos A = \frac{\text{adjacent}}{\text{hypotenuse}} = \frac{c}{b}$$

$$\tan A = \frac{\text{opposite}}{\text{adjacent}} = \frac{a}{c}$$

Note that:

$$\frac{\sin A}{\cos A} = \frac{\frac{a}{b}}{\frac{c}{b}} = \frac{a}{b} \times \frac{b}{c} \text{ (by Rule 2)}$$

$$\text{i.e., } \frac{\sin A}{\cos A} = \frac{a}{c} = \tan A$$

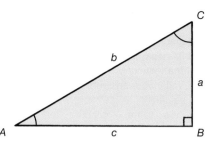

Fig. A.5 A right-angled triangle. See text for definition of sine, cosine and tangent of an angle.

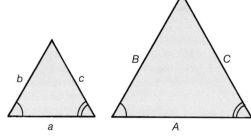

Fig. A.7 Two similar triangles.

EXERCISE A.8

a. Write down expressions for sin C, cos C and tan C from Fig. A.5.
b. What is the value of $\sin^2 A + \cos^2 A$?

The sine function occurs frequently throughout this book, for example, in the geometry of triangles and in alternating current theory (Chapter 5). Its graphical form is shown in Fig. A.6. This graph is known as a *sine wave*, and always lies between +1 and −1. Also, the shape of the curve is cyclical, repeating itself every 360 degrees.

A.9.2   Similarity of triangles

The two triangles shown in Fig. A.7 are said to be 'similar' because one is just a bigger version of the other, while retaining the same shape. Thus the corresponding angles of the two triangles are equal, but the lengths of the corresponding sides need not necessarily be so.

However, if one side has a length which is double (say) that of the corresponding side of the other triangle, then *all* the sides will be doubled compared with the other triangle. Generally, then, we may write:

$$\frac{A}{a} = \frac{B}{b} = \frac{C}{c}$$ **Equation A.5**

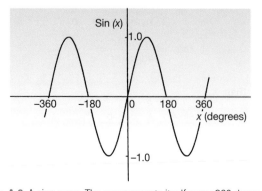

Fig. A.6 A sine wave. The curve repeats itself every 360 degrees.

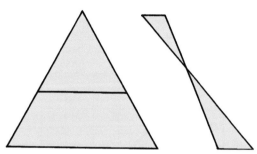

Fig. A.8 Further examples of similar triangles.

In many practical examples in radiography, however, the similar triangles look more like those shown in Fig. A.8.

A.10   POCKET CALCULATORS AND CALCULATIONS IN EXAMINATIONS

Because the price of pocket calculators now puts them within the range of even the most impoverished student, the purchase of such a calculator is strongly recommended. 'Scientific' pocket calculators have the advantage that they can perform calculations which involve trigonometrical and logarithmic functions and so will be found especially useful. Many such calculators are also 'programmable' which means that formulae may be inserted into the calculator memory to allow it to perform certain calculations by simply inserting the appropriate data—a formula for Ohm's law could be inserted so that when the program is invoked the calculator will automatically calculate the resistance from the value of the potential and the current. It should also be noted that applications providing the functionality of a 'good' scientific calculator are available for use on-line, downloadable to tablets and also embedded within common computer operating systems, for example, Microsoft Windows and Apple MacOS.

If you are to use a pocket calculator in examinations or if you are about to buy one, here are some suggestions which you might find helpful:

- Consider the types of calculations which you require from the calculator and do not buy one with lots of unnecessary functions—these simply increase your chance of error.
- Try out a calculator before you buy it (if possible) and, if you are about to use one in an examination, make sure you are familiar with its layout and functions.
- Find out the policy regarding the use of calculators in examinations at your university. Some universities will issue calculators for the purpose of examinations whereas others have specific regulations regarding programmable calculators.
- Remember that the calculator will give the correct answer only if the correct information is keyed into it. Remember indices and also try to get some 'feel' for the magnitude of the correct answer.

A.11   LOGARITHMS

Although few students would now undertake calculations using logarithms as the chosen method —thanks to the ease of use of the pocket calculator or computer software—it is nevertheless helpful to have a basic grasp of the theory of logarithms to explain certain functions in radiography; for example, it may be easier to understand the exponential equations in their logarithmic form or the use of exposure indices which, for some manufacturers, are presented as logarithms.

> **DEFINITION**
>
> The logarithm of a number to a given base is the power by which the base must be raised to give the number.

Thus, the logarithm of 100 to the base 10 is 2 as $10^2 = 100$. This would normally be written as $\log_{10}100 = 2$.

The base can be any number but, in practice, logarithms are usually to the base 10 or to the base e where e is the exponential number and is approximately equal to 2.7183.

Consider a situation where we wish to multiply two numbers a and b. If $a = 10^x$ and $b = 10^y$ then:

$$a \times b = 10^x \times 10^y = 10^{(x+y)}$$

Thus from our initial definition of logarithms we can say:

$$\log_{10}\left(\frac{a}{b}\right) = \log_{10}a - \log_{10}b$$

By a similar argument it can be shown that:

$$\log_{10}\left(\frac{a}{b}\right) = \log_{10}a - \log_{10}b$$

The main use of logarithms in radiography is to allow the simplification of complex formulae —if we consider the intensity of a beam of radiation which has travelled a distance x through a medium, this is given by the equation:

$$I_x = I_0 e^{-\mu x}$$

where I_x is the intensity of the radiation after a thickness x, I_0 is the initial intensity of the radiation, e is the exponential number and μ is the linear attenuation coefficient – these are all explained in Chapter 13. This equation is quite complicated to use in the above form but is much easier to use in its logarithmic form:

$$\log_e I_x = \log_e I_0 - \mu x$$

A.12   VECTOR QUANTITIES

In vector quantities, the quantity concerned has direction as well as dimension. Thus in vector addition we need to take both these factors into account. This is probably best illustrated by two simple examples:

1. A man walks 30 metres in an easterly direction and then walks 20 metres in a northerly direction. How far must he walk in a straight line to get back to where he started? The situation may be visualised using Fig. A.9. By applying Pythagoras' theorem to this we can calculate that the distance from C to A is 36 metres.
2. Forces $F_1 = 1$ newton, $F_2 = 4$ newtons and $F_3 = 2$ newtons are applied to a point source as shown in Fig. A.10.

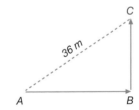

Fig. A.9 Distances walked for calculation.

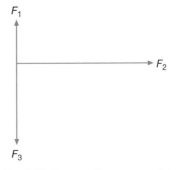

Fig. A.10 Forces acting upon a point.

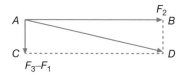

Fig. A.11 Vector addition of forces.

What is the resultant force and what is its direction? Because F_1 and F_3 are in opposite directions, the resultant force is the difference between F_1 and F_3 and is in the direction of F_3 as this is the larger of the two forces. We can now do vector addition (see Fig. A.11), where AB represents force F_2 and BD represents $(F_3 - F_1)$. The resultant force is represented by AD. By application of Pythagoras' theorem, the length of this line is 4.12 newtons. Tan A is BD/AB and thus A can be calculated as approximately 14 degrees.

Thus we can say that the resultant force measures 4.12 newtons and is in a direction 14 degrees below the horizontal.

APPENDIX SUMMARY

- If we multiply or divide two +s or two −s, we get a +.
- If we multiply or divide a + and a − sign, we get a −.
- When dividing by a fraction, we can get the same result if we multiply by the fraction inverted (the fraction turned upside down).
- The following mathematical relationships have been established:

$$x^a \times x^b = x^{(a+b)}$$

$$\frac{x^a}{x^b} = x^{(a-b)}$$

$$x^{-a} = \frac{1}{x^a}$$

$$x^{1/2} = \sqrt{x}$$

$$\frac{x^a}{y^a} = \left(\frac{x}{y}\right)^a$$

- In direct proportion, $y \propto x$ or $y = kx$ whereas in inverse proportion, $y \propto 1/x$ or $y = c/x$ where k and c are constants of proportionality.
- Sin θ = opposite/hypotenuse; cos θ = adjacent/hypotenuse and tan θ = opposite/adjacent.
- Sine and cosine functions are cyclical, repeating themselves every 360 degrees.
- When drawing graphs, use a manageable scale, use a ruler, label both axes and use a title.

- Similar triangles have the ratio of their corresponding sides being equal.
- There are certain factors to consider when purchasing or using a pocket calculator.
- The basic theory of logarithms tells us that if $y = x^n$ then $\log_x y = n$.
- $\log_{10}(x \times y) = \log_{10}x + \log_{10}y$.
- $\log_{10}(x/y) = \log_{10}x - \log_{10}y$.
- In vector addition, we can get the resultant vector by joining the vectors end to end. The resultant vector is from the origin to the tip of the last vector.

ANSWERS TO EXERCISES

Exercise A.1

a. $\dfrac{11}{12} - \dfrac{5}{6} = \dfrac{11-10}{12} = \dfrac{1}{12}$

b. $\dfrac{7}{9} + \dfrac{2}{3} = \dfrac{7+6}{9} = \dfrac{13}{9} = 1\dfrac{4}{9}$

c. 30% of $50 = \dfrac{30}{100} \times 50 = 15$

d. $\dfrac{2}{3} - \dfrac{1}{4} + \dfrac{3}{5} = \dfrac{40-15+36}{60} = \dfrac{61}{60} = 1\dfrac{1}{60}$

e. $\dfrac{7}{11} + \dfrac{2}{9} - \dfrac{2}{3} = \dfrac{63+22-66}{99} = \dfrac{19}{99}$

f. Percentage change $= 100 \times \dfrac{(90-80)}{80}$
$$= 100 \times \dfrac{10}{80} = 12.5\%$$

Exercise A.2

a. $28 \div 7 = 4$

b. $\dfrac{-36}{6} = -6$

c. $\dfrac{144}{-4} = -36$

d. $-13 \times -3 = 39$

e. $-7 \times \dfrac{-8}{-2} = -7 \times 4 = -28$

Exercise A.3

a. $\dfrac{\frac{-4}{11}}{\frac{7}{22}} = \dfrac{-4}{11} \times \dfrac{22}{7} = \dfrac{-8}{7} = -1\dfrac{1}{7}$

b. $\dfrac{\frac{2}{9}}{\frac{7}{3} \times \frac{-2}{11}} = \dfrac{2}{9} \times \dfrac{3}{7} \times \dfrac{11}{-2} = \dfrac{-11}{21}$

c. $\dfrac{\dfrac{1}{3} \times \dfrac{2}{9}}{\dfrac{9}{1} \times \dfrac{1}{2}} \times \dfrac{\dfrac{2}{27}}{\dfrac{9}{2}} = \dfrac{2}{27} \times \dfrac{2}{9} \times \dfrac{4}{243}$

Exercise A.4

a. $7a - 4(a - 2) = 7a - 4a + 8 = 3a + a$
b. $-6(- x + y - 3) = 6x - 6y + 18$
c. $2(3a - 4) - 3(- a + 6) = 6a - 8 + 3a - 18 =$
   $9a - 26$

Exercise A.5

a. $\dfrac{2}{3}x = 4$

   $2x = 12$

   $x = 6$

b. $\dfrac{7}{9}y - 1 = 13$

   $7y - 9 = 117$

   $7y = 126$

   $y = 18$

c. $q + \dfrac{3}{10} = \dfrac{5}{12}q$

   $12q + \dfrac{36}{10} = 5q$

   $12q - 5q = \dfrac{-36}{10}$

   $q = \dfrac{-36}{70}$

   $q = \dfrac{-18}{35}$

d. $3\dfrac{3}{5}z - 12\dfrac{4}{5} = 1\dfrac{5}{5}z - \dfrac{7}{10}$

   $3\dfrac{3}{5}z - 1\dfrac{2}{5}z = 12\dfrac{4}{5} - \dfrac{7}{10}$

   $2\dfrac{1}{5}z = 12\dfrac{1}{10}$

   $\dfrac{11}{5}z = \dfrac{121}{10}$

   $110z = 605$

   $z = \dfrac{605}{110} = 5\dfrac{1}{2}$

Exercise A.6

a. 50 mA
b. 125 kVp
c. 65 µF
d. 0.00000055 m

Exercise A.7

a. From the graph you should obtain the following readings:
   - When $x = 1.5$, $y = 0.3$
   - When $x = 9.5$, $y = 1.9$
   - When $x = 12$, $y = 2.4$
   - When $x = 0.5$, $y = 0.1$
b. From the graph you should obtain the following readings:
   - When $x = 1.5$, $y = 0.45$
   - When $x = 9.5$, $y = 18.05$
   - When $x = 12$, $y = 28.8$
   - When $x = 0.5$, $y = 0.05$

Exercise A.8

a. From Fig. A.5:
   $\sin C = c/b$
   $\cos C = a/b$
   $\tan C = c/a$
b. From Fig. A.5:
   $\sin^2 A + \cos^2 A = (a/b)^2 + (c/b)^2$

   $$= \dfrac{a^2 + c^2}{b^2}$$

   But $a^2 + c^2 = b^2$ by Pythagoras' theorem.
   Thus, $\sin^2 A + \cos^2 A = 1$.

Modulation transfer function

Modulation transfer function (MTF) is a mathematical method of assessing the resolving power of an imaging system, whether it be optical, radiographic or radioactive. The use of the MTF for this purpose was pioneered in the field of optics when it was discovered that a lens which was excellent at imaging the structure of very fine objects was not necessarily as good as another lens of lower resolving power when imaging coarser (i.e., larger) objects.

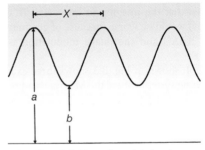

Fig. B.1 The definition of modulation (see text).

> ## DEFINITION
>
> The modulation transfer function (MTF) of an image is a numerical value determined by the division of the modulation (m_i) of the recorded image by the modulation of the stimulus (m_0):
>
> $$MTF(v) = m_i/m_0 \quad \textbf{Equation B.1}$$

B.1 MODULATION AND SPATIAL FREQUENCIES

As can be seen from the definition, the process of modulation is inherent in any description of the MTF and will therefore be considered first. Modulation is linked to spatial frequency. Consider the sine wave shown in Fig. B.1, which has a wavelength of X. The spatial frequency of this waveform is the number of cycles per unit length (say, v cycles per cm), and is therefore given by $1/X$. The modulation of the object, m_0, is defined as:

$$m_0 = \frac{(a-b)}{(a+b)} \quad \textbf{Equation B.2}$$

where a and b are the height of the peaks and the troughs of the waveform respectively.

The units in which amplitude of the sine wave is recorded will differ with the application, for example, X-ray intensity in radiography, light intensity for optical lenses, level of activity for gamma cameras or optical density for photographic film.

If it is supposed that an absorber is placed in the path of an X-ray beam such that it would produce a sinusoidal variation of intensity of the transmitted beam, then a perfect imaging system would produce a sine wave of the same modulation.

The image modulation would then be the same as the object modulation. However, in practice, the relative amplitude of the image modulation is reduced by the finite size of the focal spot; in addition, the recorded image is also affected by the characteristics of the image receptor. This tends to spread the image onto a larger area than theoretically desirable. Thus the 'peaks' of the sinusoidal exposure tend to contribute to the 'troughs', so that an overall reduction in amplitude (and therefore modulation) is experienced.

This effect of a reduction in image modulation is small when the sinusoidal object has a long wavelength (low spatial frequency) but is of increasing importance as the wavelength is reduced to about 1 mm or less (spatial frequencies of ≥10 per cm). The image modulation therefore depends upon the spatial frequency of the object, and this forms the basis of the MTF, described later.

B.2 MODULATION TRANSFER FUNCTION AND SPATIAL FREQUENCY

As seen, the MTF (Equation B.1) is defined as:

$$\mathrm{MTF}(v) = m_i/m_0$$

In a perfect imaging system, the image is an exact copy of the object and so has the same modulation at all spatial frequencies. The MTF is therefore always unity for such a system. However, as the spatial frequency increases, it is to be expected that the imaging of fine detail (high spatial frequencies) would be worse (because of geometric distortion [Fig. B.2A]) and the image modulation is reduced (Fig. B.2B).

The graph shown in Fig. B.3 shows three examples: an 'ideal' imaging system, where the MTF is 1 and is independent of the spatial frequency; a curve where the MTF is reduced at the higher frequencies because of geometric unsharpness (U_g) only and, lastly, a curve obtained when using a film-screen recording medium (U_g + screens).

The MTF is particularly useful in separating the individual causes of image degradation. MTFs, because of each

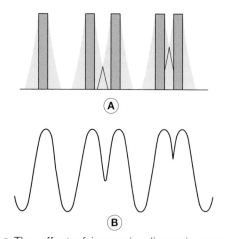

Fig. B.2 The effect of increasing line-pairs per centimeter on spatial frequency. (A) Increasing geometric distortion as line-pairs per millimeter increase; (B) the sine wave plot of the densities produced.

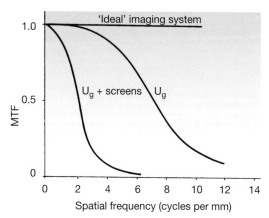

Fig. B.3 The variation of the modulation transfer function (MTF) with spatial frequency for an ideal system, that due to geometric unsharpness (Ug), and that due to geometric unsharpness and screens (Ug + screens).

cause, may be measured separately (MTF_1, etc.) and may be combined to produce the overall MTF of the system:

$$\mathrm{MTF} = \mathrm{MTF}_1 \times \mathrm{MTF}_2 \ldots \qquad \textbf{Equation B.3}$$

It thus becomes possible to predict the response of the overall system with various combinations of focal spot size, film-screen combinations, etc. if the MTF of each is known.

B.3 OBJECTS AS SPATIAL FREQUENCIES

A 'sinusoidal' object does not bear much similarity to the objects which are normally radiographed. However, it may be shown that the shape of any object may be obtained from the summation of sine and cosine waves of different amplitudes and frequencies (Fourier's theorem). Thus if the MTF of the X-ray unit is known at each frequency, the overall response to the object may be determined.

As an example of the summation of amplitudes of different frequencies forming a shape, consider the flat-topped object shown by the dashed lines in Fig. B.4A. The height of the object may be considered to represent the degree of absorption of the X-rays by the object, and its width as the physical size of the object. It may be shown that such a shape may be obtained by adding an infinite series of cosine waves (which are just sine waves displaced by 90 degrees) of increasing frequency (f), where the amplitudes are given by:

$$g = \frac{\sin(\pi f d)}{(2\pi f)} \qquad \textbf{Equation B.4}$$

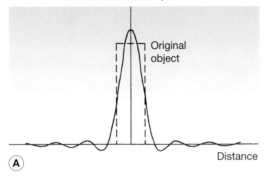

Summation of all amplitudes

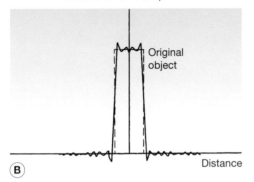

Fig. B.4 The representation of a "square" object (dashed lines) by the summation of the frequencies of different amplitudes. (A) 500 terms; (B) 2500 terms. An infinite number of terms reproduces the object exactly.

The sum of the first 500 terms of such amplitudes is shown in Fig. B.4A. The effect of including 2500 terms (i.e., containing higher frequencies) is shown in Fig. B.4B, where a closer approximation to the square shape is obtained. The agreement is exact when an infinite number of terms is included. However, the higher spatial frequencies present in the object are poorly reproduced in the image, because the MTF is low at high frequencies. Because the high frequencies are responsible for the 'squareness' of the corners for objects such as shown in Fig. B.3, sharp objects will be shown as being slightly blurred or out of focus. This is in accordance with the concept of unsharpness, as discussed earlier, and the two approaches are just two ways of looking at the same thing. The MTF is more mathematically rigorous as a complete description of the imaging properties of the X-ray unit, but even this does not consider other problems such as statistical 'noise' within the image, known as *quantum mottle*.

B.4 MEASUREMENT OF MODULATION TRANSFER FUNCTION

In practice it is difficult to manufacture sinusoidal objects in the numbers and wavelengths required and it would also be very time consuming to measure the image modulation for every combination of frequency, position of absorber and image receptor for every object recorded. Fortunately, there is no need to do this: an intensity curve can be obtained by 'shining' an X-ray beam through a very narrow slit (see Fig. B.5).

Because the width of the slit is known, the blur or line spread function (LSF) of these images can be calculated, after taking into consideration all other factors affecting the 'blur' produced. These calculations are carried out by complex computer programs, the explanation of which is beyond the scope of this book. Once the LSF is known, it can in turn be used to calculate the MFT of the recorded image.

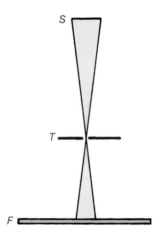

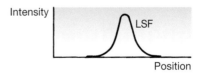

Fig. B.5 The line spread function (LSF). F, image recording medium; S, source of X-rays; T, test object with narrow slit.

Signal-to-noise ratio

A factor termed 'signal-to-noise ratio' (SNR) impacts very greatly on the quality of diagnostic images, including conventional X-ray as well as computed tomography (CT) and magnetic resonance imaging (MRI). Within the imaging process, we wish to acquire signal, which provides a true representation of structures such as body anatomy, while reducing noise. Noise can be defined as random fluctuations in signal which do not relate to true structural features within the image. Noise may be caused by small changes in current within electrical circuits and imaging detectors, as well as by random statistical variations in X-ray photon density, which can become particularly apparent at low exposure values. This latter feature is often termed *quantum mottle* because the effects of individual X-ray quanta (tiny packets of energy) may be apparent at low exposure values.

The relative sizes of signal and noise in any digital image are referred to as the SNR. This has a big effect on diagnostic images because a poor SNR value can reduce image contrast and resolution. SNR is defined as the relative powers of the signal and noise in a detector, as shown by Fig. C.1.

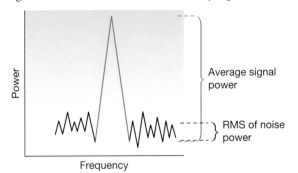

Fig. C.1 This graph shows the larger power peak that normally results from true signal in an image, as well as the fluctuating and smaller signal that may be attributed to background noise. Noise tends to map across a wider range of signal frequencies in the data, as shown. Note that overall noise power is usually expressed as a root mean square value (*RMS*). This provides a more realistic 'average' measure when negative as well as positive numerals may be encountered, for example, in a fluctuating voltage or signal.

It might be thought that very small pixels and voxels would be beneficial to an image, by providing fine detail and resolution. In practice this might not be the case because small pixels and voxels provide less signal because of their smaller area or volume and hence random statistical noise may degrade the image. This point is illustrated by Fig. C.2, in which one of the two images has a more 'noisy' or 'grainy' appearance caused by signal variations that affect pixel brightness. Doubling the width of a square pixel will provide a four-fold increase in surface area and hence a fourfold increase in signal. In imaging, SNR may often be defined as the ratio between the mean signal value in a pixel or voxel and its standard deviation (a measure of spread each side of the mean).

It is quite easy to understand how a poor SNR will reduce image resolution or sharpness, because a grainy or mottled image will be less able to show boundaries between structures clearly. There is also a reduction in contrast because contrast in fact consists of signal differences between two structures. Hence any deterioration in SNR will in turn affect contrast and the contrast-to-noise ratio (CNR). For example, this can occur because of the overall image 'fog' which can result from X-ray scatter. Scatter can be considered to be a source of image noise.

Noise in an image becomes more of problem as signal decreases. This is in fact a statistical issue and can be explained in terms of the following analogy. Let's imagine that we are aiming to calculate the average height of people in a sample. With a large sample of 1000 people, the random effects of very tall or very short people on the result will tend to get averaged out. But in a small sample of only 10 people, the effect of just one very tall person would be to skew the result much more. In the same way, as the sample of X-ray photons arriving at an image detector decreases, statistical variations in these X-rays may have more of an effect on the overall signal level received by that detector. Digitally, the brightness of a pixel or voxel is based on the signal received by it.

SNR may be increased by repeated sampling of image data. This tends to average out the random statistical

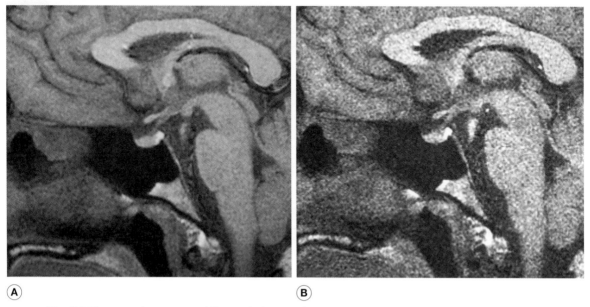

Fig. C.2 These two images are midline sagittal magnetic resonance imaging scans of the brain. In (A), the choice of larger voxels has produced a much better signal-to-noise ratio than in the very 'noisy' image of (B). Note how image (B) has a grainy 'salt and pepper' signal appearance which reduces image resolution and contrast.

variations in signal which we refer to as noise. A good example of signal averaging can be found in MRI, where the averaging process is referred to as number of excitations (NEX) or number of signal averages (NSA). In this case, the SNR increases according to the square root of the number of averages. This gives a 1.4 increase in SNR for 2 signal averages.

In digital plain radiography, the exposure index (see Chapter 16) should be set sufficiently high to avoid the appearance of noise within the diagnostic image. Noise may become more apparent if the mAs value (which is a major factor influencing the number of X-ray photons produced) is set too low.

International System of base units

International System of Units (SI) base units were discussed in Chapter 4. Here are the precise definitions of these units.

D.1 MASS

The unit of mass is the kilogram. The mass of one kilogram is equal to the mass of the international platinum–iridium prototype of the kilogram.

D.2 LENGTH

The unit of length is the metre. The metre is the length equal to 1,650,763.73 wavelengths in a vacuum of the radiation corresponding to the transition between the levels $2p_{10}$ and $5d_5$ of the krypton-86 atom.

D.3 TIME

The unit of time is the second. The second is the duration of 9,192,631,770 periods of the radiation corresponding to the transition between the two hyperfine levels of the ground state of the caesium-133 atom.

D.4 ELECTRIC CURRENT

The unit of electric current is the ampere. The ampere is the constant current which, if maintained in two straight parallel conductors of infinite length, of negligible circular cross-section and placed 1 metre apart in a vacuum, would produce between these conductors a force equal to 2×10^{-7} newtons per metre of length.

D.5 TEMPERATURE

The unit of temperature is the kelvin. The kelvin is the fraction 1/273.16 of the thermodynamic temperature of the triple point of water.

D.6 LUMINOUS INTENSITY

The unit of luminous intensity is the candela. The candela is the luminous intensity, in the perpendicular direction, of the surface of 1/600,000 square metre of a black body at the temperature of freezing platinum under a pressure of 101,325 newtons per square metre.

D.7 AMOUNT OF SUBSTANCE

The unit of amount of substance is the mole. The mole is the amount of substance of a system which contains as many elementary entities as there are atoms in 0.012 kg of carbon-12.

Powers of 10

Prefix	Symbol	Name	Common notation	Factor
Exa	E	Quintillion	1 000 000 000 000 000 000	10^{18}
peta	P	Quadrillion	1 000 000 000 000 000	10^{15}
Tera	T	Trillion	1 000 000 000 000	10^{12}
giga	G	Billion	1 000 000 000	10^{9}
mega	M	Million	1 000 000	10^{6}
kilo	k	Thousand	1 000	10^{3}
hecto	h	Hundred	100	10^{2}
deca	da	Ten	10	10^{1}
deci	d	One tenth	0.1	10^{-1}
centi	c	One hundredth	0.01	10^{-2}
milli	m	One thousandth	0.001	10^{-3}
micro	μ	One millionth	0.000 001	10^{-6}
nano	n	One billionth	0.000 000 001	10^{-9}
pico	p	One trillionth	0.000 000 000 001	10^{-12}
femto	f	One quadrillionth	0.000 000 000 000 001	10^{-15}
atto	a	One quintillionth	0.000 000 000 000 000 001	10^{-18}

Physical constants

Quantity	Value
Avogardro's number, N_A	6.02×10^{23} mol^{-1}[a]
Velocity of light in a vacuum, c	3.00×10^8 m.s^{-1}
Permittivity of a vacuum, ε_0	8.8×10^{-12} F.m^{-1}
Permeability of a vacuum, μ_0	1.26×10^{-6} Hm^{-1}
Electron rest mass, m_e	9.11×10^{-31} kg
Proton rest mass, m_p	1.672×10^{-27} kg
Neutron rest mass, m_n	1.675×10^{-27} kg
Planck's constant, h	6.63×10^{-34} J.s
Electronic charge, e	-1.60×10^{-19} C

[a]Or 6.02×10^{26} (kg. mol)$^{-1}$.

TABLE C

Important conversion factors

Quantity	Conversion factor
1 atomic mass unit (amu)	$= 1.66 \times 10^{-27}$ kg
1 electron volt (eV)	$= 1.60 \times 10^{-19}$ J
1 joule (J)	$= 6.24 \times 10^{18}$ eV
Electron mass	$= 0.511$ MeV
Proton mass	$= 938$ MeV
Neutron mass	$= 940$ MeV
1 angstrom (Å)	$= 0.1$ nm

Greek symbols and their common usage

Name	Symbol Capital	Symbol Lower case	Usage
Alpha	A	α	α-Particle (He nucleus); also lower-case (α) is the flip angle in MRI
Beta	B	β	β-Particle (electron or positron)
Gamma	Γ	γ	γ-Rays; also gyromagnetic ratio in MRI
Delta	Δ	δ	Δx or δx used to indicate change in x
Epsilon	E	ε	
Zeta	Z	ζ	
Eta	H	η	
Theta	Θ	θ	Used to represent angle
Iota	I	ι	
Kappa	K	κ	
Lambda	V	λ	(λ) Wavelength; radioactive decay constant
Mu	M	μ	(μ) Total linear attenuation coefficient
Nu	N	ν	(ν) Frequency of electromagnetic radiation
Xi	Ξ	ξ	
Omicron	O	o	
Pi	Π	π	(π) Linear attenuation coefficient for pair production
Rho	P	ρ	(ρ) Density of matter; resistivity
Sigma	Σ	σ	(σ) Linear attenuation coefficient for Compton effect
Tau	T	τ	(τ) Linear attenuation coefficient for photoelectric absorption
Upsilon	Y	υ	
Phi	Φ	φ	Used to represent angle
Chi	X	χ	
Psi	Ψ	ψ	
Omega	Ω	ω	(Ω) Symbol used for resistance or impedance in ohm; (ω) used for precessional frequency in MRI

MRI, Magnetic resonance imaging.

The periodic table of elements

Group →	1	2	3	4	5	6	7	8	9	10	11	12	13	14	15	16	17	18
Period ↓																		
1	H 1																	He 2
2	Li 3	Be 4				Transition elements							B 5	C 6	N 7	O 8	F 9	Ne 10
3	Na 11	Mg 12											Al 13	Si 14	P 15	S 16	Cl 17	Ar 18
4	K 19	Ca 20	Sc 21	Ti 22	V 23	Cr 24	Mn 25	Fe 26	Co 27	Ni 28	Cu 29	Zn 30	Ga 31	Ge 32	As 33	Se 34	Br 35	Kr 36
5	Rb 37	Sr 38	Y 39	Zr 40	Nb 41	Mo 42	Tc 43	Ru 44	Rh 45	Pd 46	Ag 47	Cd 48	In 49	Sn 50	Sb 51	Te 52	I 53	Xe 54
6	Cs 55	Ba 56	La 57	Hf 72	Ta 73	W 74	Re 75	Os 76	Ir 77	Pt 78	Au 79	Hg 80	Ti 81	Rb 82	Bi 83	Po 84	At 85	Rn 86
7	Fr 87	Ra 88	Ac 89	Rf 104	Db 105	Sg 106	Bh 107	Hs 108	Mt 109	Ds 110	Rg 111	Cn 112	Nh 113	Fl 114	Mc 115	Lv 116	Ts 117	Og 118

Lanthanoids*	*	Ce 58	Pr 59	Nd 60	Pn 61	Sm 62	Eu 63	Gd 64	Tb 65	Dy 66	Ho 67	Er 68	Tm 69	Yb 70
Actinoids**	**	Th 90	Pa 91	U 92	Np 93	Pu 94	Am 95	Cm 96	Bk 97	Cf 98	Es 99	Fm 100	Md 101	No 102

- Reactive non-metals
- Alkali metals
- Alkaline earth metals
- Metalloids
- Post transition elements
- Halides
- Inert gases (18th column)

Electron configuration of the elements

Element	Atomic number	Symbol	Number of electrons in shell						
			K	L	M	N	O	P	Q
Hydrogen	1	H	1						
Helium	2	He	2						
Lithium	3	Li	2	1					
Beryllium	4	Be	2	2					
Boron	5	B	2	3					
Carbon	6	C	2	4					
Nitrogen	7	N	2	5					
Oxygen	8	O	2	6					
Fluorine	9	F	2	7					
Neon	10	Ne	2	8					
Sodium	11	Na	2	8	1				
Magnesium	12	Mg	2	8	2				
Aluminium	13	Al	2	8	3				
Silicon	14	Si	2	8	4				
Phosphorus	15	P	2	8	5				
Sulphur	16	S	2	8	6				
Chlorine	17	Cl	2	8	7				
Argon	18	Ar	2	8	8				
Potassium	19	K	2	8	8	1			
Calcium	20	Ca	2	8	8	2			
Scandium	21	Sc	2	8	9	2			
Titanium	22	Ti	2	8	10	2			
Vanadium	23	V	2	8	11	2			
Chromium	24	Cr	2	8	13	1			
Manganese	25	Mn	2	8	13	2			
Iron	26	Fe	2	8	14	2			
Cobalt	27	Co	2	8	15	2			
Nickel	28	Ni	2	8	16	2			
Copper	29	Cu	2	8	18	1			
Zinc	30	Zn	2	8	18	2			
Gallium	31	Ga	2	8	18	3			
Germanium	32	Ge	2	8	18	4			
Arsenic	33	As	2	8	18	5			
Selenium	34	Se	2	8	18	6			

(Continued)

Element	Atomic number	Symbol	Number of electrons in shell						
			K	L	M	N	O	P	Q
Bromine	35	Br	2	8	18	7			
Krypton	36	Kr	2	8	18	8			
Rubidium	37	Rb	2	8	18	8	1		
Strontium	38	Sr	2	8	18	8	2		
Yttrium	39	Yt	2	8	18	9	2		
Zirconium	40	Zr	2	8	18	10	2		
Niobium	41	Nb	2	8	18	12	1		
Molybdenum	42	Mo	2	8	18	13	1		
Technetium	43	Tc	2	8	18	14	1		
Ruthenium	44	Ru	2	8	18	15	1		
Rhodium	45	Rh	2	8	18	16	1		
Palladium	46	Pd	2	8	18	18			
Silver	47	Ag	2	8	18	18	1		
Cadmium	48	Cd	2	8	18	18	2		
Indium	49	In	2	8	18	18	3		
Tin	50	Sn	2	8	18	18	4		
Antimony	51	Sb	2	8	18	18	5		
Tellurium	52	Te	2	8	18	18	6		
Iodine	53	I	2	8	18	18	7		
Xenon	54	Xe	2	8	18	18	8		
Caesium	55	Cs	2	8	18	18	8	1	
Barium	56	Ba	2	8	18	18	8	2	
Lanthanum	57	La	2	8	18	18	9	2	
Cerium	58	Ce	2	8	18	20	8	2	
Praseodymium	59	Pr	2	8	18	21	8	2	
Neodymium	60	Nd	2	8	18	22	8	2	
Promethium	61	Pm	2	8	18	23	8	2	
Samarium	62	Sm	2	8	18	24	8	2	
Europium	63	Eu	2	8	18	25	8	2	
Gadolinium	64	Gd	2	8	18	25	9	2	
Terbium	65	Tb	2	8	18	26	9	2	
Dysprosium	66	Dy	2	8	18	28	8	2	
Holmium	67	Ho	2	8	18	29	8	2	
Erbium	68	Er	2	8	18	30	8	2	
Thulium	69	Tm	2	8	18	31	8	2	
Ytterbium	70	Yb	2	8	18	32	8	2	
Lutetium	71	Lu	2	8	18	32	9	2	
Hafnium	72	Hf	2	8	18	32	10	2	
Tantalum	73	Ta	2	8	18	32	11	2	
Tungsten	74	Wo	2	8	18	32	12	2	
Rhenium	75	Re	2	8	18	32	13	2	
Osmium	76	Os	2	8	18	32	14	2	
Iridium	77	Ir	2	8	18	32	15	2	
Platinum	78	Pt	2	8	18	32	17	1	
Gold	79	Au	2	8	18	32	18	1	
Mercury	80	Hg	2	8	18	32	18	2	
Thallium	81	Tl	2	8	18	32	18	3	

Element	Atomic number	Symbol	Number of electrons in shell						
			K	L	M	N	O	P	Q
Lead	82	Pb	2	8	18	32	18	4	
Bismuth	83	Bi	2	8	18	32	18	5	
Polonium	84	Po	2	8	18	32	18	6	
Astatine	85	At	2	8	18	32	18	7	
Radon	86	Rn	2	8	18	32	18	8	
Francium	87	Fr	2	8	18	32	18	8	1
Radium	88	Ra	2	8	18	32	18	8	2
Actinium	89	Ac	2	8	18	32	18	9	2
Thorium	90	Th	2	8	18	32	18	10	2
Protactinium	91	Pa	2	8	18	32	20	9	2
Uranium	92	U	2	8	18	32	21	9	2
Neptunium	93	Np	2	8	18	32	23	8	2
Plutonium	94	Pu	2	8	18	32	24	8	2
Americium	95	Am	2	8	18	32	25	8	2
Curium	96	Cm	2	8	18	32	25	9	2
Berkelium	97	Bk	2	8	18	32	27	8	2
Californium	98	Cf	2	8	18	32	28	8	2
Einsteinium	99	Es	2	8	18	32	29	8	2
Fermium	100	Fm	2	8	18	32	30	8	2
Mendelevium	101	Md	2	8	18	32	31	8	2
Nobelium	102	No	2	8	18	32	32	8	2
Lawrencium	103	Lw	2	8	18	32	32	9	2
Rutherfordium	104	Rf	2	8	18	32	32	10	2
Dubnium	105	Dd	2	8	18	32	32	11	2
Seaborgium	106	Sg	2	8	18	32	32	12	2
Bohrium	107	Bh	2	8	18	32	32	13	2
Hassium	108	Hs	2	8	18	32	32	14	2
Meitnerium	109	Mt	2	8	18	32	32	15	2
Darmstadtium	110	Ds	2	8	18	32	32	17	1
Roentgenium	111	Rg	2	8	18	32	32	18	1
Copernicium	112	Cn	2	8	18	32	32	18	2
Ununtrium	113	Uut	2	8	18	32	32	18	3
Ununquadium	114	Uuq	2	8	18	32	32	18	4
Ununpentium	115	Uup	2	8	18	32	32	18	5
Ununquadium	116	Uuh	2	8	18	32	32	18	6
Ununseptium	117	Uus	2	8	18	32	32	18	7
Ununoctium	118	Uuo	2	8	18	32	32	18	8

SELF-TEST QUESTIONS

CHAPTER 1

1. State the imaging modalities (methods) that are available in medical imaging.
2. Explain the difference between transmission and emission imaging.
3. Which imaging methods have a functional depiction capability?
4. Briefly explain the key difference between medical imaging and radiotherapy.

CHAPTER 2

1. State the meaning of the terms *atomic number* and *mass number*.
2. What is an isotope?
3. Why are some isotopes radioactive?
4. Define the term *binding energy*.
5. Explain *ionic bonds* and *covalent bonds*.
6. Define *atoms*, *molecules* and *compounds*.

CHAPTER 3

1. State the Law of Conservation of Matter.
2. Does this law always hold true in medical imaging physics?
3. What is the significance of the law of conservation of energy for medical imaging physics?
4. Why does a mole of a substance always contain the same number of molecules?
5. Name two temperature scales used in science.
6. Give an example of specific heat capacity in medical imaging practice.
7. What are the three ways in which heat may be lost from an object?

CHAPTER 4

1. State the SI units for acceleration, force, energy and power.
2. Explain the concept of potential energy.

3. What is the meaning of mAs and keV?
4. Express the following terms as powers to the base of 10—micro, milli, centi, kilo, mega, giga.

CHAPTER 5

1. What influences the magnitude of the force between two electric charges?
2. State the definition of electrical potential difference and give its units.
3. Define the *volt*.
4. What is a capacitor?
5. What are the electrical properties of a conductor?
6. Define the *ampere* (amp).
7. What factors increase the resistance of a conductor?
8. State Ohm's law.
9. What is the difference between direct current and alternating current?

CHAPTER 6

1. State TWO sources of magnetic fields.
2. What are the strengths of the earth's magnetic field and the magnetic fields used in magnetic resonance imaging (MRI)?
3. Define *diamagnetic*, *paramagnetic* and *ferromagnetic* materials.
4. Define *electromagnetic induction*.
5. Give some practical examples of applications of Faraday's laws of electromagnetic induction.

CHAPTER 7

1. What is a *generator* as found in an X-ray room?
2. Why do transformers work best when supplied by alternating current?
3. Give the advantages of high frequency generators.
4. What is the purpose of rectifiers in an X-ray circuit?
5. What is a semiconductor?
6. Explain the difference between *P*- and *N*-type semiconductors.

CHAPTER 8

1. State the key differences between the laws of modern physics and classical physics.
2. State the equation of mass-energy equivalence.
3. State the equation which gives the energy of an X-ray photon.

CHAPTER 9

1. List the regions of the electromagnetic spectrum in order of increasing energy.
2. State the common properties of electromagnetic radiations.
3. What equation links wave frequency and wavelength?
4. Give examples of the use of electromagnetic radiations in medical imaging.

CHAPTER 10

1. Explain why some naturally occurring nuclei are radioactive.
2. Define the unit of *radioactivity*.
3. State the difference between beta minus (negative) and beta plus (positive) decay.
4. Give an example of a commonly used radioisotope which emits only gamma rays.
5. What is *branching decay*?
6. Explain the process of nuclear fission.

CHAPTER 11

1. State the TWO processes that result in X-ray production.
2. Which of these two processes is the most important?
3. What are the differences between the two X-ray production processes?
4. What factors affect the quantity of Bremsstrahlung X-ray production?
5. At an X-ray tube kVp of 100, what would be the most common (most prevalent) energy range of the X-rays found in the continuous spectrum?
6. Why are X-ray energies expressed in keV?
7. What happens to the continuous X-ray spectrum when (i) mA is increased and (ii) kVp is increased?

CHAPTER 12

1. What are the required properties of an X-ray tube housing (shield)?
2. State the differences between stationary and rotating anode X-ray tube designs.
3. Why is tungsten a good material to use in an X-ray tube target?
4. Explain the *line focus principle*.

5. What is the *anode heel effect*?
6. Describe *thermionic emission*.
7. Define the *rating* of an X-ray unit.
8. Why are modern X-ray tube inserts often made of metal?

CHAPTER 13

1. Define X-ray *attenuation*.
2. Define the *linear attenuation coefficient*.
3. The linear attenuation coefficient is based on specific requirements—what are these?
4. Explain the differences between photoelectric absorption and Compton scatter.

CHAPTER 14

1. Define the *intensity* of an X-ray beam.
2. Define the *quality* of an X-ray beam.
3. Explain half-value thickness (HVT).
4. What is the effect of filtration on an X-ray beam?
5. Define the *inverse square law*.

CHAPTER 15

1. Define the term *pixel*.
2. Define the term *matrix*.
3. State the three stages of converting an analogue signal into a digital signal using an *analogue-to-digital* converter.
4. State a typical material used in the phosphor layer of a computed radiography (CR) imaging plate.
5. State the name of the X-ray absorbing layer in a direct digital radiography (DDR) imaging receptor.
6. State the purpose of thin film transistors (TFTs) in a DDR imaging system.

CHAPTER 16

1. State the factors which commonly affect the attenuation of the X-ray beam as it travels through the patient.
2. State TWO common methods in which the scatter to an X-ray image can be limited.
3. State the equation for describing the *grid ratio*.
4. State the name of the graphical relationship between optical density of an image and the incident air kerma used to generate it.
5. Define the terms *density* and *contrast*.
6. Explain the term *radiographic speed* with respect to an imaging system.

CHAPTER 17

1. State ONE key feature of a mobile X-ray unit which distinguishes it from a portable X-ray unit.
2. State ONE limitation of a capacitor-discharge mobile X-ray unit.
3. Explain how the X-ray field size and centring is achieved when using an intra-oral dental X-ray unit.
4. State TWO locations for the material tungsten within a dental X-ray tube.
5. Explain the main principle of the function of an OPG X-ray unit.
6. Describe the purpose of the aluminium wedge filter in a lateral cephalostat examination.

CHAPTER 18

1. State the TWO materials commonly used as the X-ray tube target material in mammography.
2. State a typical kV range used in digital mammography examinations.
3. Explain why a very small focal spot size is necessary in mammography X-ray units.
4. State the metric that is used to provide a precise estimate of the radiation dose to the examined breast during mammography.
5. Explain what happens during a digital breast tomosynthesis examination.
6. State TWO benefits of applying compression during mammography.

CHAPTER 19

1. Provide a *brief* definition of the term *fluoroscopy*.
2. Within an image intensifier, state <u>both</u> the material used and the purpose of the *photocathode*.
3. Explain the terms *vignetting* and *pincushion image distortion*.
4. State the TWO types of flat-panel (solid-state) fluoroscopy systems that are currently available.
5. Explain the purpose of the *automatic brightness control (ABC)* device.
6. State THREE methods for reducing the radiation dose from fluoroscopy examinations.

CHAPTER 20

1. Describe *briefly* the benefit of using 'slip-ring' technology within a CT scanner.
2. Describe *briefly* the modifications to the X-ray tube anode that occur within a CT scanner.

3. Explain why mobile CT scanners might be useful if integrated into the back of emergency response vehicles (ambulances).
4. Explain the THREE methods for varying the X-ray tube voltage during spectral CT acquisitions.
5. Explain briefly the differences between *filtered back projection* and *iterative reconstruction*.
6. State the typical window width and level for an abdominal (soft tissue) CT examination.

CHAPTER 21

1. State the units of absorbed dose and equivalent dose.
2. State TWO advantages of using thermoluminescent dosimeters (TLDs) in radiation dosimetry.
3. State in full the abbreviation MOSFET.
4. Explain the term *Radiation Protection Advisor* (RPA).
5. Explain the term *Radiation Protection Supervisor* (RPS).
6. State the dose limits to the eye lens and skin for employees and trainees (18+years).

CHAPTER 22

1. What are the three key components of a gamma camera?
2. What are the functions of a collimator?
3. Describe the process of scintillation.
4. Name the most common isotope used in RNI and explain how it is produced?

CHAPTER 23

1. Briefly explain how gamma rays are produced in positron emission tomography (PET).
2. What are coincidence detectors?
3. What radionuclides are commonly used in PET imaging and what practical issues can be associated with their use?
4. What is the key working principle of SPECT scanning?

CHAPTER 24

1. What are the physical differences between sound and X-rays?
2. What is meant by acoustic impedance and why is it important?
3. What is a longitudinal wave?
4. What is the Doppler Effect?
5. How are sound waves produced in an ultrasound machine?
6. What are the differences between A mode and B mode scans?

CHAPTER 25

1. Explain what is meant by the term *resonance* in MRI?
2. What are the implications of the Larmor equation in clinical MRI?
3. What is longitudinal recovery?
4. What are the differences between T1 and T2 images?
5. What is a spin echo sequence?
6. How does MR spectroscopy differ from MRI?
7. How can the hazards of MRI be reduced?

CHAPTER 26

1. What types of hybrid scanner are available for clinical use?
2. What advantages do hybrid scanners provide?
3. What practical difficulties may be faced by hybrid scanners?
4. What is the purpose of an attenuation correction scan in PET-CT?

CHAPTER 27

1. Explain *briefly* the function of the *Hospital Information System (HIS)*.
2. Explain briefly the function of the *Radiology Information System (RIS)*.
3. Explain briefly the function of the *Picture Archiving and Communications Systems (PACS)*.
4. State in full the abbreviation *DICOM*.

5. Describe *briefly* the main function of *dose management software.*
6. State the principal focus of *artificial intelligence (AI)* in radiology.

CHAPTER 28

1. What are the biological hazards that may be encountered by patients in MRI and CT?
2. Explain briefly the effects of time-varying magnetic fields on the human body.
3. What is a thermal index?
4. What possible hazards can be associated with the use of contrast media in MRI?
5. What are the possible risks of MRI and ultrasound in pregnancy?

CHAPTER 29

1. How do X-ray examinations provide visual signal differences between body tissues?
2. What is the most important tissue depiction capability of CT scanning?
3. Why is MRI a powerful means of showing body tissues?
4. What aspects of body function can be shown with medical imaging?

SELF-TEST ANSWERS

CHAPTER 1

1) Available medical imaging modalities include conventional X-ray, computed tomography (CT), magnetic resonance imaging (MRI), radionuclide imaging (RNI) and ultrasound.
2) In transmission imaging such as X-ray and CT, an image is formed when X-rays are differentially absorbed (some rays are absorbed while some are transmitted right through) when interacting with the human body. In emission imaging, such as RNI, an image is formed when gamma rays are emitted from within the body by radionuclides that are concentrated in areas of increased metabolic activity.
3) RNI procedures (such as PET) and also MRI have powerful functional imaging abilities. Ultrasound and CT have some functional imaging capability.
4) In medical imaging, low level radiations are used to diagnose disease. In radiotherapy, high level radiations are used to kill tumour cells.

CHAPTER 2

1) Atomic number describes the number of protons in an atomic nucleus. Chemical elements always have a set number of protons. For example carbon has 6 and lead has 82. Mass number describes the number of protons and neutrons in an atomic nucleus and affects the mass of an atom.
2) Chemical elements, with a fixed number of protons, can be found with different mass numbers (different numbers of neutrons). These are termed isotopes of that element.
3) In nature, an isotope is radioactive if it is unstable. This instability is due to an excessive number of neutrons relative to protons, so that the forces which hold the nucleus together no longer function well. Some artificially produced isotopes, used in PET scanning, are unstable due to an excessive number of protons relative to neutrons.
4) Binding energy refers to the energy that must be given to an electron orbiting the atomic nucleus in order to eject that electron from the atom. Innermost electrons, found in the K-shell, have the highest binding energy. Outer shell electrons are less tightly bound.

5) Ionic bonds are found between atoms that have a very different affinity for electrons. In such cases the atom with less electron affinity will donate an electron to the atom with greater affinity. This forms a pair of ions, negative and positive. Ionic bonds exist due to the electrostatic attraction between the oppositely charged ions. Ionic bonds are found in crystalline compounds. Covalent bonds are found between atoms that have a similar affinity for electrons. In such cases the atoms share electrons. This sharing forms a strong bond, found between atoms in molecules, for example in organic compounds.
6) An atom is the smallest chemical unit and consists of a central nucleus surrounded by electrons. It is electrically neutral since the numbers of protons and electrons are equal. A molecule consists of two or more atoms, bound together by covalent bonds. These atoms may be of the same or different elements. A compound consists of two or more elements, present in a fixed ratio.

CHAPTER 3

1) Matter is neither created nor destroyed, but it may change its chemical form as the result of a chemical reaction.
2) The law almost always holds true, but in positron emission tomography (PET), the masses of a positively charged electron and a negatively charged electron are converted into energy in the form of two gamma rays.
3) The law states that energy is always retained but may be converted from one form into another. For example in an X-ray tube, the kinetic energy of a fast moving electron is converted into heat, light and X-rays.
4) A mole is defined as the molecular weight of a substance, expressed in grams. For example one mole of carbon (mass number 12) is 12 grams. One mole of common salt, sodium chloride, consists of sodium (mass number 23) plus chlorine (mass number 35), totalling 58 grams. In each case, the heavier the molecule, the greater the weight of substance, but the number of molecules is the same.
5) The centigrade or Celsius scale, expressed as degrees C, and the kelvin scale, expressed as K. Absolute zero temperature, 0 K, is −273° C.
6) The specific heat capacity of the anode of an X-ray tube is a measure of how much heat it can retain.
7) Conduction, convection and radiation.

333

CHAPTER 4

1) Acceleration—metres per second, force—Newton, energy—joule, power—watt.
2) Potential energy refers to energy that is possessed by entities such as physical objects and charged particles by virtue of their position. This energy can be released, for example when a physical object held high is dropped or a circuit switch is opened to allow an electron to flow.
3) mAs refers to electrical current in milliamps multiplied by time in seconds. It is a measure of the total number of electrons that flow through the X-ray circuit and strike the X-ray tube anode during an exposure. Hence it also relates to the number of X-rays produced during the exposure. keV is a measure of X-ray energy. This energy relates to the charge on an electron (e) which is accelerated across an electrical potential difference (kilovolts—kV).
4) Micro—10^{-6}, milli—10^{-3}, centi—10^{-2}, kilo—10^3, mega—10^6, giga—10^9

CHAPTER 5

1) The size of the charges, the medium between them and the inverse of the square of the distance between them.
2) The potential difference between two points is the work done on a unit positive charge in moving it from one point to the other. The unit is the volt.
3) 1 volt of potential difference exists between two points if 1 joule of work is performed in moving 1 coulomb of positive charge from one point to the other.
4) A device for storing electric charge.
5) A conductor contains free moving electrons in a conduction band, which overlaps across atoms.
6) An electric current of 1 ampere (A) flows at a point if a charge of 1 coulomb (C) flows past that point per second.
7) Small cross sectional area, material of low electrical conductivity, raised temperature.
8) The current flowing through a metallic conductor is proportional to the potential difference which exists across it provided that all physical conditions remain constant. $V = I \times R$.
9) Direct current flows in one direction only, while alternating current switches direction repeatedly and regularly over time.

CHAPTER 6

1) Magnetic fields are produced by permanent magnets, flowing electrical currents and by the earth.
2) The earth's magnetic field is about 0.5 gauss (0.5×10^{-4} tesla). MRI magnets may be found from 2,000 (0.2 tesla) to 30,000 gauss (3 tesla) in strength.

3) Diamagnetic—weakly oppose a magnetic field. Paramagnetic—weakly reinforce a magnetic field. Ferromagnetic—strongly reinforce a magnetic field.
4) Electromagnetic induction is the production of electricity by the interlinking of a conductor with a changing magnetic field, or moving a conductor relative to a stationary magnetic field.
5) Moving a conductor within a magnetic field will induce electricity—as in an electrical generator. A changing magnetic field will induce electricity in a conductor—as in an electrical transformer. Also, a flowing electrical current within a magnetic field will produce motion in the conductor—as in an electrical motor.

CHAPTER 7

1) A device for producing a high voltage supply for X-ray production. Traditionally transformers have been a key component.
2) Alternating current provides a large magnetic flux change, thus inducing a lot of electrical current in the transformer windings.
3) Compact, unaffected by type of power supply, reduced cooling demands, linear output, precise control of voltage and current output.
4) Rectifiers permit current flow in one direction only, in other words DC (direct current). This permits current flow to be always from the cathode to the anode in an X-ray tube and not in the reverse direction.
5) A semiconductor will conduct electricity only when certain conditions are met. This enables it to function in an on/off mode, as in a switch, or to permit the flow of electricity in one direction only, as in a rectifier.
6) Both are forms of extrinsic semiconductor, which have impurities added to a base substance such as silicon. In an N-type semiconductor, flow of electrons occurs. In a P-type semiconductor, movement of positive 'holes' in the electron structure occurs.

CHAPTER 8

1) In modern physics, mass and energy are regarded as convertible from one to another. They are not separate entities, as was the case in classical physics. Also in modern physics, X-rays can be regarded both as waves and as particles (photons). Likewise electrons can be regarded as particles and waves. These concepts were separated in classical physics.
2) $E = mc^2$, where E is energy, m is mass and c is a constant, the speed of light.
3) $E = hv$ or $E = hf$, where E is the energy of the X-ray photon, v or f is frequency and h is Planck's constant.

CHAPTER 9

1) Radio, microwave, infrared, visible, ultraviolet, X-ray and gamma ray.
2) Travel at the speed of light (300,000 km/s), travel in straight lines, have electric and magnetic field components, may be considered as photons (packets of energy) and as waves.
3) Velocity = frequency × wavelength. Since velocity is a constant for electromagnetic radiations, it follows that frequency and wavelength are inversely related.
4) Radio waves—in MRI. Infrared—heat emissions in an X-ray tube. Visible light—emissions from phosphor materials and scintillation crystals, lasers used in CR image processing and for patient positioning. Ultraviolet—emissions from some phosphor materials. X-rays—from X-ray tubes. Gamma rays—emissions from isotopes in RNI.

CHAPTER 10

1) Radioactivity occurs when unstable nuclei change to a more stable state, resulting in the emission of particle and/or electromagnetic radiations. As elements increase in atomic number, more neutrons are needed to bind the nuclear particles together. In the case of heavy elements such as radon and uranium, this 'nuclear glue' is often insufficient and the nucleus decays with the emission of an alpha particle, thereby reducing its size and improving stability. In lighter radioactive nuclei, there is usually an excess of neutrons relative to protons. Such nuclei, such as carbon-14, decay via the conversion of a neutron to a proton, with the emission of a beta minus particle.
2) The unit is the Becquerel (Bq) which is defined as radioactive decay at a rate of one nuclear disintegration per second. An older unit was the Curie (Ci) which is 3.7×10^{10} Bq.
3) Beta minus decay involves the transformation of a neutron to a proton with the emission of a negatively charged (i.e., standard) electron or negatron. The nucleus increases in atomic number by 1. Beta plus decay involves the transformation of a proton to a neutron with the emission of a positively charged (i.e., antimatter) electron or positron. The nucleus decreases in atomic number by 1. The positron is rapidly annihilated on contact with a negatron, resulting in the formation of two 511 keV gamma rays.
4) Technetium-99m. The 'm' term means metastable.
5) Branching decay means that a radioactive nucleus may decay via more than one route.

6) Fission occurs when large nuclei are split, either spontaneously or during bombardment by neutrons. This results in the emission of huge amounts of energy. Fission takes place in nuclear power stations and weapons but not in medical imaging.

CHAPTER 11

1) Bremsstrahlung (braking radiation) and characteristic X-ray production
2) Bremsstrahlung accounts for about 90% of diagnostic X-rays. At a kVp below 69 it is the only process (i.e., 100% of rays) when tungsten X-ray targets are used—characteristic X-rays from tungsten are only produced above 69 kVp.
3) Bremsstrahlung occurs when electrons become braked (slowed) when passing close to an atomic nucleus in the X-ray tube target. Characteristic X-rays form when an electron from the X-ray tube filament ejects a K-shell electron from an atomic nucleus in the X-ray tube target. Bremsstrahlung results in X-rays with a wide range of energies, forming a continuous spectrum. Characteristic X-rays are produced only at fixed energies, giving a line spectrum.
4) The atomic number of the X-ray tube target, the square of the tube voltage (kVp^2) and of course the mA across the X-ray tube.
5) The largest proportion of continuous spectrum X-rays are emitted at keV values ranging from a third to a half of the peak keV. Thus for a kVp of 100, many X-rays will have energies of 30-50 keV.
6) The keV is a unit of X-ray energy. Energy is equal to the charge on an electron (e) that is accelerated by a voltage (kilovolts or kV) across the X-ray tube.
7) mA increase causes the number of X-rays produced to increase across all energies in the continuous spectrum. But the maximum and average energies remain unchanged. Thus the penetrating ability of the X-ray beam is unaffected. kVp increase results in an increase in the maximum and average values of the X-ray energies produced. The beam becomes more penetrating. Also an increase in kVp results in a large increase in the number of X-rays produced. In fact the number of X-rays is proportional to kVp^2.

CHAPTER 12

1) Good electrical insulation (no possibility of giving the operator an electric shock). Prevention of leakage radiation.
2) In a stationary anode, the target is set in a solid block of anode metal, such as copper. The rating (exposure capacity) of such a design is poor. Such designs may be used for low output applications such as portable

machines or dentals. In a rotating anode, the target is a circular strip set in an anode disc which rotates at high speed. This improves the rating of the anode.

3) High melting temperature, permitting good heat properties. High atomic number, maximising Bremsstrahlung X-ray production. Good electrical conductor. Does not easily vaporise. Easily machined into required shape.

4) The line focus principle means that the X-ray beam appears to emerge from a fairly small area on the X-ray tube target, giving a small focal spot and good image resolution. This is due to geometry—the steep angulation of the X-ray target face.

5) The anode heel effect means that steep target angulation results in some X-rays which are produced in the anode direction being absorbed in the target material. This results in a 'fade out' of X-ray beam intensity towards the anode end of the X-ray beam.

6) Thermionic emission occurs when electrons are ejected from the tungsten filament of the X-ray tube into the vacuum. This heat results from electrical resistance to the flow of current in the filament.

7) The rating of an X-ray unit is the combination of exposure settings which the unit can withstand without incurring unacceptable damage.

8) Metal inserts are electrically insulated at both ends and thus a build-up of tungsten vapour on the inside of the insert does not cause electrical arcing as it would in the case of a glass insert. Earthing prevents the accumulation of static electrical charges, which are conducted away. Metal inserts are also strong and durable.

CHAPTER 13

1) Attenuation is the reduction in the intensity of an X-ray beam which occurs as it passes through matter.

2) The linear attenuation coefficient is the fraction of X-rays removed from a beam per unit thickness of the attenuating medium.

3) It requires that the X-ray beam is of a single energy (monochromatic) and the attenuating material is homogeneous (uniform in composition).

4) Photoelectric absorption results in the complete removal of an X-ray photon from the beam and the transfer of its energy to an electron orbiting an atom. The electron is ejected from the atom. Photoelectric absorption is affected by the atomic number and density of matter. It predominates at < 70 kVp.

   Compton scatter results in an X-ray photon being deflected from its original course by interaction with an electron orbiting an atom. The deflected X-ray has a reduced energy. Compton scatter is affected by the electron density of matter. It predominates at > 70 kVp.

CHAPTER 14

1) Intensity is the amount of X-ray energy passing through unit cross sectional area per second. It is often expressed in terms of the exposure (due to ionisations) recorded in an exposure meter. However in radiography the term 'intensity' is also sometimes expressed as the number of X-ray photons in an exposure.

2) A measure of the penetrating ability of an X-ray beam. It is often expressed in terms of half-value thickness (HVT).

3) That thickness of a homogeneous material such as copper or aluminium which will reduce the intensity of an X-ray beam by 50%.

4) Filtration preferentially removes low energy X-ray photons from a beam. Thus it increases the half-value thickness and quality of that beam, by increasing the average X-ray energy. It also reduces a patients' skin radiation dose.

5) The intensity of radiation in an X-ray beam is inversely proportional to the square of the distance from the X-ray source. Thus a doubling of distance reduces beam intensity to a quarter of its original value. The law only applies in air, not in the human body nor in a metal absorber.

CHAPTER 15

1) The smallest element of a digital image is termed a 'pixel'. A pixel (picture element) is a small square-shaped element of the image and can vary in its density or shade of grey.

2) A digital image is made of pixels arranged in rows and columns which form an image matrix.

3) Scanning, quantization and coding are the three stages of converting an analogue signal into a digital signal using an analogue-to-digital converter.

4) Barium fluorohalide doped with europium is an example of a phosphor layer material used in computed radiography.

5) The X-ray absorbing layer of a direct digital imaging receptor is manufactured from amorphous selenium (a-Se).

6) Thin film transistors (TFTs), used in DDR, act as switches which send the signals from the amorphous selenium layer to the processing system.

CHAPTER 16

1) The attenuation of the X-ray beam is affected by the atomic number, density and the thickness of the material that the X-ray beam is passing through.

2) Limiting the amount of scatter formed and stopping any scatter reaching the image receptor are the two main methods for limiting scatter on the X-ray image.

3) The equation for describing the grid ratio (r) is the ratio of the height of the grid strips (h) to the width between them (D).
4) The *characteristic curve* is the term used to describe the graphical relationship between optical density and the incident air kerma.
5) The *density* is the term for the degree of image darkening seen on an image. The *contrast* refers to the ability of an imaging system to discriminate objects with small differences in density.
6) The term *radiographic speed* refers to the inverse of the radiation exposure necessary to produce net optical density equal to 1.

CHAPTER 17

1) A mobile X-ray unit is generally larger and heavier than a portable X-ray unit and is typically confined to a single location. Also the power output of a mobile unit is usually greater.
2) Capacitor-discharge X-ray units require access to a wall power outlet and cannot be used during a power failure. Such systems also lack motorised movements and must be manually moved.
3) The centring cone provides a means of limiting the X-ray field size and also acts as a guide for aiming the primary radiation beam during intra-oral dental radiography.
4) The material tungsten is located in the tube filament and also at the anode focus.
5) An OPG X-ray unit is designed to produce a panoramic 'single image' of the whole mouth and dentition.
6) The aluminium wedge filter is designed to reduce the radiation exposure to the image receptor from X-ray photons transmitted through the anterior facial soft tissues (i.e., nose/lips).

CHAPTER 18

1) Tungsten and molybdenum are commonly used materials in the X-ray tube target.
2) Mammograms are commonly acquired using a kV range of between 24 and 32 kV.
3) In mammography, a very small focal spot size is necessary to reduce geometric unsharpness and maximise resolution.
4) Mean glandular dose (MGD) provides a precise estimate of the radiation dose received by the examined breast.
5) Digital breast tomosynthesis is a relatively new technique where multiple 2D projections are acquired throughout the breast.
6) Compression helps reduce blurring from patient motion and improves the visualisation of the tissues near the anterior chest wall.

CHAPTER 19

1) The term 'fluoroscopy' refers to a radiographic technique used to produce images of moving structures.
2) The photocathode is typically comprised of caesium antimony and emits electrons from its surface when light is absorbed.
3) Vignetting refers to the phenomenon relating to the geometry of an imaging system where the centre of the image field appears brighter than the periphery. Pincushion image distortion refers to a characteristic of an image where an image is more magnified towards its edges.
4) Direct and indirect flat-panel fluoroscopy systems are currently available.
5) The automatic brightness control (ABC) monitors the light output from the image intensifier and increases X-ray output if light levels fall and vice versa.
6) Increasing the X-ray tube potential (kV), reducing the tube current (mA) and reducing the screening time are methods for reducing the radiation dose from a fluoroscopy examination.

CHAPTER 20

1) Slip-ring technology eliminated the need for the X-ray tube to return to its starting position before it commenced another rotation and was a forerunner to the development of a helical CT scanner.
2) An X-ray tube in a CT scanner has a much larger and thicker anode.
3) Mobile CT scanners, if integrated into an emergency response vehicle (ambulance), can be potentially useful for evaluating patients suspected of acute strokes in remote locations.
4) During spectral CT, the X-ray tube voltage can be varied by having two X-ray tubes operating at two different energy levels. Alternatively, a single X-ray tube can be rapidly pulsed between different voltages or the CT scanner can incorporate specially designed detectors which can record different kV levels during a scan.
5) Traditional filtered back-projection is based on several assumptions where projectional attenuation data from the CT scanner is reconstructed into individual linear attenuation coefficients for each voxel contained within a single CT slice. Iterative reconstruction works by revisiting an image over and over with multiple iterations to clear up artefacts clarifing the image pixel by pixel.
6) Typical window width and window level settings for an abdominal CT scan (soft tissue) are 400 and 40 HU, respectively.

CHAPTER 21

1) The units of absorbed dose and equivalent dose are gray (Gy) and sievert (Sv), respectively.
2) TLDs are radiolucent and do not show up on X-ray images. They also have the ability to measure radiation doses across a wide range (μGy to kGy).
3) MOSFET refers to Metal Oxide Semiconductor Field Effect Transistors.
4) The RPA is an accredited, medically qualified physicist who is appointed by the employer to advise on radiation safety and compliance with regulations.
5) Every area of an institution in which ionising radiation is used must have an RPS. The RPS is responsible to the employer for ensuring the safety measures are implemented and maintained.
6) According to the Ionising Radiation Regulations 2017, the dose limits to the eye lens and skin are 20 and 500 mSv, respectively.

CHAPTER 22

1) The collimator, crystal and photomultipliers.
2) The collimator prevents scattered gamma rays from entering the crystal detector. Different collimators may be used, depending on the energy of the gamma rays emitted by the radionuclide being used. Also high and standard resolution collimators are available.
3) In the process of scintillation, gamma rays are absorbed by sodium iodide crystals with thallium impurities. This results in short flashes of emitted light. The light results from changes in energy level affecting electrons in the material.
4) The most common isotope is technetium-99m ('m' means metastable). This has a suitable half-life of 6 hours and emits 140 keV gamma rays. It is obtained from molybdenum-99 in a 'generator' (not to be confused with an electrical generator) at the clinical site.

CHAPTER 23

1) Some artificially produced radionuclides can have an excess of protons in the atomic nucleus. This is unstable and hence a proton decays to form a neutron plus a positively charged electron (positron). When this positron meets a standard negatively charged electron, the two particles annihilate to form two 511 keV gamma rays. This is an example of conversion of mass into energy.
2) In PET, a pair of gamma rays are produced which emerge in opposite directions and strike a detector array which surrounds the patient. Since the gamma rays travel at the speed of light (extremely fast) they will strike the detectors at almost exactly the same instance in time. This near simultaneous signal in the detectors is called a coincidence and so the two gamma rays can be regarded as arising from the same positron-negatron annihilation. This enables the true location of their emission to be calculated.
3) Fluorine-18, Gallium-68, Rubidium-68. They all have short half-lives, meaning that they must be transported rapidly to the imaging department from the cyclotron source or produced on site.
4) In SPECT, a gamma camera or pair of gamma cameras is rotated around the patient. This permits sectional images to be obtained, of greater detail than would be obtained with planar (2D) MRI.

CHAPTER 24

1) X-rays can also be considered as little packets of energy (photons) which have particle-like properties. Sound can be considered as waves, but not as particles. Sound travels relatively slowly, while X-rays travel at a fantastic speed—the speed of light.

   Sound requires a medium (a solid, liquid or gas) to travel in, as it consists of mechanical oscillations in the particles of that medium. X-rays can travel through a medium and also through a vacuum—they consist of oscillating electrical and magnetic fields (electromagnetic radiations) which are self-perpetuating.
2) Acoustic impedance refers to the 'opposition' presented by materials to the passage of sound waves through them. Impedance affects the strength of sound passing through a material, and also the amount of sound wave reflection occurring at boundaries between materials. Where there are large differences in acoustic impedance, there is a lot of sound reflection (giving a strong echo) but little or no sound transmission to deeper structures.
3) A longitudinal wave (such as sound) consists of periodic oscillations of amplitude in the direction of travel. A transverse wave (such as all electromagnetic radiations including X-rays and light) consists of periodic oscillations of amplitude perpendicular to the direction of travel.
4) The Doppler Effect occurs when a speeding source of wave energy produces waves with an altered frequency, due to the motion of the source relative to an observer. When a source is moving towards an observer, the frequency (or pitch) of the waves increases—the waves become 'bunched up'. When a source is moving away from an observer, the frequency (or pitch) decreases—the waves become 'drawn out'. This phenomenon is used in ultrasound to measure the speed and direction of movement of a tissue or flowing blood.

5) In an ultrasound probe, a piezoelectric crystal material vibrates in response to a changing electrical current applied across it. This mechanical vibration results in compressions and rarefactions of the particles in any medium touching the probe. Sound transmission is improved by a using a gel applied to the patient's skin.

6) An 'A mode' or amplitude modulated ultrasound scan produces a simple plot of echo amplitudes from different depths in the body. A 'B mode' or brightness modulated ultrasound scan produces a two-dimensional section through a patient, in which the brightness of echoes corresponds to the magnitude of sound reflections at tissue boundaries. Anatomy is more recognizable in a B mode scan and the resulting real-time but 'fuzzy' picture is the type of ultrasound display familiar to most people.

CHAPTER 25

1) Within a powerful magnetic field, the magnetic dipole moments of individual hydrogen nuclei are rotating (precessing) at a high frequency. If a radiofrequency field is applied to the nuclei at precisely this frequency and at 90 degrees to the main magnetic field, energy is transferred to the nuclei. This is known as magnetic resonance and is a key step in the MRI process. The efficient transfer of energy from one system to another at a set frequency, at which the amplitude of an oscillation increases, is known more generally in science as resonance.

2) According to the Larmor equation, the precessional frequency of the magnetic dipole moments of nuclei in a strong magnetic field is proportional to the strength of that field. Resonance will only occur when radiofrequency energy is applied at precisely that frequency. This means that any local variations in magnetic field will reduce the MRI signal. This can be the case in poor quality scanners. Also, if the strength of the magnetic field is altered in a linear and controlled way via magnetic 'gradients', the precessional frequency of the magnetic dipole moments of nuclei will also vary. This fact can be used in anatomical slice selection within a patient and for other purposes too. Slight 'chemical shifts' of radiofrequency signal occur in magnetic resonance spectroscopy due to the different magnetic effects of different chemical environments within molecules.

3) Longitudinal recovery occurs when the overall magnetisation of a patient's hydrogen nuclei gradually returns to an orientation parallel to the main magnetic field after a radiofrequency pulse is applied. The speed of recovery is fast in fat and slow in water. The process is the basis of T1 weighted imaging and is also called spin-lattice relaxation or recovery.

4) In a T1 weighted image, fat appears bright and fluid appears dark. The time to repetition (TR) and time to echo (TE) are relatively short. Thus this type of imaging is relatively fast. Gadolinium contrast agent enhancement can be used with T1 weighting. In a T2 weighted image, fat appears grey and fluid appears bright (one slight complication is that fat can appear quite bright on T2 weighted fast spin echo images). The time to repetition (TR) and time to echo (TE) are relatively long. Thus T2 weighted imaging is relatively slow and more prone to motion artefacts. Iron oxide contrast agent signal depression (negative contrast) can be used with T2 weighting. It should be noted that all MR images contain both T1 and T2 components—an image is 'weighted' to be more biased towards one or the other.

5) A spin echo sequence is one of the most basic 'pulse sequences' used in MRI to apply RF energy to nuclei and focus the returning signal in order to produce an image. In its most basic form, it consists of a single 90-degree RF excitation pulse followed by a single 180-degree refocusing pulse. This results in a spin echo (signal) after a time period termed the time to echo (TE). The overall magnetization of the hydrogen nuclei is 'flipped' to 90 degrees or 180 degrees relative to the main magnetic field by the RF pulses. The larger the flip angle, the greater the magnitude and/or duration of the RF pulse. There are many variations on the basic spin echo sequence, such as fast spin echo (turbo spin echo) which gives a rapid image acquisition, and inversion recovery, which increases image contrast between tissues.

6) Magnetic resonance spectroscopy (MRS), unlike magnetic resonance imaging (MRI), results in a chemical spectrum, not an image of the human body. Within this spectrum, the amplitude of individual peaks relates to the amounts of chemicals present and the frequency of their signals relates to the identity of these chemicals. MRS may use various nuclei, such as hydrogen-1, fluorine-19, phosphorus-31, while MRI only uses hydrogen-1 normally. MRS depends upon the chemical shift effect, which is often regarded as an annoying image artefact in MRI.

7) MRI hazards can be reduced by remembering that not all patients are suitable for MR scanning. Those with pacemakers, ferromagnetic implants and other devices affected by strong magnetic fields should be excluded. This highlights the importance of patient screening questionnaires. No ferromagnetic objects should be brought into the magnet room, due to the risk of 'projectile effect'. The room should not provide open access and there should be a 5 gauss exclusion zone. MR operating parameters should be restricted to avoid undue overheating of patients' body tissues or production of large induced currents. MRI is not recommended in

the first trimester of pregnancy, due to potential (but unproven) concerns about the effects of strong magnetic fields on the human embryo. Patients should wear ear protection should sound levels be excessive (flexing of the magnet coils results in a lot of noise during scanning). Attention should be paid to patients who suffer from claustrophobia when superconducting magnets (which have quite enclosed apertures) are used.

CHAPTER 26

1) SPECT-CT, PET-CT and PET-MRI.
2) Fusion of anatomical data (CT or MRI) with metabolic data (SPECT or PET). This provides a very powerful way to visualise tumours and the heart.
3) Patient movement between the two scans must be minimised or else an accurately fused image will not result (anatomy and metabolic activity will not coincide properly). In PET-MRI, some PET scanner components are sensitive to magnetic fields and thus design changes are needed.
4) In PET, the high energy gamma rays arising from radioactive decay are to some extent attenuated by the anatomy of the human body. A CT scan provides a map of the attenuation properties of the body, which can be used to correct the PET data.

CHAPTER 27

1) A Hospital Information System (HIS) is an information management system used in hospitals/healthcare facilities.
2) Radiology Information Systems (RIS) provide opportunities for collecting data around imaging examinations.
3) A Picture Archiving and Communications System (PACS) is a complex system for managing medical images and related data in a DICOM compliant manner.
4) The term DICOM stands for Digital Imaging and Communications in Medicine and is an international standard for the exchange, storage and communication of digital medical images and related media.
5) Dose Management Software can automatically gather and analyse information on a patient's exposure to ionising radiation facilitating the optimisation of such examinations.
6) The principal focus of AI within radiology is in diagnosis.

CHAPTER 28

1) In MRI, there are many possible biological hazards. The 'projectile effect' can cause ferromagnetic objects to move, potentially causing injury. Other possible effects include tissue heating, induced electrical currents, alterations in the cardiac ECG waveform, burns and claustrophobia. In ultrasound, possible hazards are heating and cavitation (bubble formation and collapse).
2) Time-varying (altering) magnetic fields arise from gradient coils in MRI. These changes induce electrical currents in body tissues and particularly in any metallic substances such as coils of wire. The currents can cause tingling and muscle spasm, as well as burns. An additional effect is the high noise level that can arise from the flexing of the gradient coils.
3) A thermal index is used in ultrasound as a means of quantifying and controlling the amount of heat produced in the human body during a scan. It is expressed as the amount of acoustic power being applied compared with that acoustic power which would cause a tissue temperature rise of 1° C.
4) Possible hazards of contrast media include osmotoxicity (due to movement of water from the tissues into the circulation), nephrotoxicity (kidney injury) and anaphylaxis (severe allergic reactions). However the risk of these effects is less than that arising from iodinated contrast media in CT.
5) MRI is not recommended during the first trimester of pregnancy, since some animal studies have suggested fetal effects arising from strong and varying magnetic fields. However studies of MRI in human pregnancy do not seem to indicate harm. MRI is much safer than CT in pregnancy. In ultrasound, there may be potential heating effects on the fetus during high power procedures such as Doppler and so power levels are constrained. However no studies have yet provided convincing evidence of developmental detriment arising from the routine use of ultrasound.

CHAPTER 29

1) X-ray examinations use the attenuation properties of body tissues in order to depict them. Any visual differences are due to the atomic numbers, densities and thicknesses of these tissues.
2) CT amplifies signal differences (contrast) between body tissues. It achieves this by avoiding superimposition of tissues (by taking sections), reducing scatter and employing the Hounsfield scale.
3) MRI can image several characteristics of human tissues, such as hydrogen density (proton density), T1 and T2 properties (which can show fat and water, respectively, as bright signals), magnetic susceptibility and chemical shift (which is used in spectroscopy).
4) Blood perfusion to tissues (in CT, MRI and RNI). Water diffusion in tissues (in MRI). Metabolic activity (in RNI, especially PET). Blood flow (in MRI and ultrasound). Tissue elasticity (in ultrasound). Neuronal activation (in functional MRI). Chemical composition (in MR spectroscopy).

INDEX